New Developments in Medical Research

Medicine & Health
New York

New Developments in Medical Research

Botulinum Toxin: Therapeutic Uses, Procedures and Efficacy
James C. Lark (Editor)
2022. ISBN: 978-1-68507-817-1 (Hardcover)
2022. ISBN: 978-1-68507-826-3 (eBook)

Evidence-Based Medicine: From the Clinician and Educator Perspective
Sowdhamini Wallace, DO, MS (Editor)
Ganga Gokulakrishnan, MD, MS (Editor)
2022. ISBN: 978-1-68507-546-0 (Hardcover)
2022. ISBN: 978-1-68507-700-6 (eBook)

COVID-19 by Cases: A Pandemic Review
Sujanthy S. Rajaram, MD, MPH, FACP, FAASM, FCCM (Editor)
Anthony Longo, MD (Editor)
Nicole Burak, MD (Editor)
2021. ISBN: 978-1-68507-099-1 (Hardcover)
2021. ISBN: 978-1-68507-262-9 (eBook)

Respiratory Care in Non Invasive Mechanical Ventilatory Support: Principles and Practice
Antonio M. Esquinas, M.D, PhD (Editor)
Mohammed Alahmari, PhD (Editor)
2021. ISBN: 978-1-53619-702-0 (Hardcover)
2021. ISBN: 978-1-53619-902-4 (eBook)

Platelet-Rich Plasma: Myths vs. Reality, Health Effects, and Risks
Pietro Gentile, MD, PhD
2021. ISBN: 978-1-53619-722-8 (eBook)

More information about this series can be found at https://novapublishers.com/product-category/series/new-developments-in-medical-research/

Soner Şahin and Kenan Demir
Editors

Autoimmunity and Cancer

Nova Medicine & Health
New York

DOI: https://doi.org/10.52305/GHGD5301.

Library of Congress Cataloging-in-Publication Data

Names: Şahin, Soner, editor. | Demir, Kenan, editor.
Title: Autoimmunity and cancer / Soner Şahin, PhD (editor), Professor, Faculty of Medicine, Department of Neurosurgery, Nisantasi University, Turkey, Kenan Demir, MD (editor), Health Sciences University, Samsun Training and Research Hospital, Samsun Eğitim ve Araştırma, Hastanesi, İlkadım, Turkey.
Description: New York : Nova Science Publishers, [2022] | Series: New developments in medical research | Includes bibliographical references and index. |
Identifiers: LCCN 2022027573 (print) | LCCN 2022027574 (ebook) | ISBN 9781685079376 (hardcover) | ISBN 9798886970777 (adobe pdf)
Subjects: LCSH: Cancer--Immunological aspects. | Autoimmune diseases.
Classification: LCC RC268.3 .A85 2022 (print) | LCC RC268.3 (ebook) | DDC 616.99/4079--dc23/eng/20220711
LC record available at https://lccn.loc.gov/2022027573
LC ebook record available at https://lccn.loc.gov/2022027574

Published by Nova Science Publishers, Inc. † New York

Contents

Preface

Today, the importance of autoimmune diseases is increasing day by day. Cancer, on the other hand, is an important cause of mortality for which no definitive treatment has been found yet. Cancer can occur for many reasons. Studies have shown that autoimmunity underlies some types of cancer. On the contrary, antitumor immune responses may become cross-reactive with their own tissues, resulting in the development of autoimmunity. Further investigation of the relationship between autoimmunity and cancer will open new horizons for diagnosis and treatment of both groups of disease. This book presents studies of potential mechanisms linking autoimmunity and cancer and the relationship of malignancies with autoimmune disorders.

Acknowledgments

As the editors, we would like to thank Nişantaşı University for their support.

Chapter 1

Introduction to Autoimmunity

Çetin Kürşad Akpınar[1,*], MD
and Hasan Doğan[2], MD
[1]Department of Neurology, Samsun University, Samsun, Turkey
[2]Sinop Ataturk Public Hospital, Sinop, Turkey

Abstract

The immune system represents a complex system that works to protect the organism against foreign substances. The immune system activated by antigens attempts to eradicate the antigen either by phagocytosis directly with leukocytes or with lymphocytes and antibodies. Immune tolerance is the non-responsiveness of the immune system whose main purpose is to work against foreign antigens, against the organism's own antigens. Loss of immune tolerance causes the development of autoantibodies, resulting in tissue damage and autoimmunity. Autoimmunity mostly causes damage to the self-antigens of the immune system and, accordingly, tissues through antibodies.

Keywords: immune system, autoimmunity, immune tolerance, central tolerance, peripheral tolerance

Introduction

The immune system, also known as the defense system of an organism, can be examined under two headings as innate immunity and acquired immunity.

---

* Corresponding Author's Email: cetin.akpinar@samsun.edu.tr.

In: Autoimmunity and Cancer
Editors: Soner Şahin and Kenan Demir
ISBN: 978-1-68507-937-6

While innate immunity works with relatively simple mechanisms such as phagocytosis, acquired immunity has a more complicated mechanism involving antibodies and activated lymphocytes (Radi & Wynn, 2020). The healthy functioning of the immune system is extremely important since its insufficient functioning causes susceptibility to infection and inappropriate overfunctioning against its own body tissues leads to autoimmune diseases (Parkin & Cohen, 2001; Smith & Germolec, 1999).

Autoimmune diseases constitute an important public health problem due to the morbidity they cause, influencing 7.6% to 9.4% of the population. There are many studies that reveal the pathogenesis of autoimmunity. The immune system's response to self-antigens makes up the basis of autoimmunity. The normally functioning immune system does not respond to self-antigens due to immune tolerance. As a result of the impairment of this immune tolerance, a series of immunological reactions occur against self-antigens, and thus different clinical pictures are formed according to the affected organ and system (Cooper et al., 2009).

In this chapter, the normal functioning of the immune system will be first presented in a short summary, then the concepts of immune tolerance and autoimmunity will be discussed.

Natural Functioning of the Immune System

The immune system, the defense system of the body, can be examined under two headings, innate and acquired immune systems. Cells involved in the immune system perform phagocytosis and can be grouped as antigen-presenting cells (APC), T lymphocytes, and B lymphocytes.

Innate immunity includes a quicker response to antigens with effectors such as neutrophils, monocytes, the complement system, and cytokines. When leukocytes, such as neutrophils, encounter an antigen stimulating the immune system, their number increases through cytokines and chemokines and they phagocytize the relevant antigen. On the other hand, the complement system consisting of a high number of glycoproteins is amplified and activated. Thus, the innate immune response is formed quickly (Parkin & Cohen, 2001).

The acquired immune response starts with the presentation of an antigen to T and B lymphocytes and its recognition. Antigens enter the lymphoid organs both directly through the lymphatic route and by phagocytizing by phagocytic cells such as dendritic cells and are presented to lymphocytes here. Dendritic cells can present both self and foreign antigens, but the presentation of foreign antigens causes the release of inflammatory mediators by stimulating a second receptor, called TLR (Casciola-Rosen et al., 1999).

After activated dendritic cells enter the lymph nodes, Th1, Th2, $CD4^+$ T lymphocytes, and antigen-reactive B lymphocyte differentiation are provided with a reaction called the germinal center reaction in the lymphoid follicle. Antigens brought by antigen-presenting cells are presented to $CD4^+$ T lymphocytes via MHC, or intracellular antigens are presented to $CD8^+$ T lymphocytes via MHC-I. The presentation of MHC-I antigens to $CD8^+$ T lymphocytes mediates cell destruction with a cytotoxic response, while the presentation of antigens to $CD4^+$ T lymphocytes with MHC-II causes the release of cytokines and the activation of different cells. B lymphocytes activated by T lymphocytes leave the lymphoid tissue as plasma cells to synthesize antibodies. Activated T and B lymphocytes exhibit the appropriate effector response to foreign antigens in combination with other systems, and the immune response is terminated (Parkin & Cohen, 2001; Vinuesa et al., 2016).

Immune Tolerance

The normal-functioning immune system should not respond to self-antigens. Immune tolerance is the inactivity of the immune system against self-antigens while the appropriate immune response against foreign antigens continues. Despite its controversial background, immune tolerance, which is thought to be multifactorial, can be examined under two main headings as central and peripheral tolerance (Mackay, 2000; Van Parijs & Abbas, 1998).

Central Tolerance

Both T and B lymphocytes, the components of the acquired immune system, are produced by the bone marrow. While B lymphocytes mature in the bone marrow, T lymphocytes arrive in the thymus to mature. T lymphocytes arriving in the thymus acquire the appropriate receptors and turn into $CD8^+$ or $CD4^+$ T lymphocytes, pass through positive selection and enter the thymic medulla. It is tested by presenting self-antigens to T lymphocytes in the thymus medulla, and T lymphocytes sensitive to self-antigens are destroyed by apoptosis. $CD4^+$ $CD8^+$ and regulatory T (Treg) lymphocytes are formed after positive and negative selection. This system, which does not allow the passage of T lymphocytes sensitive to self-antigens into peripheral blood, is called central tolerance (Thapa & Farber, 2019).

The central tolerance of B lymphocytes is not so clear. B lymphocytes, whose maturation continues in the bone marrow, are exposed to some self-antigens, and although they are eliminated, the central tolerance here is not considered very successful, since they do not encounter all self-antigens (Mackay, 2000).

Peripheral Tolerance

Although central tolerance is formed by a relatively simple and understandable mechanism, peripheral tolerance has more complex and multiple mechanisms. Central tolerance can work only with 70% efficiency in terms of autoreactive T lymphocytes. Peripheral tolerance is of critical importance to prevent autoimmunity caused by lymphocytes that escape central tolerance.

Peripheral tolerance can be addressed under different subheadings (ElTanbouly & Noelle, 2021):

1. Quiescence: Naive T cells separated from the thymus are kept with a small cell size and reduced metabolic activity. Despite different views on the mechanism of this situation, regardless of the mechanism, these naive T cells are silent, which contributes to tolerance (Tu et al., 2018; Zhang et al., 2018).
2. Ignorance: The destruction of T lymphocytes reactive to self-antigens in the thymus was mentioned in central tolerance. However, it is known that some self-antigens are not present in the thymus, but only in the relevant tissue. Hence, T lymphocytes are unaware of these antigens and are called ignorant T lymphocytes. Ignorant T cells cannot see their specific self-antigens in a sufficient amount to induce an immune response, and thus an autoimmune response is not formed. This system is one of the essential control points for peripheral tolerance (Parish et al., 2008).
3. Anergy: T lymphocytes that encounter the antigen and are adequately stimulated become the final effector by proliferating and differentiating. Despite T cell receptor (TCR) and antigen binding, this response does not occur if there is no additional costimulatory stimulation. This tolerance system, in which the T lymphocyte that encounters the antigen is not functional but remains hyporesponsive

due to the lack of costimulation and more detailed biochemical and immunological mechanisms in the event of encountering the self-antigen, is called anergy (Kuklina, 2013; Schwartz, 2003).

4. Exhaustion: T lymphocytes are exposed to constant stimulation in conditions such as chronic infections and malignancy. As a result of this continuous stimulation, the effector function of T lymphocytes gradually decreases, the number of inhibitory receptors increases, and transcriptional changes occur. This condition, when no adequate immune response is produced, is called T lymphocyte exhaustion (Wherry & Kurachi, 2015).
5. Senescence: Lymphocytes are cells that continuously reproduce as a result of the signals they receive. After these proliferations, telomere shortening and phenotypic changes take place in the cell. In this case, called T cell senescence, the lack of an adequate immune response comes to the forefront. It has been demonstrated that patients with chronic viral infections and cancer patients have high levels of senescent T cells (Crespo et al., 2013).
6. Peripheral deletion: Similarly to the mechanism in central tolerance, T cells reactive to self-antigens are also directed toward apoptosis in the periphery. The FAS pathway has been stated to be important in the apoptosis of T lymphocytes stimulated repeatedly with the same stimulus (Xing & Hogquist, 2012).

The tolerance systems mentioned above are, in summary, to ensure the unresponsiveness or destruction of the self-reactive immune system cells of the organism. Despite all these control mechanisms, autoimmunity can be triggered.

Autoimmunity and Triggering of Autoimmunity

Although autoimmune diseases are not very common, they represent important conditions due to their colorful clinical images and the mortality and morbidity they cause. Despite different views on their incidence and prevalence, it has been accepted that they are more common in women (Wang et al., 2015).

The familial characteristic of autoimmune diseases has been known for a long time. Monogenic autoimmune diseases caused by a single gene are rare; mainly environmental factors play a role in the foundation of autoimmunity based on multiple genetic factors (Marson et al., 2015). Human Leukocyte Antigen (HLA) draws attention in studies on genetic factors. Although genetic factors are important, non-genetic factors constitute 70% of the risk of developing autoimmune disease (Rosen, 2008).

It is known that infections trigger autoimmunity. There are three different mechanisms for this. If the antigen of the source of infection is similar to the body antigen, the antibody formed against the microorganism will cross-react against self-antigens, thus triggering autoimmune reactions. This is called molecular mimicry. Guillain-Barre syndrome, caused by the reaction of antibodies that develop against microorganism antigens after Campylobacter jejuni infection to peripheral nervous system myelin, is one of the best examples of molecular mimicry (Rojas et al., 2018).

Second, autoimmunity resulting from infection or molecular mimicry will cause tissue damage. Post-tissue damage and inflammation will lead to the emergence and processing of new epitopes. Thus, the activation of T lymphocytes reactive against a self-peptide occurs, which is called epitope spreading. The presentation and recognition of self-antigens increases in the inflammatory region caused by infection, thus further increasing T lymphocytes. Therefore, autoimmunity can be triggered by autoreactive T lymphocytes formed through infection (Vanderlugt & Miller, 2002).

B and T lymphocytes are connected through BCR and TCR and create specific responses. The activation of B and T lymphocytes without these connections is called bystander activation. In this case, which occurs through the mediation of cytokines and chemokines, non-antigen-specific lymphocytes are activated. It has been reported that bystander activation is important in the onset and recurrence of autoimmune diseases such as multiple sclerosis and autoimmune hepatitis (Pacheco et al., 2019).

Vaccines that target the delivery of the microorganism antigen to the body and the formation of an immune response to it may trigger autoimmunity by the mechanisms mentioned above (De Martino et al., 2013).

Vitamin D is known to play a role in calcium metabolism, cell proliferation, and the immune system. With the nuclear receptor for vitamin D, pro-inflammatory cells are suppressed, and tolerogenic regulators are supported. Studies report that low vitamin D levels cause a decrease in immunological tolerance and therefore are essential in autoimmunity (Harrison et al., 2020).

Apart from infections, it has been stated that inorganic substances such as mercury may also trigger autoimmunity. Another element, iodine, is known to be important in the pathogenesis of autoimmune thyroiditis (Pollard et al., 2019; Rose et al., 2002).

It has been known for a long time that some drugs cause autoimmune diseases in humans. Drug-induced autoimmunity is a non-allergic condition caused by autoantibodies or a cellular reaction. Drugs may trigger autoimmunity by impairing central or peripheral tolerance. Drugs are usually small molecules and are not immunogenic; drugs binding to carrier molecules become immunogenic, and the antibodies formed may be self-reactive. Drugs such as hydralazine, methyldopa, and procainamide are known to trigger systemic lupus erythematosus (Chang & Gershwin, 2010).

Mechanism of Autoimmune Diseases

In the healthy functioning of the immune system, self-reactive lymphocytes are expected to be inactive due to central and peripheral tolerance mechanisms. However, these tolerance systems do not work perfectly. Hence, there are autoreactive T cells in the body, but they do not cause pathology. In order for these T lymphocytes to cause pathology, they must be activated, proliferate, and become effectors. Activated T lymphocytes can help with antibody formation or cause tissue damage through macrophages and cytotoxic T cells. Considering all of these, T lymphocytes and antigen-presenting cells play a critical role in the pathogenesis of autoimmunity (Verhasselt & Goldman, 2001).

For the occurrence of autoimmune disease, a self-antigen or another antigen similar to the self-antigen must be presented to the immune system and introduced, and thus antibodies must be formed. These antibodies can be against cell surface antigens such as in neuromuscular junction disorders, against intracellular enzymes such as in primary biliary cirrhosis, and against nuclear components such as in lupus. In addition to these, as in multiple sclerosis, cytotoxic cells may be primarily responsible for pathogenesis (Rosen, 2008).

One of the most important pathological mechanisms of antibodies is cell destruction with or without complement activation after binding to the cell surface. In cellular-dependent cytotoxicity, natural killer cells, which direct the antibody-bound cell to direct lysis, play a prominent role. The rates of autoreactive T lymphocytes in the target tissue region are high. Autoreactive T lymphocytes recognize a cell here through MHC-I and TCR. After this stage, it damages the recognized cell through mechanisms such as fragmentation of the cell membrane, directing to apoptosis through the Fas-Fas ligand, and increasing cytokine release (Wang et al., 2015).

Conclusion

It is expected that the immune system will be unresponsive to autoantigens due to the deletion of T lymphocytes that may be self-reactive in the thymus with central tolerance and peripheral tolerance mechanisms, but these tolerance systems are not perfect. The autoimmune response can be triggered by infections, vaccines, certain drugs, iodine, and heavy metals. Furthermore, there is an association of vitamin D deficiency with an autoimmune response.

Molecular mimicry, epitope spreading, and bystander activation draw attention as important factors in triggering autoimmunity. The process that starts with the recognition of autoantigens and the presentation of autoantigens to T lymphocytes by antigen-presenting cells proceeds in two ways. After the presentation of intracellular antigens such as viral infections and malignancy with MHC-I, cell lysis is provided with the activation of cytotoxic T cells. On the other hand, after antigens presented to $CD4^+$ T lymphocytes by MHC-II, T lymphocyte proliferation and activation, B lymphocyte activation and B lymphocytes turning into plasma cells and producing antibodies continue.

Antibodies formed after the recognition of antigens are extremely important for autoimmune diseases. While contributing to diagnosis, antibodies also constitute the most significant point in pathogenesis. These antibodies can be directed against the cell surface, intracellular enzymes, and cell nucleus components. When the antibody binds to its target antigen, it leads to tissue damage or impaired function. This tissue damage may remain organ-specific, or it may also influence different systems depending on the characteristics of the antigen initiating autoimmunity.

Research on the pathogenesis of autoimmunity is still ongoing. With increased clarification of the pathogenesis, new hopes emerge for treating autoimmune diseases.

References

Casciola-Rosen, L., Andrade, F., Ulanet, D., Wong, W. B., & Rosen, A. (1999). Cleavage by Granzyme B is strongly predictive of autoantigen status: implications for initiation of autoimmunity. *The Journal of Experimental Medicine*, 190(6), 815. https://doi.org/10.1084/JEM.190.6.815.

Chang, C., & Gershwin, M. E. (2010). Drugs and autoimmunity - A contemporary review and mechanistic approach. *Journal of Autoimmunity*, 34(3), J266-J275. https://doi.org/10.1016/j.jaut.2009.11.012.

Cooper, G. S., Bynum, M. L. K., & Somers, E. C. (2009). Recent insights in the epidemiology of autoimmune diseases: improved prevalence estimates and understanding of clustering of diseases. *Journal of Autoimmunity*, 33(3-4), 197. https://doi.org/10.1016/J.JAUT.2009.09.008.

Crespo, J., Sun, H., Welling, T. H., Tian, Z., & Zou, W. (2013). T cell anergy, exhaustion, senescence and stemness in the tumor microenvironment. *Current Opinion in Immunology*, 25(2), 214. https://doi.org/10.1016/J.COI.2012.12.003.

De Martino, M., Chiappini, E., & Galli, L. (2013). Vaccines and autoimmunity. *International Journal of Immunopathology and Pharmacology*, 26(2), 283-290. https://doi.org/10.1177/039463201302600201.

ElTanbouly, M. A., & Noelle, R. J. (2021). Rethinking peripheral T cell tolerance: checkpoints across a T cell's journey. *Nature Reviews Immunology*, 21(4), 257-267. https://doi.org/10.1038/s41577-020-00454-2.

Harrison, S. R., Li, D., Jeffery, L. E., Raza, K., & Hewison, M. (2020). Vitamin D, autoimmune disease and rheumatoid arthritis. *Calcified Tissue International*, 106(1), 58-75. https://doi.org/10.1007/S00223-019-00577-2.

Kuklina, E. M. (2013). Molecular mechanisms of T-cell anergy. *Biochemistry. Biokhimiia*, 78(2), 144-156. https://doi.org/10.1134/S000629791302003X.

Mackay, I. R. (2000). Science, medicine, and the future: Tolerance and autoimmunity. *BMJ : British Medical Journal*, 321(7253), 93. https://doi.org/10.1136/BMJ.321.7253.93.

Marson, A., Housley, W. J., & Hafler, D. A. (2015). Genetic basis of autoimmunity. *The Journal of Clinical Investigation*, 125(6), 2234. https://doi.org/10.1172/JCI78086.

Pacheco, Y., Acosta-Ampudia, Y., Monsalve, D. M., Chang, C., Gershwin, M. E., & Anaya, J. M. (2019). Bystander activation and autoimmunity. *Journal of Autoimmunity*, 103(June), 102301. https://doi.org/10.1016/j.jaut.2019.06.012.

Parish, I. A., Heath, W. R., & Hall, E. (2008). Too dangerous to ignore: self-tolerance and the control of ignorant autoreactive T cells. *Immunology and Cell Biology*, 86, 146-152. https://doi.org/10.1038/sj.icb.7100161.

Parkin, J., & Cohen, B. (2001). Overview of the immune system. *The Lancet*, 357, 1777-1789. https://doi.org/10.1016/B978-0-323-39981-4.00004-X.

Pollard, K. M., Cauvi, D. M., Toomey, C. B., Hultman, P., & Kono, D. H. (2019). Mercury-induced inflammation and autoimmunity. *Biochimica et Biophysica Acta. General Subjects*, 1863(12), 129299. https://doi.org/10.1016/J.BBAGEN.2019.02.001.

Radi, Z. A., & Wynn, T. A. (2020). Toxicologic pathology forum opinion on immune tolerance therapeutic development. *Toxicologic Pathology*, 48, 712-717. https://doi.org/10.1177/0192623320948805.

Rojas, M., Restrepo-Jiménez, P., Monsalve, D. M., Pacheco, Y., Acosta-Ampudia, Y., Ramírez-Santana, C., Leung, P. S. C., Ansari, A. A., Gershwin, M. E., & Anaya, J. M. (2018). Molecular mimicry and autoimmunity. *Journal of Autoimmunity*, 95, 100-123. https://doi.org/10.1016/J.JAUT.2018.10.012.

Rose, N. R., Bonita, R., & Burek, C. L. (2002). Iodine: An environmental trigger of thyroiditis. *Autoimmunity Reviews*, 1(1-2), 97-103. https://doi.org/10.1016/S1568-9972(01)00016-7.

Rosen, A. (2008). Mechanisms of autoimmunity. *Clinical Immunology*, 1, 739-747. https://doi.org/10.1016/B978-0-323-04404-2.10050-8.

Schwartz, R. H. (2003). T cell anergy. *Annual Review of Immunology*, 21, 305-334. https://doi.org/10.1146/annurev.immunol.21.120601.141110.

Smith, D. A., & Germolec, D. R. (1999). Introduction to immunology and autoimmunity. *Environmental Health Perspectives*, 107 (Suppl 5), 661-665. https://doi.org/10.1289/EHP.99107S5661.

Thapa, P., & Farber, D. L. (2019). The role of the thymus in the immune response. *Thoracic Surgery Clinics*, 29(2), 123-131. https://doi.org/10.1016/J.THORSURG. 2018.12.001.

Tu, E., Chia, C. P. Z., Chen, W., Zhang, D., Park, S. A., Jin, W., Wang, D., Alegre, M. L., Zhang, Y. E., Sun, L., & Chen, W. J. (2018). T cell receptor-regulated TGFβ type I receptor expression determines T cell quiescence and activation. *Immunity*, 48(4), 745. https://doi.org/10.1016/J.IMMUNI.2018.03.025.

Van Parijs, L., & Abbas, A. K. (1998). Homeostasis and self-tolerance in the immune system: turning lymphocytes off. *Science (New York, N. Y.)*, 280(5361), 243-248. https://doi.org/10.1126/SCIENCE.280.5361.243.

Vanderlugt, C. L., & Miller, S. D. (2002). Epitope spreading in immune-mediated diseases: Implications for immunotherapy. *Nature Reviews Immunology*, 2(2), 85-95. https://doi.org/10.1038/nri724.

Verhasselt, V., & Goldman, M. (2001). New concepts on the pathogenesis of autoimmune disease. *Israel Medical Association Journal*, 3(8), 599-602.

Vinuesa, C. G., Linterman, M. A., Yu, D., & Maclennan, I. C. M. (2016). Follicular helper T cells. *Annual Review of Immunology*, 34 (February), 335-368. https://doi.org/10.1146/annurev-immunol-041015-055605.

Wang, L., Wang, F. S., & Gershwin, M. E. (2015). Human autoimmune diseases: a comprehensive update. *Journal of Internal Medicine*, 278(4), 369-395. https://doi.org/10.1111/JOIM.12395.

Wherry, E. J., & Kurachi, M. (2015). Molecular and cellular insights into T cell exhaustion HHS Public Access. *Nat. Rev. Immunol.*, 15(8), 486-499. https://doi.org/10.1038/nri3862.

Xing, Y., & Hogquist, K. A. (2012). T-cell tolerance: central and peripheral. *Cold Spring Harbor Perspectives in Biology*, 4(6), 1-15. https://doi.org/10.1101/CSHPERSPECT.A006957.

Zhang, S., Zhang, X., Wang, K., Xu, X., Li, M., Zhang, J., Zhang, Y., Hao, J., Sun, X., Chen, Y., Liu, X., Chang, Y., Jin, R., Wu, H., & Ge, Q. (2018). Newly generated CD4 + T cells acquire metabolic quiescence after thymic egress. *The Journal of Immunology*, 200(3), 1064-1077. https://doi.org/10.4049/JIMMUNOL.1700721/-/DCSUPPLEMENTAL.

Chapter 2

Introduction to Cancer

Nur Ekimci Gürcan, Berfin Uzunkaya and Ömer Faruk Bayrak*, PhD

Department of Medical Genetics,
Yeditepe University School of Medicine,
Istanbul, Turkey

Abstract

Cancer is one of the most complex human diseases with a highly adaptable nature and dynamic features. In the era of worldwide accessible high-throughput omics data, scientists were never more equipped for 'the war on cancer.' Now we know that understanding the mechanisms and motivation behind these complexities will provide us with the most promising weapon in this battle. In this chapter, the epidemiology and causes of cancer, characteristic properties of cancer cells, prevention, diagnosis, and treatment options will be portrayed as a brief summary.

Keywords: cancer, cancer epidemiology, cancer susceptibility, cancer characteristics, cancer treatment

Introduction

We have not slain our enemy, the cancer cell, or figuratively torn the limbs from his body. In our adventures we have only seen our monster more clearly

* Corresponding Author's Email: ofbayrak@yeditepe.edu.tr.

In: Autoimmunity and Cancer
Editors: Soner Şahin and Kenan Demir
ISBN: 978-1-68507-937-6

and described his scales and fangs in new ways – ways that reveal a cancer cell to be, like Grendel, a distorted version of our normal selves.

Harold E. Varmus, Nobel Prize Acceptance Speech (Stockholm, 1989).

The concept of cancer, which is far too complex to be considered as a single disease, is the encompassing term for more than 200 diseases with "abnormal cell growth" as a common denominator. In 2020, approximately 19 million new cancer cases and 10 million cancer-related deaths were recorded worldwide (Ferlay et al., 2021).

It is reported that one out of every five people in the world is diagnosed with cancer during his lifetime, and 1 out of every 11 women and 1 out of every 8 men die from cancer.

Worldwide, the total number of cancer patients alive within 5 years of being diagnosed with cancer is estimated to be 50.6 million. The overall incidence of cancer in transitioned countries is 2 to 3 times higher for both men and women compared to transitioning countries, while mortality rates vary less than 2 times for men and little for women (Sung et al., 2021). According to the annual reports of the *National Institutes of Health* (NIH), as of 2019, the economic burden associated with cancer care in the US alone is estimated at more than 21 billion dollars (Yabroff et al., 2021).

Carcinogenesis is driven by distinctive capabilities and enabling characteristics acquired during the malignant transformation of cancer cells. These acquired features provide cancer cells with high adaptation and survival capabilities in the processes of tumor development and metastatic spread. Exposure to radiation and harmful chemicals, infectious agents, and hereditary factors are the main causes of carcinogenesis.

In addition to classical treatment approaches such as surgery and chemotherapy, contemporary targeted options such as gene therapy, smart drugs, and immunotherapy are also gaining diversity with increasing studies in this area. Considering the severity of the disease, early diagnosis of cancer is very important at this point in saving lives.

Nevertheless, we know today that Andrew von Eschenbach, former director of NCI, did not achieve his goal of eliminating suffering and death due to cancer by 2015; the fact that we are progressing more and more rapidly in the all-out assault on cancer should not be ignored (von Eschenbach, 2003).

Epidemiology of Cancer

Cancer, also known as abnormal cell growth, is a ramous disorder that includes more than 200 different subtypes. These undisciplined cells start to proliferate in any part of the body and can penetrate other adjacent tissues or spread to other organs found in the body. The subsequent metastasis process is the leading cause of cancer-related deaths (Schulz, 2005). According to the *World Health Organization* (WHO), cancer leads to 10 million deaths in the world in 2020 and is responsible for approximately 1 in every 6 deaths.

Cancers with the highest incidence rates in 2020 include breast, lung, colon, and rectum, prostate, skin, and stomach. Additionally, as indicated in Figure 1, lung cancer is the leading cause of death in the world. According to GLOBOCAN data, while the risk of breast cancer is approximately 20% until the age of 45, after this age, the rate of breast cancer drops to 11,5% in both sexes. On the contrary, statistics indicate that the rate of lung cancer increases to 13,5% after the age of 45. In most cases, the risk of cancer increases in direct proportion to age.

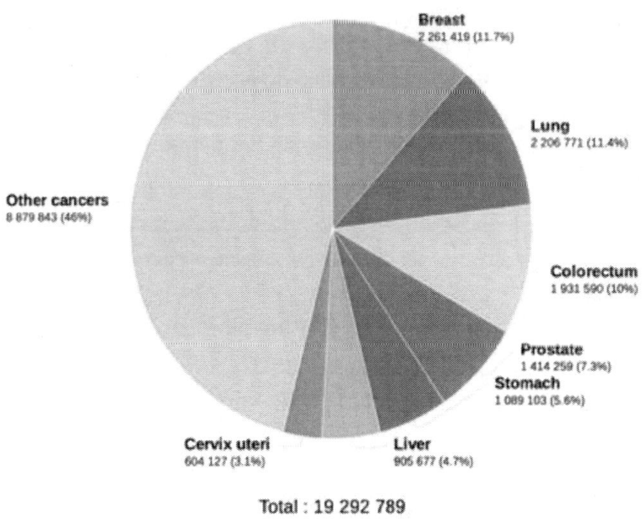

Figure 1. Estimated number of new cases in 2020, worldwide, for both sexes and all ages, according to the World Health Organization.

This complicated disease must be characterized to facilitate understanding of the process. Therefore, two ways are used for cancer characterization, the histological classification and the primary site of the cancer where it initially appeared. Histological classification, according to the *National Cancer Institute* (NCI), which indicates the type of tissue in which the cancer arises, is divided into 6 major groups. These groups are named as carcinoma, sarcoma, myeloma, leukemia, lymphoma, and mixed types.

Carcinomas are the most common cancers, representing more than 80% of cases and arise from epithelial cells. This comprehensive cancer group is divided into 2 groups in itself, which are adenocarcinoma and squamous cell carcinoma. Adenocarcinoma arises in glands or organs, while squamous cell carcinoma develops in the squamous epithelium. Adenocarcinoma encompasses most breast cancers, prostate cancers, colorectal cancers with 96% and pancreatic cancer with similar rates, and has also developed from other parts of the body such as the stomach, esophagus, and lungs. Due to its origin in the glands, adenocarcinoma can spread to other parts of the body, including the liver, lungs, brain, bone marrow, and lymph nodes. Squamous cells are found on the surface of organs such as the lungs, thyroid, throat, respiratory tracts, digestive tracts, and skin. Uncontrollable cell division in these squamous cells causes squamous cell carcinoma, which is the second most frequent type of skin cancer. In addition, head and neck squamous cell cancer (HNSCC) and non-small cell lung cancer (NSCLC) are the common types of squamous cell cancers (Cooper and Hausman, 2000; Kawase et al., 2011; Johnson et al., 2020; Sabbula and Anjum, 2021).

Sarcomas describe a variety of malignancies that originate in supportive and connective tissues, including bones, cartilage, tendons, fat, blood vessels, and muscles. The most common type of sarcoma develops in the bones, a sarcoma that arises in the bones, also called osteosarcoma (Prater and McKeon, 2019).

Myeloma that is also termed multiple myeloma originates in plasma cells in the bone marrow and accumulates there. This phenomenon causes forcing out healthy blood cells, so aberrant proteins produced by cancer cells cause problems (Fairfield et al., 2016).

Leukemia is another cancer group that originated in the bone marrow and is also called liquid cancer because it is blood cancer. The overproduction of immature white blood cells is frequently associated with leukemia. Due to the insufficient function of these infection fighters, patients are frequently infected (Addisia et al., 2022).

While leukemia occurs in the bone marrow, flows into the bloodstream, and circulates through the body, lymphoma, on the other hand, arises in the lymphatic system and includes glands, nodes, and organs, particularly the spleen, thymus, and tonsils. Lymphomas consisting of Hodgkin lymphoma and non-Hodgkin lymphoma are solid cancers, unlike leukemia. Lymphoma could occur in some specific organs, including the breast, stomach, and brain, and is called extranodal lymphomas (Singh et al., 2020).

Categorizing cancer according to its cell type does not mean that human cancer will occur in a single cell type. There are other cancer categories that include multiple cell types and, in general, are called mixed types. Adenosquamous carcinoma is an example of this mixed type cancer that contains gland-like cells and squamous cells. These mixed types of cancers show a more aggressive character compared to a single cell type (Chirieac and Attanoos, 2017). Moreover, teratocarcinoma is another mixed-type example, which is a cancerous germ tumor type. The constituent of undifferentiated embryonal carcinoma (EC) and differentiated derivatives that encompass three germ layers that are endoderm, ectoderm, and mesoderm compose these cancers (Yu and Thomson, 2014).

Causes of Cancer

Considering the causes of such a complicated disease plays an important role in the prevention and resolution of the disease. Several causes emerge in cancer in direct proportion to its complexity. The population is increasing day by day, and the different changes in the world population in certain regions and the change in incidence of individual cancers show that environmental exposures give rise to cancer. Environmental cancer-causing factors include exposures that occur naturally, pollution, lifestyle factors, and materials that people use in their jobs. According to the *National Cancer Institute* (NCI), radiation and lifestyles as cancer-causing exposures may be avoidable. One of the main sources of UV radiation is sunlight, and UV rays in sunlight increase the risk of melanoma, a type of skin cancer according to the *American Cancer Society*.

The lifestyle of people also affects cancer. For instance, in high-income countries, tobacco usage is diminished by the campaigns against smoking, but in low-income countries, the tobacco epidemic is still in its early stages (Lee and Hashibe, 2014). Another crucial example is obesity in the lifestyles of people that occurs mostly in high-income countries. Obesity leads to tumorigenesis due to the accumulation of excess phosphate by dysregulated endocrine metabolism of dietary phosphate that mediates the link between obesity and cancer (Brown, 2022).

Infectious agents that comprise bacteria, viruses, and parasites are categorized under naturally occurring exposures and increase the risk of cancer due to disrupting cell signaling, making the immune system weak and leading to chronic inflammation. The majority of viruses including Human Papillomavirus (HPV), Human Immunodeficiency Virus (HIV), Hepatitis B, Hepatitis C, and Epstein-Barr virus (EBV) are related with a higher risk of cancer due to the transfer from one person to another via body fluids. In order to prevent this transmission for reducing infection, vaccination becomes significant at this point (Liao, 2006). For example, HPV is responsible for almost all cervical cancers, mainly in low-income countries, and vaccination globally can reduce the risk of cervical cancer by at least 70% in the world (Martel et al., 2017). Due to the proximity of the genital and anal regions, vaccination decreases the viral load in the genital area and prohibits the occurrence or completely eliminates contaminant genital-anal HPV infections (Eer et al., 2022).

In addition, carcinogens, including chemical, physical, and biological processes and endogenous processes, lead to uncontrollable cell division in the human body. According to the WHO, carcinogens are classified into 4 groups as noncarcinogenic, possibly, probably, and carcinogenic. On this scale, tobacco use is classified as carcinogenic, which causes lung and mouth cancers, and smoking is responsible for one in five cancer deaths. Furthermore, the conditions people are exposed to, such as economic, psychological, and social conditions, also give rise to the change of the normal mechanism of cells.

In addition to these causes mentioned in this part of the chapter, hereditary factors also play an important role in cancer development due to the possibility of carrying inherited faulty genes (Pomerantz and Freedman, 2011). Especially in prostate and breast cancer, knowledge of family history and examination of hereditary cancer genes are of great importance in the prevention of the disease (Kalish et al., 2000; Pharoah et al., 1997). Recent analyzes reveal that between 55% and 72% of women are at risk of breast cancer due to the BRCA1 mutation, while from 45% to 69% of women are at risk of breast cancer due to carrying the mutant BRCA2 gene with increasing age (Kuchenbaecker et al., 2017; Antoniou et al., 2003; Chen and Parmigiani, 2003).

Last but not least, early diagnosis is highly significant in cancer. However, as the world struggles with COVID-19 infection, the diagnosis of cancer is delayed among people (Corley et al., 2021; İlgün and Özmen, 2022). The Netherlands Cancer Registry reported that between 24 February 2020 and 12

April 2020, there was a nearly 25% reduction in cancer diagnosis (Dinmohamed et al., 2020; Hamilton et al., 2021). In addition to that, in the UK, due to the COVID-19 pandemic, mortality rates caused by cancer have increased (Maringe, 2020).

Characteristics of Cancer Cells

Across the spectrum between Occam's Razor to Hickam's Dictum, it is crucial to understand both simple common characteristics and complex distinctive enabling mechanisms that are interpreted uniquely by each cancer in order to develop an effective battle strategy against this dynamic process.

Self-Sufficiency in Growth Signals and Avoiding Growth Suppressors

Cell proliferation is the title mechanism in several physiological processes to maintain homeostasis from embryogenesis to tissue repair, and due to its substantial role and potential, it is precisely regulated in normal cells. The initial steps of progressive conversion of normal human cells into cancer cells are associated with increased proliferative activity due to acquired self-sufficiency in growth signals (Witsch et al., 2010). There are various mechanisms that cancer cells deceive to establish an independent proliferation capability from external growth stimuli. Such as increasing autocrine mitotic stimulation factors, stimulating tumor microenvironment to synthesize growth factors for paracrine stimulation or upregulating receptor abundance to enhance response even to low stimulus levels. Mitotic signals, which are necessary for the initiation of cell division, can be externally catalyzed via soluble growth factors, the tumor microenvironment, and mechanisms controlling cell-to-cell connection/adhesion. Growth factors are transmitted to the cell to initiate the mitotic cascade by binding to membrane receptors that typically contain an intracellular tyrosine kinase domain. Alternatively, ligand-independent receptor activation via mutations that alter downstream pathways can also provoke proliferative signaling. AKT, MAPK and mTOR signaling pathways which constitute upstream regulators of cellular growth, proliferation, and/or survival mechanisms are highly dysregulated in cancers (Dhillon et al., 2007; Mundi et al., 2016; Zou et al., 2020). Furthermore, acquisition of insensitivity to negative feedback mechanisms also provides an important advancement in increasing the growth rate, which is the next capability acquired in the carcinogenesis process.

Aberrant cellular growth mechanisms in cancer cells involve mutations that include the suppression of genes that prevent growth (tumor suppressors), as well as mutation and inducement of genes involved in driving cell growth (oncogenes). A widely known analogy for the tumor suppressor and oncogene function is the 'gas-brake mechanism' (Gaiani et al., 2021). The promoting function of oncogenes on proliferation is like stepping on a gas that increases the expression that is functional on cellular metabolism. In contrast, tumor suppressors are like applying the break, only functional when used to limit an active mechanism that inhibits cellular growth and proliferation. Therefore, loss of function mutations and loss of tumor suppressor genes cause abnormal replication and growth.

Deceiving anti-proliferative mechanisms as important as accession and sustaining growth signals to promote malignancies. Environmental factors can lead to DNA damage and genetic alterations. Growth suppressor mechanisms, which are often regulated by tumor suppressor genes, can inhibit proliferation of damaged/mutated cells by cell cycle halt and induce senescence or programmed cell death mechanisms (R. Huang & Zhou, 2021). Loss of growth control mechanisms permits mutated cells to acquire unlimited replicative ability and circumvent elimination, growth arrest, and senescence which accelerate the malign transformation of cancer cells. Tumor cells may use genetic and epigenetic mechanisms to bypass tumor suppressors. Chromosome deletions, loss or inhibition of the suppressor gene and/or its downstream and upstream regulators; DNA methylation, histone methylation, and acetylation are effector factors in growth inhibition (Amin et al., 2015).

Resisting Cell Death and Enabling Replicative Immortality

Programmed cell death (PCD) mechanisms are genetically predetermined processes for the targeted elimination of redundant, irrecoverably impaired, and/or potentially harmful cells to maintain organismal homeostasis. PCD mechanisms not only function by removing redundant or potentially harmful cells, but also warn the organism of a potential hazard over the substances released by dying cells (Galluzzi et al., 2018).

Apoptosis, which is triggered in response to cellular stress conditions such as overexpression of oncogenic signaling and DNA damage associated with hyperproliferation, has both intrinsic and extrinsic initiator factors. The extrinsic apoptotic pathway can be induced by extracellular death signals (for example the Fas ligand/Fas receptor), the intrinsic pathway can be triggered by a variety of signals of intracellular origin, for example, substantial levels of DNA breaks and other chromosomal abnormalities. Cancer cells employ a variety of maneuvers to evade or cease apoptosis during initiation or promotion of tumorigenesis, such as mutation or loss of tumor suppressor gene, upregulating antiapoptotic regulators or survival signals, down-regulating pro-apoptotic proteins, or short-circuiting the extrinsic ligand-induced death pathways.

Autophagy is a programmed death response induced by cellular stress that allows cells to repurpose deconstructed cellular organelles for biosynthesis and energy metabolism. Autophagic morphology is characterized by cytoplasmic vacuolization followed by phagocytosis and subsequent lysosomal degradation, similar to apoptosis (Levine & Kroemer, 2008; Mizushima, 2007). However, when cancer cells are under extreme stress conditions such as starvation, exposure to radiation or cytotoxic agents, the autophagy program preserves the cell in a reversible dormancy phase and serves as a resistance mechanism for the death of cancer cells. In other words, depending on the context, autophagy can function as a tumor suppressor in the early stages of tumor initiation and later as a tumor promoter (Apel et al., 2009; White & DiPaola, 2009).

Unlike apoptosis and autophagy, the necrotic cell membrane ruptures and releases its cellular content and pro-inflammatory signals into the surrounding tissue microenvironment, recruiting the inflammatory response necessary to delineate the damaged area and remove the scattered cellular content (Grivennikov et al., 2010). This successive inflammatory response may facilitate tumor progression, which will be covered later in this chapter, through its ability to promote angiogenesis, cancer cell proliferation, and invasiveness. Lastly, necrotic cells can release paracrine factors that stimulate neighboring viable cells to proliferate, which can facilitate malignant progression (Galluzzi et al., 2018).

Under physiological conditions, healthy cells have limited replicative cycle capacity which is called the Hayflick Limit (Hayflick, 1965). After undergoing between 40 and 60 divisions, cell growth slows down and eventually first faces cellular senescence and then, if the cells can pass this barrier, to a crisis path and apoptosis. This process, also known as cellular aging, is an autonomous prevention mechanism to avoid the increased risk of mutagenesis due to endless cycles of DNA replication by limiting the multiplication. However, cancer cells circumvent this limit and continue to replicate indefinitely as part of the growth of preneoplastic and neoplastic cells in tumors. The main regulators of this process are telomeres and the enzyme telomerase.

Telomeres, which are repetitive DNA regions at the end of chromosomes, function as a protective shield to prevent loss of chromosomal content. Telomerase is a DNA polymerase that extends the telomere ends by adding telomere repeats to the ends of telomeric DNA. As a result of the gradual loss of telomeric regions after each cycle, telomeres lose their ability to protect the ends of chromosomal DNA. Exposed chromosome ends become impaired, which activates the DNA damage response, which eventually results in senescence and cell cycle arrest. Achieving to pass the arrest and subsequent chromatin loss eventually leads the chromosome ends to fuse with each other, causing irreversible damage and initiating the apoptotic process; the cell enters a crisis and eventually dies (Hoare & Narita, 2018). Cancer cells avoid senescence and persist in proliferation via continual extension of the telomeres by telomerase activity. Normal cells, other than stem cells and fetal cells, do not have a frequent replication cycle, making them less needy for telomerase function. However, it is crucial to reassess replicative senescence due to excessive proliferation. Cancer cells maintain telomere ends through increased expression of telomerase, which is unusual in normal cells. Many oncoproteins have the ability to upregulate telomerase expression, while most tumor suppressors restrict it. Another detrimental factor that affects the length of the telomere is oxidative stress. The DNA repair mechanisms that are responsible for maintaining oxidative stress-induced DNA damage are less effective in the telomeric regions on chromosomes. Therefore, telomeres are especially vulnerable to oxidative stress.

Enabling replicative immortality is a critical point in malignant progression and also leads to accumulation of detrimental mutations, which also explains the increase in cancer prevalence with age.

Senescence

Senescence is a protective negative feedback mechanism that contributes to embryological development, wound healing, and aging in healthy tissues. The mechanism is also known as an autonomous tumor suppressor and can be induced by extensive oncogenic signaling, loss of tumor suppressors, or anticancer therapies. Oncogene-induced senescence is often driven by the inhibitory activity of the RAS/MAPK/PI3K pathways as a negative feedback mechanism (Hoare & Narita, 2018). However, recent studies revealed the diverse range of autonomous and non-autonomous features of senescence with tumor suppressor and promoting effects on adjacent cancer cells and other stromal cells in the tumor microenvironment.

One of the tumor-promoting features of senescence is the creation of a cancer cell phenotype with transient and reversible cell cycle arrest. Cancer cells in transient senescence can escape from their non-proliferative senescence-associated secretory phenotype (SASP), exhibit a dormancy state that avoids therapeutic targeting of proliferating cancer cells, which is observed as resistance to treatment. When the unfavorable circumstances disappeared, residual dormant cancer cells return to a mitotic phenotype and can recover their oncogenic capabilities back (De Blander et al., 2021).

Stromal cells of the tumor microenvironment in senescence also have a regulatory effect that is driven by SASP through paracrine or juxtacrine signaling. Stromal SASP can stimulate plasticity, modulate tumor microenvironment, mediate fibrosis, and stimulate tumor neovasculature. These cells can also initiate their own immune-mediated death; and if this mechanism is disrupted, residual senescent cells can become tumorigenic. Eventually, these non-autonomous effects, depending on the signal receiving cell, could be tumor suppressive or pro-oncogenic (Hoare & Narita, 2018).

Promoting Angiogenesis

During tumorigenic progression, preexisting blood vessels become insufficient to meet increasing demands for nutrients and oxygen supply, and to remove metabolic waste and carbon dioxide produced due to increased consumption. In order to meet this expectation, the "angiogenic switch," which is in a quiescent state in adults, is kept active for tumor associated neoangiogenesis. Various pro-angiogenic and antiangiogenic factors operate in concert to control angiogenesis. Several substances released by tumor cells and reactive cells in the tumor microenvironment encourage the migration and proliferation of these endothelial cells to form new blood capillaries and lymph arteries. Proangiogenic Vascular Endothelial Growth Factor (VEGF), Fibroblast Growth Factor (FGF), Hypoxia inducible factor (HIF), platelet-derived growth factor (PDGF), as well as antiangiogenic thrombospondin (TSP), angiostatin, and endostatin are known angiogenesis regulator protein families with opposite functions (Nyberg et al., 2005).

VEGF expression, involved in neovascularization during embryogenesis and endothelial cell homeostasis in adults, can be upregulated by both hypoxia and oncogene signaling. Chronically upregulated expression of the FGF protein family has been linked to maintaining tumor angiogenesis (Carmeliet, 2005; Gabhann & Popel, 2008). TSP-1 is an endogenous angiogenesis inhibitor that acts as a physiological modulator in transitory angiogenesis during wound healing, as well as a hindering mechanism for nascent neoplasia-induced angiogenesis (Baeriswyl & Christofori, 2009).

In addition to oncogenic expression that upregulates angiogenic factors, inductive signals secreted by some bone marrow-derived immune cells can also contribute to tumor angiogenesis. Immune inflammatory cells that have infiltrated the peritumoral regions can help to activate the angiogenic switch indirectly to sustain the ongoing angiogenesis associated with tumor growth and facilitate local invasion (Ferrara, 2010), which will be discussed in detail throughout this book. The 'angiogenic switch' is activated frequently during or prior to invasion in primary tumors. In metastases, it may indicate the critical shift from micrometastases to exponentially growing lesions.

Activating Invasion and Metastatic Cascade

The expansion and penetration of cancer cells into nearby environments is called invasion. Whereas metastasis refers to the process in which cancer cells leave their primary site of growth and migrate by blood or lymph to distant regions to form malignant neoplasia. These two multifactorial and reciprocal processes are definitive criteria that distinguish benign tumors from malignant ones. Furthermore, metastatic spread with tumor cachexia and immune suppression is the main cause of cancer-related mortality (Guan, 2015).

During metastatic progression, cancer cells first invade locally into different layers of the primary sites of growth. Projections of sprouting cells erode the basement membrane by pressurizing neighboring connective and muscular tissues, creating malignant tumors without clear boundaries. In order to translocate systemically, cancer cells need to expand and intravasate into the lumina of blood vessels or lymph channels. The surviving cells in the stream then halt at a distant site and extravasate into the organ parenchyma. If a migrating cell is able to adapt to the new environment, it may remain dormant or form multicellular micrometastases and eventually establish apparent metastatic tumors, which is called colonization (Massagué & Obenauf, 2016).

The complex colonization process after the invasion and migration cascade, which requires massive restructuring of tissue structure, is a multistep process maintained by tumor cells and accompanying stromal immune and inflammatory cells in the tumor microenvironment. Furthermore, the preferred migration route is also a fate determining factor for the new region where the metastatic tumor arises next. In particular, while hematogenic metastases usually increase the probability of migration to a distant organ, lymphogenic metastasis often results in metastases in lymph nodes that drain the region where the cancer originated (Valastyan & Weinberg, 2011).

Increased Genomic Instability and Mutations

Maintenance of genomic integrity is a highly conserved and monitored process in the cell. This machinery is responsible for detecting and minimizing the risk of somatic mutations that may occur during each cell cycle at the lowest possible rate (Negrini et al., 2010). However, the malign transformation process of cancer cells is achieved by accumulation of genetic and epigenetic alterations. The increased susceptibility of these alterations in each cell cycle is called genomic instability, which includes minor alterations such as base pair mutations or microsatellite instability, as well as chromosomal instability resulting from numerical or structural chromosomal abnormalities. Both mutational changes induced by loss of tumor suppressor gene function or oncogene-driven mitotic activation, and non-mutational changes altering gene expression patterns like histone modification or DNA methylation are effective mechanisms that result in the formation of cancer cells with mutant genotype.

Genomic integrity checkpoint control mechanisms, which are precisely controlled throughout the cell cycle, are responsible for detecting possible spontaneous mutations that may occur during DNA replication and chromosomal segregation promptly (Potapova & Gorbsky, 2017). These mechanisms, also known as caretakers, ensure the detection of damage in the genome and activation of the DNA repair mechanisms; and in the event of irreversible impairment, induce cell cycle arrest and apoptosis. Deteriorations in DNA damage checkpoints, DNA repair machinery, and mitotic checkpoint surveillance mechanisms often result in the continuation of the lineage with a mutant phenotype, rather than abolition via senescence and apoptosis. Once genomically unstable cells evade cytostatic controls, their increased growth rate favors cancer cells, making the mutant genotype dominant in the population while contributing to the accumulation of more mutations and increasing genomic instability (Yao & Dai, 2014).

Reprogramming Cellular Metabolism

Cancer cells are known to have elevated biosynthesis and energy demand in conjunction with an increase in mitotic rate. However, reprogramming metabolism to favor 'Aerobic glycolysis,' while normal cells implement only when subjected to hypoxic conditions or mitochondrial dysfunction, is the major energy production mechanism in cancer. This phenomenon that increased oxygen consumption and preferential lactate production of cancer cells, even in the presence of oxygen, is called the Warburg effect (Racker, 1972; Warburg et al., 1926). There are various motivations behind the preference of cancer cells, which have a much higher energy deficit than a normal cell, for anaerobic glycolysis, which yields far less ATP compared to oxidative phosphorylation.

Due to the catastrophic neoangiogenic network developed during tumor growth, low oxygenation in dense regions of solid tumors is inevitable. Eliminating the need for high oxygen concentrations required for oxidative phosphorylation gives cancer cells the advantage to sustain metabolic activity even under hypoxic conditions. Increased glycolysis in cancer cells facilitates the biosynthesis of cellular macromolecules, such as nucleic acids, proteins, and lipids, for assembly of new cells by allowing recycling of metabolic intermediates of interrupted TCA cycle (Kroemer & Pouyssegur, 2008; Lunt & Vander Heiden, 2011).

Disabling the oxidative phosphorylation pathway eliminates mitochondrial dependence. Considering the regulator role of mitochondria in the intrinsic apoptotic pathway, and its limiting effects on ROS accumulation in cells, the absence of mitochondrial functions also contributes to carcinogenesis by affecting downstream cell signaling pathways (Iommarini et al., 2017; Izzo et al., 2016; Wallace, 2012). Additionally, elevated lactic acid levels act as a metabolite of glycolysis and fermentation, HIF-1α drives angiogenesis via VEGF expression, thereby providing more nutrient access to tumor cells (Goodwin et al., 2015).

Two-Faced Sword: Antitumor Immunity and Tumor-Promoting Inflammation

Antitumor immunity is the innate and adaptive immune responses developed to restrict tumor growth. Adequacy of the antitumor response is managed by a series of complex mechanisms. Basically, tumor–immune system interface includes antigen processing and secretion by antigen-presenting cells (APCs), interaction with T lymphocytes, following cytotoxic T-cell activation, regulation of antigen-specific effector cells, and inevitably eradication of the target cancer cell by the activated effector T cell (Teng et al., 2008).

Immune surveillance mechanisms are responsible for the immune system to detect and remove possible malignancies as early as possible by keeping neoplastic cells under constant surveillance. In this context, tumors that became clinically detectable are those that have managed to avoid immune surveillance or limited the scope of immunological killing actions. In fact, since highly immunogenic cancer cells are eliminated by the immune response of the immunocompetent host, weakly immunogenic cells constitute the majority of the tumor, which is referred to as immunomodulation. Deficiencies in the development or functioning of immune cells responsible for the antitumor response cause an increase in tumor incidence, increasing the susceptibility of primary and even secondary malignancies. Furthermore, immunogenic (hot) tumors may evade immune system-related destruction by secreting inhibitory cytokines themselves or by recruiting highly immune-suppressive cells into the tumor microenvironment (TME), such as regulatory T cells (Tregs), myeloid-derived suppressor cells (MDSCs), cancer-associated fibroblasts, and M2 macrophages (TAMs), to abolish the cytotoxic effects of lymphocytes (Campesato et al., 2020).

Infiltrating immune cells in neoplastic lesions was only interpreted as an antitumor defense mechanism for many years. However, as is known today, inflammation also has tumor-promoting functions (DeNardo et al., 2010; Goswami et al., 2017; Man et al., 2013). In fact, both tumor-promoting inflammation and antitumor response occur simultaneously but at different stages of tumorigenesis, in order that environmental and microenvironmental variables govern the balance (Bui & Schreiber, 2007; Swann et al., 2008). A set of distinct strategies to avoid detection and elimination by antitumor immunity mechanisms is called immune escape (Beatty & Gladney, 2015). Both stimulating and obstructing functions of tumor-infiltrating immune cells suggest that inflammation is a conditionally variable response to tumor immunity (Grivennikov et al., 2010). *Exempli gratia*, inflammation-derived metabolites, and cytokines secreted in the tumor microenvironment can contribute to neoplastic progression by secretion of growth factors that sustain mitotic activity, survival factors to resist programmed cell death mechanisms, proangiogenic factors for the formation of neovascularization within the tumor mass, and induction of epithelial to mesenchymal transition factors to facilitate the invasion-metastasis cascade (Karnoub & Weinberg, 2006; Multhoff et al., 2012; Qian & Pollard, 2010). Furthermore, reactive oxygen species released by inflammatory cells have pro- tumorigenic effects on cancer cells, which accelerates the malign progression by inducing proliferation, survival, and adaptation to hypoxia. Ergo, inflammation can be regarded as a facilitating mechanism during tumorigenesis (Reczek & Chandel, 2017).

The cancer-immunology relationship, which is one of the most prominent topics in cancer research of the last quarter century, is used in the clinic to fight cancer with various tools such as vaccines, nonspecific immune-therapies, adoptive cell therapy, and immune checkpoint inhibitors. This subject, which will be evaluated in detail in the following parts of the book, stands out as one of the most powerful weapons we have against cancer today.

Phenotypic Plasticity in Cancer Cell Populations

Cellular plasticity is the ability to adapt in response to an external stimulus without genetic alterations along a certain phenotypic spectrum. During organogenesis, progenitor cells are driven into a specific terminal phenotype through differentiation mechanisms for the development, determination and organization of undifferentiated cells into functional tissues, which in most cases infers an antiproliferative state. Plasticity mechanisms provide cells with a phenotype switch capability that is responsible for the development and repair mechanisms in injury (Burggren, 2020).

The cellular plasticity mechanism in cancer is distorted to evade or escape from a terminally differentiated state to grant a momentous advantage of the ability to survive under environmental stress (hypoxia, starvation, chemo= therapeutic agents, etc.) via phenotype switch without any mutational dependencies. Studies suggest that cellular plasticity is a prominent mediator and promising target for premalignant progression, metastasis, and resistance to therapy (Yuan et al., 2019).

During malignant progression, disorganized differentiation mechanisms can provoke aberrations in cell fate (Hanahan, 2022). *Dedifferentiation* of mature cells into progenitor cells enables them to escape dormant state into a hyperproliferative phase, which was also proposed as a possible origin mechanism for cancer stem cells that they might be dedifferentiated somatic cells undergoing an oncogenic route (Friedmann-Morvinski & Verma, 2014; Yamada et al., 2014). *Blocking the differentiation* of progenitor cells into a terminally differentiated state via suppression of differentiation factors can facilitate tumorigenesis. Furthermore, partially or undifferentiated cancer stem cells/progenitor cells remained in niches as dormant, while carrying the potential for reinitiation of proliferative expansion, and constitute as an overlooked threat, which can survive after a 'successful' therapy of primary tumor and regenerate to cause a relapsed or metastatic disease (Phan & Croucher, 2020). *Transdifferatiation* of one differentiated cell type to another differentiated class is a form of tissue metaplasia. The process, which serves as a regeneration mechanism in healthy tissue, manifests itself in cancer as malignancies with morphologies that differ from the tissue in which it is located. One of the well-known occurrences of gross tissue metaplasia is the transdifferentiation of stratified squamous epithelium cells of the esophagus into the simple columnar epithelium, which are characteristic intestine cells, when exposed to chronic inflammation (Yuan et al., 2019). This phenomenon is known as Barrets' esophagus. Although this metaplasia is not cancerous at the beginning, dedifferentiated cells are at high risk of developing esophageal adenocarcinomas (Helm et al., 2005). Based on the cancer type, transdifferentiation could both give rise to a drug resistant cell lineage, or could be directed into a phenotype that is susceptible to therapy. EGFR-driven non-small cell lung cancers (NSLCs) transdifferentiate into small cell lung cancer (SCLC) phenotype when exposed to EGFR tyrosine kinase inhibitors; which in turn rise to an acquired resistance to therapy (Marcoux et al., 2019; Shen & Clairambault, 2020).

Non-Mutational Epigenetic Reprogramming

The term epigenetic was first used by Waddington in 1942 to introduce a mechanism to describe why all cells in the body that express different genes have the same DNA material and how cell fate specification and lineage switching work (Waddington, 1942). The model illustrates cell fate as a 'landscape' with hills and valleys. The progenitor cell, which was symbolized as a marble rolling down from a 'progeny' hill to 'specific phenotype' valleys, is committed to a lineage and this transformation is irreversible. Later, Huang proposed to add "bisurfections" between "the valleys" to this model to describe multilineage priming as seen in both erythroid and myelomonocytic lineages, which originate from common myeloid precursor cells (S. Huang et al., 2007; S. Huang, 2013).

Under normal physiological conditions, both the modulation of differentiation and organogenesis during embryonic development stages and long-term memory formation in adults are regulated by non-mutational epigenetic mechanisms, which are DNA methylation, histone modifications, chromatin remodeling, and noncoding RNAs (Klymenko & Nephew, 2018). Chromatin-level plasticity driven by epigenetic regulators, cellular-level plasticity by intracellular signaling, microenvironmental plasticity through cell-to-cell interactions, and physiological stress conditions mediate non-mutational epigenetic programming in favor of malignant transformation, which plays an important role in tumor progression and resistance in cancer cells (Shen & Clairambault, 2020). Bidirectional epigenetic crosstalk between the tumor microenvironment and cancer cells, such as structure, density, and composition of the extracellular matrix, hypoxic conditions, secretome composition of stromal cells in the tumor microenvironment, are few of the deterministic factors for tumor-promoting epigenetic changes (Hanahan, 2022).

Prevention, Diagnosis and Treatment of Cancer

As mentioned in the previous part, early diagnosis has a significant impact on cancer. Therefore, medical care includes regular control, such as self-exams, and screening is highly crucial in the prevention of cancer. Medical care is not enough to prevent cancer alone, other precautions are required to be taken as well. Avoiding tobacco use and a balanced diet with an active lifestyle also help prevent the development of cancer. As mentioned in the previous part, it is known that viral infections cause cancer, and vaccination may be helpful in avoiding cancer-causing viral infections. Avoiding exposure to the sun by restricting time under the sun can prevent the risk of skin cancer due to the limitation of exposure to ultraviolet (UV) radiation.

Cancer diagnosis is another issue that is highly crucial in handling this disease. In the early stages, it provides a chance for cure. Cancer screening becomes important at this point. Colorectal, breast and prostate cancers are common cancers which screenings are performed by using screening tests including mammogram and colonoscopy. Especially, cancer screening is highly recommended for the person who is under the risk due to the significance of family medical history. Women diagnosed with breast cancer have a 10-year survival rate of more than 70% patients, while those in the earliest stages of this invasive disease have a 10-year survival rate of over 90% patients (Jacobs and Finlayson, 2011).

Cancer is diagnosed using a variety of approaches including physical examination, laboratory tests, imaging tests, and biopsy. Depending on the location and size of the tumor, feeling the tumor by physical examination is the simplest way to diagnose cancer. The presence (existence) of high or low amounts of substances in the body can indicate the presence of cancer. As a result, laboratory tests measuring these compounds contained in body fluids, such as blood and urine, can assist doctors in making a diagnosis. Many laboratory tests check for tumor markers in blood or tissue samples. In response to cancer, cancer cells or healthy cells produce specific substances, these are called tumor markers. The majority of tumor markers are produced by both normal and cancer cells, but cancer cells produce them at considerably higher levels. To determine whether or not the tumor is present, imaging tests such as CT, PET, and MRI are used to create images of areas inside the body. For the diagnosis of cancer, the evaluation of the pathologists is important and the pathologists decide whether the removed tissue sample, which is called biopsy, is cancerous or not and determine the type of cancer, the stage of the tumor and the grade of the tumor of the cancerous tissue. The tumor stage describes the extent of the cancer, as well as whether it has spread, while the appearance of the cancerous sample describes the tumor grade. In addition to the identification of cancer, pathology reports are crucial in determining treatment options for the appropriate therapy. Several objectives come in sight about cancer treatment. Curing the disease is one of them and allows a person to live a normal life. The removal of the cancerous part from the body or the killing of cancer cells is called primary treatment. Surgery, which is one of the treatment options, is the most common primary treatment. To reduce the recurrence chance of cancer, after primary treatment, adjuvant treatment is applied to destroy any cancer cells. One of the adjuvant treatments is chemotherapy, and in this treatment option, drugs used to destroy cancer cells also have a subversive effect on healthy cells, unfortunately. At this point, targeted drug therapy comes into prominence due to focusing on proteins that control the cancer cells and not being cytotoxic to healthy cells. A smart drug delivery system that is based on nanocarriers is a good example of targeted drug therapy in current research due to the application of the drug to the specific site of the body and the release of the drug within control (Unsoy and Gunduz, 2018; Hossen et al., 2019). For example, gold nanoparticles are widely used nanocarriers due to their low toxicity, which are reduced by making surface modifications considering their size, shape, and surface chemistry (Altunbek et al., 2016).

Radiation therapy is the other type of adjuvant therapy and the human body is exposed to powerful energy beams such as protons and X-rays for destroying cancer cells. The other common adjuvant therapy is hormone therapy. In this treatment option, the removal of hormones that are used as fuel by cancer cells and blocking of their effects are intended to kill cancer cells. Hormone therapy is applied especially to patients who suffer from breast cancer and prostate cancer due to targeting hormone receptors. Another example of adjuvant therapy, which has a wide spectrum, is immunotherapy, which depends on the adjustment of immune cells, allowing them to attack cancerous cells. Immunotherapy is a newly discovered field, and research on this topic is increasing day by day due to its advantages. Compared to conventional therapies, side effects are reduced in immunotherapy. Other advantages of immunotherapy include long-term survival rate, effective treatment, and a wide range of adaptation (Tan et al., 2020). Recently, mRNA cancer vaccines, which will be discussed in next chapter, have an importance in the cancer immunotherapy researches due to providing powerful fighting for the body against cancer cells (Miao, 2021).

Gene therapy is a new, safe, and effective treatment option due to enhancing the survival rate and lifespan of patients. The principle of gene therapy regards to infect the host cell with a target gene in order to cause favorable biological activity by expressing itself (Gonçalves et al., 2017; Samaniego et al., 2020). However, the long-term risks of gene therapy are not stated in order to carry gene therapy in clinics according to *Nature Medicine*.

Due to the development of new treatment strategies, new diagnostic methods, and the provision of human health for a high-quality lifespan, clinical trials are of vital importance (Novitzke, 2008). Currently, more than 4000 clinical trials are conducted on immunotherapy and 2000 studies are conducted on gene therapy according to *Clinical Trials* data.

Since cancer, which is a complex disease, can turn into more complex states, researchers are conducting research and doing more work in this field. Cancer researchers intend to unravel the language of this disease to fight it effectively.

Conclusion

Cancer is a complex disease under the influence of various exposures such as lifestyle, environmental, hereditary, and dietary factors. Worldwide, more than 19 million new cancer cases were reported in 2020. Since the incidence of most cancers increases with age, it is expected that this rate will increase as life expectancy increases in developing countries. Every day we learn even more about cancer. Parallel to the complexity of this disorder, numerous treatment approaches are used alongside conventional treatments, including the use of immune cells as warriors against cancer. The prevention and diagnosis of cancer, as well as its treatment, are of great importance in improving quality of life.

References

Addisia, G. D., Tegegne, A. S., Belay, D. B., Muluneh, M. W., & Kassaw, M. A. (2022). Risk factors of white blood cell progression among patients with chronic lymphocytic leukemia at Felege Hiwot Referral Hospital, Bahir Dar, Ethiopia. *Cancer Informatics, 21*, 11769351211069902.

Altunbek, M., Kuku, G., & Culha, M. (2016). Gold nanoparticles in single-cell analysis for surface enhanced Raman scattering. *Molecules, 21*(12): 1617.

Antoniou, A., Pharoah, P. D., Narod, S., Risch, H. A., Eyfjord, J. E., Hopper, J. L., & Easton, D. (2003). Average risks of breast and ovarian cancer associated with BRCA1 or BRCA2 mutations detected in case series unselected for family history: a combined analysis of 22 studies. *The American Journal of Human Genetics*, *72*(5): 1117-1130.

Apel, A., Zentgraf, H., Büchler, M. W., & Herr, I. (2009). Autophagy-A double-edged sword in oncology. *International Journal of Cancer*, *125*(5): 991–995. https://doi.org/10.1002/ijc.24500.

Baeriswyl, V., & Christofori, G. (2009). The angiogenic switch in carcinogenesis. Seminars in Cancer Biology, *19*(5): 329–337. https://doi.org/10.1016/j.semcancer.2009.05.003.

Beatty, G. L., & Gladney, W. L. (2015). Immune escape mechanisms as a guide for cancer immunotherapy. *Clinical Cancer Research: An Official Journal of the American Association for Cancer Research*, *21*(4): 687–692. https://doi.org/10.1158/1078-04 3 2.CCR-14-1860.

Brown, R. B. (2022). Obesity and cancer: potential mediation by dysregulated dietary phosphate. *Obesities*, *2*(1): 64-75.

Bui, J. D., & Schreiber, R. D. (2007). Cancer immunosurveillance, immunoediting and inflammation: Independent or interdependent processes? *Current Opinion in Immunology, 19*(2): 203–208. https://doi.org/10.1016/j.coi.2007.02.001.

Burggren, W. W. (2020). Phenotypic switching resulting from developmental plasticity: fixed or reversible? *Frontiers in Physiology, 10.* https://www.frontiersin.org/article/10.3389/fphys.2019.01634.

Breasted, J.H. (1930). *The Edwin Smith Surgical Papyrus: Published in Facsimile and Hieroglyphic Transliteration with Translation and Commentary in Two Volumes.* Chicago: The University of Chicago Press.

Campesato, L. F., Weng, C.-H., & Merghoub, T. (2020). Innate immune checkpoints for cancer immunotherapy: Expanding the scope of non-T cell targets. *Annals of Translational Medicine*, *8*(16): 1031. https://doi.org/10.21037/atm-20-1816.

Carmeliet, P. (2005). VEGF as a key mediator of angiogenesis in cancer. *Oncology*, *69 Suppl 3*: 4–10. https://doi.org/10.1159/000088478.

Chen, S., & Parmigiani, G. (2007). Meta-analysis of BRCA1 and BRCA2 penetrance. *Journal of Clinical Oncology: Official Journal of the American Society of Clinical Oncology*, *25*(11): 1329.

Cooper, G. M., & Hausman, R. E. (2000). The development and causes of cancer. *The Cell: A Molecular Approach*, *2*: 719-728.

Corley, D. A., Sedki, M., Ritzwoller, D. P., Greenlee, R. T., Neslund-Dudas, C., Rendle, K. A., & Haas, J. S. (2021). Cancer screening during the coronavirus disease-2019 pandemic: a perspective from the National Cancer Institute's PROSPR Consortium. *Gastroenterology*, *160*(4): 999-1002.

De Blander, H., Morel, A. P., Senaratne, A. P., Ouzounova, M., & Puisieux, A. (2021). Cellular plasticity: a route to senescence exit and tumorigenesis. *Cancers*, *13*(18): 4561. https://doi.org/10.3390/cancers13184561.

De Martel, C., Plummer, M., Vignat, J., & Franceschi, S. (2017). Worldwide burden of cancer attributable to HPV by site, country and HPV type. *International Journal of Cancer*, *141*(4): 664-670.

DeNardo, D. G., Andreu, P., & Coussens, L. M. (2010). Interactions between lymphocytes and myeloid cells regulate pro- versus anti-tumor immunity. *Cancer Metastasis Reviews*, *29*(2): 309–316. https://doi.org/10.1007/s10555-010-9223-6.

Dhillon, A. S., Hagan, S., Rath, O., & Kolch, W. (2007). MAP kinase signalling pathways in cancer. *Oncogene*, *26*(22): 3279–3290. https://doi.org/10.1038/sj.onc.1210421.

Dinmohamed, A. G., Visser, O., Verhoeven, R. H., Louwman, M. W., van Nederveen, F. H., Willems, S. M., & Siesling, S. (2020). Fewer cancer diagnoses during the COVID-19 epidemic in the Netherlands. *The Lancet Oncology*, *21*(6): 750-751.

Fairfield, H., Falank, C., Avery, L., & Reagan, M. R. (2016). Multiple myeloma in the marrow: pathogenesis and treatments. *Annals of the New York Academy of Sciences*, *1364*(1): 32-51.

Ferlay, J., Colombet, M., Soerjomataram, I., Parkin, D. M., Piñeros, M., Znaor, A., & Bray, F. (2021). Cancer statistics for the year 2020: An overview. International Journal of Cancer. *Cancer Epidemiology, 149*(4)*:* 778-789. https://doi.org/10.1002/ijc.33588.

Ferrara, N. (2010). Pathways mediating VEGF-independent tumor angiogenesis. *Cytokine & Growth Factor Reviews*, *21*(1): 21–26. https://doi.org/10.1016/j.cytogfr.2009.11.003.

Friedmann-Morvinski, D., & Verma, I. M. (2014). Dedifferentiation and reprogramming: Origins of cancer stem cells. *EMBO Reports*, *15*(3): 244–253. https://doi.org/10.1002/embr.201338254.

Gabhann, F. M., & Popel, A. S. (2008). Systems biology of vascular endothelial growth factors. *Microcirculation*, *15*(8): 715–738. https://doi.org/10.1080/1073968080209 5964.

Gaiani, F., Marchesi, F., Negri, F., Greco, L., Malesci, A., de'Angelis, G. L., & Laghi, L. (2021). Heterogeneity of colorectal cancer progression: molecular gas and brakes. *International Journal of Molecular Sciences*, *22*(10): 5246. https://doi.org/10.3390/ijms22105246.

Galluzzi, L., Vitale, I., Aaronson, S. A., Abrams, J. M., Adam, D., Agostinis, P., Alnemri, E. S., Altucci, L., Amelio, I., Andrews, D. W., Annicchiarico-Petruzzelli, M., Antonov, A. V., Arama, E., Baehrecke, E. H., Barlev, N. A., Bazan, N. G., Bernassola, F., Bertrand, M. J. M., Bianchi, K., Kroemer, G. (2018). Molecular mechanisms of cell death: recommendations of the nomenclature committee on cell death 2018. *Cell Death & Differentiation*, *25*(3): 486–541. https://doi.org/10.1038/s41418-017-0012-4.

Gonçalves, G. A. R., & Paiva, R. D. M. A. (2017). Gene therapy: advances, challenges and perspectives. *Einstein (Sao Paulo)*, *15*: 369-375.

Goodwin, M. L., Gladden, L. B., Nijsten, M. W. N., & Jones, K. B. (2015). Lactate and cancer: revisiting the Warburg Effect in an era of lactate shuttling. *Frontiers in Nutrition*, *1:* 27. https://www.frontiersin.org/article/10.3389/fnut.2014.00027.

Goswami, K. K., Ghosh, T., Ghosh, S., Sarkar, M., Bose, A., & Baral, R. (2017). Tumor promoting role of anti-tumor macrophages in tumor microenvironment. *Cellular Immunology*, *316*: 1–10. https://doi.org/10.1016/j.cellimm.2017.04.005.

Grivennikov, S. I., Greten, F. R., & Karin, M. (2010). Immunity, inflammation, and cancer. *Cell*, *140*(6): 883–899. https://doi.org/10.1016/j.cell.2010.01.025.

Guan, X. (2015). Cancer metastases: Challenges and opportunities. *Acta Pharmaceutica Sinica B*, *5*(5): 402–418. https://doi.org/10.1016/j.apsb.2015.07.005.

Hamilton, A. C., Donnelly, D. W., Loughrey, M. B., Turkington, R. C., Fox, C., Fitzpatrick, D., & Coleman, H. G. (2021). Inequalities in the decline and recovery of pathological cancer diagnoses during the first six months of the COVID-19 pandemic: a population-based study. *British Journal of Cancer*, *125*(6): 798-805.

Hanahan, D. (2022). Hallmarks of cancer: new dimensions. *Cancer Discovery*, *12*(1): 31–46. https://doi.org/10.1158/2159-8290.CD-21-1059.

Hayflick, L. (1965). The limited in vitro lifetime of human diploid cell strains. *Experimental Cell Research*, *37*(3): 614–636. https://doi.org/10.1016/0014-4827(65)90211-9.

Helm, J., Enkemann, S. A., Coppola, D., Barthel, J. S., Kelley, S. T., & Yeatman, T. J. (2005). Dedifferentiation precedes invasion in the progression from Barrett's metaplasia to esophageal adenocarcinoma. *Clinical Cancer Research: An Official Journal of the American Association for Cancer Research*, *11*(7): 2478–2485. https://doi.org/10.1158/1078-0432.CCR-04-1280.

Hoare, M., & Narita, M. (2018). *The Power Behind the Throne: Senescence and the Hallmarks of Cancer*. https://doi.org/10.1146/ANNUREV-CANCERBIO-030617-050352

Hossen, S., Hossain, M. K., Basher, M. K., Mia, M. N. H., Rahman, M. T., & Uddin, M. J. (2019). Smart nanocarrier-based drug delivery systems for cancer therapy and toxicity studies: A review. *Journal of Advanced Research, 15*: 1-18.

Huang, R., & Zhou, P. K. (2021). DNA damage repair: Historical perspectives, mechanistic pathways and clinical translation for targeted cancer therapy. *Signal Transduction and Targeted Therapy, 6*(1): 1–35. https://doi.org/10.1038/s41392-021-00648-7.

Huang, S. (2013). Genetic and non-genetic instability in tumor progression: Link between the fitness landscape and the epigenetic landscape of cancer cells. *Cancer Metastasis Reviews, 32*(3–4): 423–448. https://doi.org/10.1007/s10555-013-9435-7.

Huang, S., Guo, Y. P., May, G., & Enver, T. (2007). Bifurcation dynamics in lineage-commitment in bipotent progenitor cells. *Developmental Biology, 305*(2): 695–713. https://doi.org/10.1016/j.ydbio.2007.02.036.

İlgün, A. S., & Özmen, V. (2022). The impact of the COVID-19 pandemic on breast cancer patients. *European Journal of Breast Health, 18*(1): 85.

Iommarini, L., Ghelli, A., Gasparre, G., & Porcelli, A. M. (2017). Mitochondrial metabolism and energy sensing in tumor progression. *Biochimica et Biophysica Acta (BBA) - Bioenergetics, 1858*(8): 582–590. https://doi.org/10.1016/j.bbabio.2017.02.006.

Izzo, V., Bravo-San Pedro, J. M., Sica, V., Kroemer, G., & Galluzzi, L. (2016). Mitochondrial permeability transition: new findings and persisting uncertainties. *Trends in Cell Biology, 26*(9): 655–667. https://doi.org/10.1016/j.tcb.2016.04.006.

Jacobs, L., & Finlayson, C. (2010). *Early Diagnosis and Treatment of Cancer Series: Breast Cancer-E-Book: Expert Consult*. Elsevier Health Sciences.

Johnson, D. E., Burtness, B., Leemans, C. R., Lui, V. W. Y., Bauman, J. E., & Grandis, J. R. (2020). Head and neck squamous cell carcinoma. *Nature Reviews Disease Primers, 6*(1): 1-22.

Kalish, L. A., McDougal, W. S., & McKinlay, J. B. (2000). Family history and the risk of prostate cancer. *Urology, 56*(5): 803-806.

Karnoub, A. E., & Weinberg, R. A. (2006). Chemokine networks and breast cancer metastasis. *Breast Disease, 26*: 75–85. https://doi.org/10.3233/bd-2007-26107.

Kawase, A., Yoshida, J., Ishii, G., Nakao, M., Aokage, K., Hishida, T., & Nagai, K. (2011). Differences between squamous cell carcinoma and adenocarcinoma of the lung: are adenocarcinoma and squamous cell carcinoma prognostically equal? *Japanese Journal of Clinical Oncology, 42*(3): 189-195.

Klymenko, Y., & Nephew, K. P. (2018). Epigenetic crosstalk between the tumor micro-environment and ovarian cancer cells: a therapeutic road less traveled. *Cancers, 10*(9): 295. https://doi.org/10.3390/cancers10090295.

Kroemer, G., & Pouyssegur, J. (2008). Tumor cell metabolism: Cancer's Achilles' heel. *Cancer Cell, 13*(6): 472–482. https://doi.org/10.1016/j.ccr.2008.05.005.

Kuchenbaecker, K. B., Hopper, J. L., Barnes, D. R., Phillips, K. A., Mooij, T. M., Roos-Blom, M. J., & BRCA1 and BRCA2 Cohort Consortium. (2017). Risks of breast, ovarian, and contralateral breast cancer for BRCA1 and BRCA2 mutation carriers. *Jama*, *317*(23): 2402-2416.

Lanza, R., Gearhart, J., Hogan, B., Melton, D., Pedersen, R., Thomas, E. D., & Thomson, J. A. (Eds.). (2005). *Essentials of Stem Cell Biology*. Elsevier.

Lee, Y. C. A., & Hashibe, M. (2014). Tobacco, alcohol, and cancer in low and high income countries. *Annals of Global Health*, *80*(5): 378-383.

Levine, B., & Kroemer, G. (2008). Autophagy in the pathogenesis of disease. *Cell*, *132*(1): 27–42. https://doi.org/10.1016/j.cell.2007.12.018.

Liao, J. B. (2006). Cancer issue: Viruses and human cancer. *The Yale Journal of Biology and Medicine*, *79*(3-4): 115.

Lunt, S. Y., & Vander Heiden, M. G. (2011). Aerobic glycolysis: Meeting the metabolic requirements of cell proliferation. *Annual Review of Cell and Developmental Biology*, *27*: 441–464. https://doi.org/10.1146/annurev-cellbio-092910-154237.

Man, Y., Stojadinovic, A., Mason, J., Avital, I., Bilchik, A., Bruecher, B., Protic, M., Nissan, A., Izadjoo, M., Zhang, X., & Jewett, A. (2013). Tumor-infiltrating immune cells promoting tumor invasion and metastasis: existing theories. *Journal of Cancer*, *4*(1): 84–95. https://doi.org/10.7150/jca.5482.

Marcoux, N., Gettinger, S. N., O'Kane, G., Arbour, K. C., Neal, J. W., Husain, H., Evans, T. L., Brahmer, J. R., Muzikansky, A., Bonomi, P. D., del Prete, S., Wurtz, A., Farago, A. F., Dias-Santagata, D., Mino-Kenudson, M., Reckamp, K. L., Yu, H. A., Wakelee, H. A., Shepherd, F. A., Sequist, L. V. (2019). EGFR-mutant adenocarcinomas that transform to small-cell lung cancer and other neuroendocrine carcinomas: clinical outcomes. *Journal of Clinical Oncology*, *37*(4): 278–285. https://doi.org/10.1200/JCO.18.01585.

Maringe, C., Spicer, J., Morris, M., Purushotham, A., Nolte, E., Sullivan, R., & Aggarwal, A. (2020). The impact of the COVID-19 pandemic on cancer deaths due to delays in diagnosis in England, UK: a national, population-based, modelling study. *The Lancet Oncology*, *21*(8): 1023-1034.

Massagué, J., & Obenauf, A. C. (2016). Metastatic colonization. *Nature*, *529*(7586): 298–306. https://doi.org/10.1038/nature17038.

Miao, L., Zhang, Y., & Huang, L. (2021). mRNA vaccine for cancer immunotherapy. *Molecular Cancer*, *20*(1): 1-23.

Mizushima, N. (2007). Autophagy: Process and function. *Genes & Development*, *21*(22): 2861–2873. https://doi.org/10.1101/gad.1599207.

Montaño-Samaniego, M., Bravo-Estupiñan, D. M., Méndez-Guerrero, O., Alarcón-Hernández, E., & Ibáñez-Hernández, M. (2020). Strategies for targeting gene therapy in cancer cells with tumor-specific promoters. *Frontiers in Oncology*, 2671.

Multhoff, G., Molls, M., & Radons, J. (2012). Chronic inflammation in cancer development. *Frontiers in Immunology*, *2*. https://www.frontiersin.org/article/10.3389/fimmu.2011.00098.

Mundi, P. S., Sachdev, J., McCourt, C., & Kalinsky, K. (2016). AKT in cancer: New molecular insights and advances in drug development. *British Journal of Clinical Pharmacology*, *82*(4): 943–956. https://doi.org/10.1111/bcp.13021.

Negrini, S., Gorgoulis, V. G., & Halazonetis, T. D. (2010). Genomic instability—An evolving hallmark of cancer. *Nature Reviews. Molecular Cell Biology*, *11*(3): 220–228. https://doi.org/10.1038/nrm2858.

Novitzke, J. M. (2008). The significance of clinical trials. *Journal of Vascular and Interventional Neurology*, *1*(1): 31.

Nyberg, P., Xie, L., & Kalluri, R. (2005). Endogenous inhibitors of angiogenesis. *Cancer Research*, *65*(10): 3967–3979. https://doi.org/10.1158/0008-5472.CAN-04-2427.

Phan, T. G., & Croucher, P. I. (2020). The dormant cancer cell life cycle. *Nature Reviews. Cancer*, *20*(7): 398–411. https://doi.org/10.1038/s41568-020-0263-0.

Pharoah, P. D., Day, N. E., Duffy, S., Easton, D. F., & Ponder, B. A. (1997). Family history and the risk of breast cancer: a systematic review and meta-analysis. *International Journal of Cancer*, *71*(5): 800-809.

Pomerantz, M. M., & Freedman, M. L. (2011). The genetics of cancer risk. *Cancer Journal (Sudbury, Mass.)*, *17*(6): 416.

Potapova, T., & Gorbsky, G. J. (2017). The consequences of chromosome segregation errors in mitosis and meiosis. *Biology*, *6*(1): 12. https://doi.org/10.3390/biology6010012.

Prater, S., & McKeon, B. (2019). *Cancer, Osteosarcoma, Malignancy*. StatPearls.

Qian, B. Z., & Pollard, J. W. (2010). Macrophage diversity enhances tumor progression and metastasis. *Cell*, *141*(1): 39–51. https://doi.org/10.1016/j.cell.2010.03.014.

Racker, E. (1972). Bioenergetics and the problem of tumor growth. *American Scientist*, *60*(1): 56–63.

Reczek, C. R., & Chandel, N. S. (2017). The two faces of reactive oxygen species in cancer. *Annual Review of Cancer Biology*, *1*(1): 79–98. https://doi.org/10.1146/annurevcancerbio-041916-065808.

Sabbula, B. R., & Anjum, F. (2021). Squamous cell lung cancer. *StatPearls* [Internet].

Schulz, W. (2005). *Molecular Biology of Human Cancers: An Advanced Student's Textbook*. Springer Science & Business Media.

Shen, S., & Clairambault, J. (2020). Cell plasticity in cancer cell populations. *F1000-Research*, *9*, F1000 Faculty Rev-635. https://doi.org/10.12688/f1000research.24803.1.

Singh, R., Shaik, S., Negi, B. S., Rajguru, J. P., Patil, P. B., Parihar, A. S., & Sharma, U. (2020). Non-Hodgkin's lymphoma: a review. *Journal of Family Medicine and Primary Care*, *9*(4): 1834.

Sung, H., Ferlay, J., Siegel, R. L., Laversanne, M., Soerjomataram, I., Jemal, A., & Bray, F. (2021). Global cancer statistics 2020: GLOBOCAN estimates of incidence and mortality worldwide for 36 cancers in 185 countries. *CA: A Cancer Journal for Clinicians*, *71*(3): 209-249.

Swann, J. B., Vesely, M. D., Silva, A., Sharkey, J., Akira, S., Schreiber, R. D., & Smyth, M. J. (2008). Demonstration of inflammation-induced cancer and cancer immunoediting during primary tumorigenesis. *Proceedings of the National Academy of Sciences of the United States of America*, *105*(2): 652–656. https://doi.org/10.1073/pnas.0708594105.

Tan, S., Li, D., & Zhu, X. (2020). Cancer immunotherapy: Pros, cons and beyond. *Biomedicine & Pharmacotherapy*, *124*, 109821.

Teng, M. W. L., Swann, J. B., Koebel, C. M., Schreiber, R. D., & Smyth, M. J. (2008). Immune-mediated dormancy: An equilibrium with cancer. *Journal of Leukocyte Biology*, *84*(4), 988–993. https://doi.org/10.1189/jlb.1107774.

Thomas, D., & Majeti, R. (2017). Biology and relevance of human acute myeloid leukemia stem cells. *Blood, The Journal of the American Society of Hematology*, *129*(12): 1577-1585.

Unsoy, G., & Gunduz, U. (2018). Smart drug delivery systems in cancer therapy. *Current Drug Targets*, *19*(3): 202-212.

Valastyan, S., & Weinberg, R. A. (2011). Tumor Metastasis: Molecular Insights and Evolving Paradigms. *Cell*, *147*(2): 275–292. https://doi.org/10.1016/j.cell.2011.09.024.

van Eer, K., Laâbi, I., van Benthem, B. H., Steenbergen, R. D., King, A. J., Adema, D., & Pelgrim, M. (2022). The association between viral load and concurrent human papillomavirus infection at the genital and anal sites of young women and the impact of vaccination. *Tumour Virus Research*, *13*: 200233.

von Eschenbach, A. C. (2003). NCI sets goal of eliminating suffering and death due to cancer by 2015. Journal of the National Medical Association, 95(7): 637–639.

Waddington, C. H. (1942). The epigenotype. *Endeavour*, *1*: 18–20.

Wallace, D. C. (2012). Mitochondria and cancer. *Nature Reviews. Cancer*, *12*(10): 685–698. https://doi.org/10.1038/nrc3365.

Warburg, O., Wind, F., & Negelein, E. (1926). Über den Stoffwechsel von Tumoren im Körper [*About the metabolism of tumors in the body*]. *Klinische Wochenschrift*, *5*(19): 829–832. https://doi.org/10.1007/BF01726 240.

White, E., & DiPaola, R. S. (2009). The double-edged sword of autophagy modulation in cancer. *Clinical Cancer Research: An Official Journal of the American Association for Cancer Research*, *15*(17): 5308–5316. https://doi.org/10.1158/1078-0432.CCR-07-5023.

Witsch, E., Sela, M., & Yarden, Y. (2010). Roles for growth factors in cancer progression. *Physiology*, *25*(2): 85–101. https://doi.org/10.1152/physiol.00045.2009.

Yabroff, K. R., Mariotto, A., Tangka, F., Zhao, J., Islami, F., Sung, H., Sherman, R. L., Henley, S. J., Jemal, A., & Ward, E. M. (2021). Annual report to the nation on the status of cancer, part 2: patient economic burden associated with cancer care. *JNCI: Journal of the National Cancer Institute*, 113(12): 1670–1682. https://doi.org/10.1093/jnci/djab192.

Yamada, Y., Haga, H., & Yamada, Y. (2014). Concise review: dedifferentiation meets cancer development: proof of concept for epigenetic cancer. *Stem Cells Translational Medicine*, *3*(10): 1182–1187. https://doi.org/10.5966/sctm.2014-0090.

Yao, Y., & Dai, W. (2014). Genomic instability and cancer. *Journal of Carcinogenesis & Mutagenesis*, *5*: 1000165. https://doi.org/10.4172/2157-2518.1000165.

Yuan, S., Norgard, R. J., & Stanger, B. Z. (2019). Cellular plasticity in cancer. *Cancer Discovery*, *9*(7): 837–851. https://doi.org/10.1158/2159-8290.CD-19-0015.

Zou, Z., Tao, T., Li, H., & Zhu, X. (2020). mTOR signaling pathway and mTOR inhibitors in cancer: Progress and challenges. *Cell & Bioscience*, *10*(1): 31. https://doi.org/10.1186/s13578-020-00396-1.

Chapter 3

Cancer Immunity

Sukru Gulluoglu*
Department of Immunology,
School of Medicine,
Marmara University, Istanbul, Turkey

Abstract

Cancer is one of the leading causes of death worldwide. In the past, the effects of the immune system on cancer tumorigenesis and progression have been neglected since the immune system was conventionally believed to attack "non-self" cells only. Relatively recent findings have revealed that the immune system is constantly in search of neoplastic cells, and can recognize defects and threats by "self" cells as well. Both innate and adaptive immune cells are involved in various mechanisms that can detect and destroy cancer cells at any stage. However, tumor heterogeneity and subpopulation evolution in tumors make cancer find ways to escape immune pressure and even use immune cells in its favor. This chapter is about how the immune system is involved in the tumorigenesis and progression of cancer, from tumor recognition and development of the first response, inflammation and the tumor microenvironment, immune surveillance, and immune editing, and to immune escape.

Keywords: cancer, immune system, tumorigenesis, immune editing, immune escape

---

* Corresponding Author's Email: sukru.gulluoglu@marmara.edu.tr.

In: Autoimmunity and Cancer
Editors: Soner Şahin and Kenan Demir
ISBN: 978-1-68507-937-6

Introduction

Early evidence on human cancer immunity was introduced to the literature in the early 1950s (Foley, 1953). As a genetic disease, the genesis and progression of cancer is driven by a series of mutations. These mutations provide the tumor with a tremendous ability to adapt to changing situations such as hypoxia, nutrient depletion, growth towards physical limits, and attacks by the immune system (Tian et al., 2011). As the tumor faces such stress factors, the genetic diversity of the tumor subpopulations provides a selective advantage which results in genetic diversity and evolutionary fitness. Such genetic changes are driven not only by changing environmental conditions but also by factors such as genomic instability, lack of DNA replication error checking, and telomere shortening. Consequently, the more cancer cells diverge from original healthy cells, the more neoantigens they will probably produce, which makes them more immunogenic, namely more recognizable by the immune system (Boon & van der Bruggen, 1996). This is a stage in most cancers where the tumor faces a vigorous response by the immune system; however, tumors find several ways to overcome such a situation by hiding from the immune response, taming immune elements, and even using the immune response to its advantage (Dunn et al., 2002).

Tumor Recognition and Anti-Tumor Response

To initiate an immune response, first from the tumor should be recognized as non-self, or defective by the immune system. The discovery of tumor-reactive T cells that can recognize specific antigens has been a great breakthrough both in the fields of cancer science and immunology. In several human cancers, restricted MHC class I and II peptides have been identified in tumor-associated antigens (TAA), allowing researchers to investigate the relationship between tumor-associated T cells and how they target cancer cells (Haigh et al., 1999; Nestle, 2000; Zeh et al., 1999). In the case that tumorigenesis occurs and the nascent cancer cells show up, Natural Killer (NK) cells take part in distinguishing healthy cells, from tumor cells which are driven by inhibitory and stimulatory factors. The stimulatory NKG2D receptor, which is a member of the Natural Cytotoxicity Receptors family, can detect the increase in normal self-molecules, which are also extremely expressed in newly transformed cells, before a drastic accumulation in mutations occurs and produces abundantly non-self molecules (Cerwenka et al., 2000; Diefenbach et al.,

2000; Moretta et al., 2001). NKP46 has also been shown to endow NK cells with the tools to attack TRAIL-sensitive tumors (Turchinovich et al., 2018). MHC class I-like proteins MICA, MICB, and ULBP1-6 can also be listed as indicators of tumorigenesis along with other nonmicrobial challenges such as heat shock and oxidative stress that can also be detected by the immune system (Baychelier & Vieillard, 2013; Gleimer & Parham, 2003). Immunosurveillance and consequent NK cell attacks result in the dispersal of tumor neoepitopes along with other inflammatory factors to the tumor site. Macrophages, which originate from circulating monocytes, are another type of innate immune cell that plays a role in the early response to tumorigenesis and immunosurveillance. Macrophages can attack early cancer cells and suppress tumor progression. For instance, they have been found to suppress lung metastasis in mice by inducing NKs (Hanna et al., 2015). Macrophages also enhance antitumor activity by TMP195 inhibiting metastasis (Guerriero et al., 2017).

As the response to the tumor progresses, an evolutionary process takes part which results in tumor cells having more mutations; therefore, TAAs are usually overtaken by tumor-specific antigens (TSAs) (Ott et al., 2017). TSAs are neoantigens that are considerably distinct from those of the original healthy cells (Sahin et al., 2017; Yarchoan et al., 2017). These neoantigens generate a stronger immune response compared to TAAs, since in this case, T cells can escape negative selection in the thymus, which is a process aiming to suppress autoimmunity.

Antigen-presenting cells such as dendritic cells (DCs) move to the tumor site after attacks by innate immunity cells such as NKs and Macrophages. Endogenous and exogenous antigens are then presented to naïve and memory T cells that, under ideal conditions, would trigger an effector T cell response. Infiltrating DCs have been discovered in many cancers (Tran Janco et al., 2015). In cervical cancer and melanoma, CD103+ DCs play a major role in the anti-tumor immune response (Broz et al., 2014; Roberts et al., 2016). During chemotherapy, as a result of necrosis, myeloid cell differentiation occurs, which is followed by engulfment of tumor antigens by DCs which initiates an effector T-cell response (Ma et al., 2013). In a visualization study, $CD103^+$ DCs in the lung were found to directly suppress melanoma metastasis (Headley et al., 2016).

T cells take part in adaptive immunity, acting both as the main effectors and also as orchestrators (Speiser et al., 2016). During tumorigenesis followed by priming in the lymph nodes, T cells migrate to the tumor microenvironment, consequently eliminating cancer cells. Infiltrating T cells can be found in hypoxic and invasive locations of the tumor (Donadon et al., 2017; Halama et al., 2011). A high level of T cell infiltration is correlated with a better outcome in a number of cancers (Dieu-Nosjean et al., 2008; Kondo et al., 2006; Kusuda et al., 2005). The $CD8^+$ subtype of T-cells is also called cytotoxic T lymphocytes (CTLs) upon activation. This subtype is considered to be the main attack force of the immune system against unwanted cells, including transformed cells. CTLs secrete granzyme and perforin which can directly and solely destroy the target cell, without harming adjacent cells (Matsushita et al., 2012). Another subtype of T cells is the $CD4^+$ T Helper 1 cell, which can promote an antitumor response by secreting cytokines that would activate CTLs, macrophages and NKs (Pardoll & Topalian, 1998; Shankaran et al., 2018). High infiltration of T cells, especially CTLs, results in a favorable prognosis such as overall survival, disease-free survival, and lower chance of metastases in a number of cancers, including muscle-invasive urothelial carcinoma, ovarian cancer, and esophageal squamous cell carcinoma (Cho et al., 2003; Sato et al., 2005; Sharma et al., 2007).

Inflammation and the Tumor Microenvironment

The response of the immune system to the tumor causes a variety of immune cells to rush to the tumor site causing intense secretion of cytokines to the tumor microenvironment, causing tumor-associated inflammation (Mantovani et al., 2008).

Although it aims to eliminate the tumor, inflammation can have effects that favor the tumor, which is called tumor-promoting inflammation. Aside from promoting the tumor chronic inflammation is considered as one of the main causes of tumorigenesis estimated to be around 20% of all cases (Aggarwal et al., 2009). Locally, bacterial and viral infections can cause tumorigenesis (de Martel & Franceschi, 2009). As a carcinogen, tobacco can initiate cancer, but can also cause chronic inflammation that will promote the tumor (Takahashi et al., 2010).

Tumorigenesis is followed by inflammation in most solid tumor cases. The tumor surrounding can be remodeled by RAS and MYC family member proteins, which can help recruit immune cells, induce angiogenesis, and increase the secretion of pro-inflammatory factors (Soucek et al., 2007; Sparmann & Bar-Sagi, 2004). Tumor necrosis, which is common in fast-growing solid tumors, results in the release of pro-inflammatory factors such as interleukin 1 and HMBG1 (Vakkila & Lotze, 2004). Cancer therapy is another factor that promotes massive inflammation at the tumor site. Radiotherapy and chemotherapy result in necrosis that causes inflammation (Zong & Thompson, 2006). Inflammation, accompanied by cancer therapy, can have a beneficial or tumor-promoting effect (Vakkila & Lotze, 2004; Zitvogel et al., 2008). Overall inflammation can cause the recruitment of more inflammatory cells, and facilitate angiogenesis, which will aid the tumor to progress further.

The Tumor Microenvironment

The tumor microenvironment consists of fibroblasts, healthy tissue, innate immune cells, adaptive immune cells, extracellular matrix, blood vessels, fibroblasts, endothelial cells, mesenchymal cells, pericytes, and other tumor-associated cells. Tumors can influence their microenvironment by secreting factors that can promote vascularization, local tissue invasion, and immune tolerance. Additionally, other members of the tumor microenvironment can communicate by direct contact and with cytokine and chemokine secretion, which is a determining factor about how the tumor will grow. The balance between factors secreted by cells of the tumor microenvironment decides whether the immune response will cause tumor-promoting inflammation or antitumor immunity (Smyth et al., 2006). In further stage cancers, inflammation can work in favor of the tumor, and tumor regression is rarely seen without therapy. Overall, one can assume that after tumorigenesis and during tumor progression both pro and antitumor inflammation take place with the power balance shifting back and forth, with environmental factors playing a role in which direction the shift takes place (Bui & Schreiber, 2007; Swann et al., 2008).

Immune Surveillance and Immunoediting

Immune surveillance is a process in which the immune system monitors cells in the body for their infection and transformation status. Tissue-specific macrophages and immune cells patrolling the body look for deviations in tissue homeostasis by finding and destroying stressed, infected, senescent cells along with cells that have the potential to form malignant tumors (von Kobbe, 2019). In the case of a surviving tumor, despite being fully functioning, the immune system fails to destroy the tumor. This is a process that is defined as tumor immunoediting that happens in three phases: elimination, equilibrium, and escape (Dunn et al., 2004). The elimination phase occurs as a result of the successful immune surveillance of newly transformed cells with the potential to form a growing tumor. This first phase might completely remove all transformed cells, but it might also only partially remove some cells from the bunch. In such a case an equilibrium phase starts in which the tumor is neither growing, shrinking, nor escaping the constant watch of the immune system. Cells of the tumor are thought to stay dormant or continue their evolution by increasing tumor heterogeneity and mutational burden. During this process, the immune system would detect immunogenic changes in these newly evolved subpopulations and attack, exerting a selective pressure that will help the tumor evolve further. If this attack cannot completely remove the tumor, emerging evolutionary subpopulations that can be less immunogenic will become more abundant in the tumor, which can resist, avoid, or suppress the immune system. At this stage, the escape phase begins. In the escape phase, the immune system is ineffective against the tumor, unable to stop its rapid growth. This is the time when the tumor starts to appear and is diagnosed.

Immune Escape

Immune Tolerance

Immune activation and tolerance were conventionally thought to mainly depend on self and non-self discrimination by the immune system. This approach was based on the protective mechanism against autoimmunity in which the immune system would attack only "non-self" cells and spare "self" cells. Originating from the organism's own cells, cancer cells were thought to be completely unaffected by the immune system. As explained above, more research revealed that the immune system can detect problems even if the antigens were "self" originating in the case of necrotic, senescent, and neoplastic cells. Therefore the self vs. non-self concept has been modified as "harmful" vs "harmless" (Bareke et al., 2021). Interestingly, the immune system eliminates more self-antigens than non-self. Especially during tumorigenesis and early progression, cancer cells that are composed of self-antigens are under pressure from the immune system. Observations on immunosuppressed individuals and animal models with immunodeficiency point to the role of the immune system in controlling cancer (Burkholder et al., 2014). Central and peripheral immune tolerance suppress the antitumor immune response. Immune tolerance is a mechanism by which autoimmunity is prevented by the elimination of T or B lymphocytes, which are reactive against self-antigens (Romagnani, 2006). Central tolerance takes place in the thymus and bone marrow. During the process called thymic education, thymocytes in the thymus present self-antigens to T cells, followed by the elimination of those who recognize these antigens (Kyewski & Klein, 2006). A similar process occurs in the bone marrow and in this case B cells are selected for self-antigen binding (Pelanda & Torres, 2012). As a result of the central tolerance process, some self-reacting lymphocytes may still escape and move to the periphery. In this case, regulatory T cells (Tregs) destroy or pacify such cells, which means that they are only partially removed and their activation threshold is high. This means that self-reactive lymphocytes are kept in reserve in peripheral immune nodes and are activated in case of excessive exposure to self-antigens and high cytokine release environment, against neoplastic cells (Odum, 2019).

Evading the Immune System

Evading immune destruction is considered one of the emerging hallmarks of cancer (Hanahan & Weinberg, 2011). During the equilibrium phase of immune surveillance, where the tumor is under constant pressure by the immune system, the evolutionary selection of tumor subpopulations results in changes in tumor cells that can use several mechanisms to keep the attacking immune cells away. Cells in the tumor might find ways to secrete immunosuppressive cytokines, stop producing major histocompatibility complex molecules, and manage immune suppression by expressing checkpoint inhibitor proteins such as PD-L1 and CTLA-4. CTLA-4 suppresses T-cell activity by competitive binding to CD80 and CD86, which is one of the switching checkpoints in T-cell activation. PD-1 on T cells can bind to PD-L1 on the surface of cancer cells, which will suppress its activation by generating an inhibitory signal that causes the phenomenon called "T-cell exhaustion" (Chen & Mellman, 2017).

Many advanced tumors are known to have a predominantly high number of Tregs in their microenvironments, which would suppress CTLs. Another immune regulator that can be recruited by tumors is myeloid-derived suppressor cells (MDSCs) (Wing et al., 2019). Tregs use a repertoire of mechanisms to suppress CTL activity. They can promote apoptosis by death receptors or cytolysis by secreting granzyme B/perforin. Tregs can deplete IL-

2, which is a cytokine that can activate T helper cells and CTLs, from the tumor microenvironment. Tregs can also suppress dendritic cell activation (Arce-Sillas et al., 2016). MDSCs, which reside in the bone marrow under normal conditions, become available under various physiological conditions in blood, spleen, peripheral lymphoid tissues, and the tumor micro-environment, preventing immune cells from functioning (Condamine & Gabrilovich, 2011). MDSCs can carry out immune suppression in the tumor microenvironment by mechanisms such as Treg recruitment, tryptophan depletion, introduction of reactive oxygen species, and direct cell contact (Bronte & Zanovello, 2005; Kusmartsev et al., 2004; Yang et al., 2015). Both MDSCs and Tregs are associated with a poor prognosis in cancer (Ai et al., 2018; Zahran et al., 2021; Zhou et al., 2017). These findings summarize the fact that tumors can exploit the mechanisms available to prevent autoimmune responses by using them as a shield to stop an antitumor immune response.

Hot Tumors vs. Cold Tumors

Depending on the immune pressure against them and perhaps also on their origins, tumors can be highly inflamed, which is called a hot tumor, or non-inflamed, which is called a cold tumor. Hot tumors tend to have infiltration of a large number of immune cells in their parenchyma or the invasive margin (Rizvi et al., 2015; Woo et al., 2015). Immune cell abundance is accompanied by pro-inflammatory interferons and interleukins. In cold tumors, immunosuppressive cytokines are abundant. Immunosuppressive cells such as Tumor-Associated Macrophages, Tregs, or MDSCs can also be available in a cold tumor. Antigen-presenting cell recruitment or antigen presentation mechanisms can be defective (Sharma et al., 2017). Cancer-associated fibroblast activation can make the tumor microenvironment impenetrable to CTLs (Mariathasan et al., 2018). Antigen loss is another feature of cold tumors in which prolonged antitumor immune pressure causes the emergence of subpopulations lacking immunogenic antigens (Ferris et al., 2005).

Conclusion

The immune system is constantly at watch against both self and non-self threats throughout the body. In the case of cancer, there is a fine balance between eliminating the newly formed tumor and promoting it. Not very long ago, the role of the immune system against cancer has been neglected, since researchers in the field were assuming that only non-self antigens were targeted by the immune system. The following studies revealed that self-antigens are also under scrutiny by the immune system. Today, tremendous knowledge has accumulated about the mechanisms behind anti-tumor immunity and immune surveillance which can help the tumor evolve to become more aggressive. This knowledge is currently being utilized by clinicians in cancer immunotherapy, which has proven to be successful when used along with or without conventional cancer therapies. Many speculate that the future of cancer therapy will be based on orchestrating the immune system against the tumor.

References

Aggarwal, B. B., Vijayalekshmi, R. V., & Sung, B. (2009). Targeting inflammatory pathways for prevention and therapy of cancer: short-term friend, long-term foe. *Clin Cancer Res*, *15*(2), 425-430. https://doi.org/10.1158/1078-0432.CCR-08-0149.

Ai, L., Mu, S., Wang, Y., Wang, H., Cai, L., Li, W., & Hu, Y. (2018). Prognostic role of myeloid-derived suppressor cells in cancers: a systematic review and meta-analysis. *BMC Cancer*, *18*(1), 1220. https://doi.org/10.1186/s12885-018-5086-y.

Arce-Sillas, A., Alvarez-Luquin, D. D., Tamaya-Dominguez, B., Gomez-Fuentes, S., Trejo-Garcia, A., Melo-Salas, M., Cardenas, G., Rodriguez-Ramirez, J., & Adalid-Peralta, L. (2016). Regulatory T cells: molecular actions on effector cells in immune regulation. *J Immunol Res*, *2016*, 1720827. https://doi.org/10.1155/2016/1720827.

Bareke, H., Juanes-Velasco, P., Landeira-Vinuela, A., Hernandez, A. P., Cruz, J. J., Bellido, L., Fonseca, E., Niebla-Cardenas, A., Montalvillo, E., Gongora, R., & Fuentes, M. (2021). Autoimmune responses in oncology: causes and significance. *Int J Mol Sci*, *22*(15). https://doi.org/10.3390/ijms22158030.

Baychelier, F., & Vieillard, V. (2013). The modulation of the cell-cycle: a sentinel to alert the NK cells of dangers. *Front Immunol*, *4*, 325. https://doi.org/10.3389/fimmu.2013.00325.

Boon, T., & van der Bruggen, P. (1996). Human tumor antigens recognized by T lymphocytes. *J Exp Med*, *183*(3), 725-729. https://doi.org/10.1084/jem.183.3.725.

Bronte, V., & Zanovello, P. (2005). Regulation of immune responses by L-arginine metabolism. *Nat Rev Immunol*, *5*(8), 641-654. https://doi.org/10.1038/nri1668.

Broz, M. L., Binnewies, M., Boldajipour, B., Nelson, A. E., Pollack, J. L., Erle, D. J., Barczak, A., Rosenblum, M. D., Daud, A., Barber, D. L., Amigorena, S., Van't Veer, L. J., Sperling, A. I., Wolf, D. M., & Krummel, M. F. (2014). Dissecting the tumor myeloid compartment reveals rare activating antigen-presenting cells critical for t cell immunity. *Cancer Cell*, *26*(6), 938. https://doi.org/10.1016/ j.ccell.2014.11.010.

Bui, J. D., & Schreiber, R. D. (2007). Cancer immunosurveillance, immunoediting and inflammation: independent or interdependent processes? *Curr Opin Immunol*, *19*(2), 203-208. https://doi.org/10.1016/j.coi.2007.02.001.

Burkholder, B., Huang, R. Y., Burgess, R., Luo, S., Jones, V. S., Zhang, W., Lv, Z. Q., Gao, C. Y., Wang, B. L., Zhang, Y. M., & Huang, R. P. (2014). Tumor-induced perturbations of cytokines and immune cell networks. *Biochim Biophys Acta*, *1845*(2), 182-201. https://doi.org/10.1016/j.bbcan.2014.01.004.

Cerwenka, A., Bakker, A. B., McClanahan, T., Wagner, J., Wu, J., Phillips, J. H., & Lanier, L. L. (2000). Retinoic acid early inducible genes define a ligand family for the activating NKG2D receptor in mice. *Immunity*, *12*(6), 721-727. https://doi.org/10.1016/s1074-7613(00)80222-8.

Chen, D. S., & Mellman, I. (2017). Elements of cancer immunity and the cancer-immune set point. *Nature*, *541*(7637), 321-330. https://doi.org/10.1038/nature21349.

Cho, Y., Miyamoto, M., Kato, K., Fukunaga, A., Shichinohe, T., Kawarada, Y., Hida, Y., Oshikiri, T., Kurokawa, T., Suzuoki, M., Nakakubo, Y., Hiraoka, K., Murakami, S., Shinohara, T., Itoh, T., Okushiba, S., Kondo, S., & Katoh, H. (2003). CD4+ and CD8+ T cells cooperate to improve prognosis of patients with esophageal squamous cell carcinoma. *Cancer Res*, *63*(7), 1555-1559. https://www.ncbi.nlm.nih.gov/pubmed/12670904.

Condamine, T., & Gabrilovich, D. I. (2011). Molecular mechanisms regulating myeloid-derived suppressor cell differentiation and function. *Trends Immunol*, *32*(1), 19-25. https://doi.org/10.1016/j.it.2010.10.002.

de Martel, C., & Franceschi, S. (2009). Infections and cancer: established associations and new hypotheses. *Crit Rev Oncol Hematol*, *70*(3), 183-194. https://doi.org/10.1016/j.critrevonc.2008.07.021.

Diefenbach, A., Jamieson, A. M., Liu, S. D., Shastri, N., & Raulet, D. H. (2000). Ligands for the murine NKG2D receptor: expression by tumor cells and activation of NK cells and macrophages. *Nat Immunol*, *1*(2), 119-126. https://doi.org/10.1038/77793.

Dieu-Nosjean, M. C., Antoine, M., Danel, C., Heudes, D., Wislez, M., Poulot, V., Rabbe, N., Laurans, L., Tartour, E., de Chaisemartin, L., Lebecque, S., Fridman, W. H., & Cadranel, J. (2008). Long-term survival for patients with non-small-cell lung cancer with intratumoral lymphoid structures. *J Clin Oncol*, *26*(27), 4410-4417. https://doi.org/10.1200/JCO.2007.15.0284.

Donadon, M., Hudspeth, K., Cimino, M., Di Tommaso, L., Preti, M., Tentorio, P., Roncalli, M., Mavilio, D., & Torzilli, G. (2017). Increased infiltration of natural killer and t cells in colorectal liver metastases improves patient overall survival. *J Gastrointest Surg*, *21*(8), 1226-1236. https://doi.org/10.1007/s11605-017-3446-6.

Dunn, G. P., Bruce, A. T., Ikeda, H., Old, L. J., & Schreiber, R. D. (2002). Cancer immunoediting: from immunosurveillance to tumor escape. *Nat Immunol*, *3*(11), 991-998. https://doi.org/10.1038/ni1102-991.

Dunn, G. P., Old, L. J., & Schreiber, R. D. (2004). The three Es of cancer immunoediting. *Annu Rev Immunol*, *22*, 329-360. https://doi.org/10.1146/annurev.immunol.22.012703.104803.

Ferris, R. L., Hunt, J. L., & Ferrone, S. (2005). Human leukocyte antigen (HLA) class I defects in head and neck cancer: molecular mechanisms and clinical significance. *Immunol Res*, *33*(2), 113-133. https://doi.org/10.1385/IR:33:2:113.

Foley, E. J. (1953). Antigenic properties of methylcholanthrene-induced tumors in mice of the strain of origin. *Cancer Res*, *13*(12), 835-837. https://www.ncbi.nlm.nih.gov/pubmed/13116120.

Gleimer, M., & Parham, P. (2003). Stress management: MHC class I and class I-like molecules as reporters of cellular stress. *Immunity*, *19*(4), 469-477. https://doi.org/10.1016/s1074-7613(03)00272-3.

Guerriero, J. L., Sotayo, A., Ponichtera, H. E., Castrillon, J. A., Pourzia, A. L., Schad, S., Johnson, S. F., Carrasco, R. D., Lazo, S., Bronson, R. T., Davis, S. P., Lobera, M., Nolan, M. A., & Letai, A. (2017). Class IIa HDAC inhibition reduces breast tumours and metastases through anti-tumour macrophages. *Nature*, *543*(7645), 428-432. https://doi.org/10.1038/nature21409.

Haigh, P. I., Difronzo, L. A., Gammon, G., & Morton, D. L. (1999). Vaccine therapy for patients with melanoma. *Oncology (Williston Park)*, *13*(11), 1561-1574; discussion 1574 passim. https://www.ncbi.nlm.nih.gov/pubmed/10581603.

Halama, N., Michel, S., Kloor, M., Zoernig, I., Benner, A., Spille, A., Pommerencke, T., von Knebel, D. M., Folprecht, G., Luber, B., Feyen, N., Martens, U. M., Beckhove, P., Gnjatic, S., Schirmacher, P., Herpel, E., Weitz, J., Grabe, N., & Jaeger, D. (2011). Localization and density of immune cells in the invasive margin of human colorectal cancer liver metastases are prognostic for response to chemotherapy. *Cancer Res*, *71*(17), 5670-5677. https://doi.org/10.1158/0008-5472.CAN-11-0268.

Hanahan, D., & Weinberg, R. A. (2011). Hallmarks of cancer: the next generation. *Cell*, *144*(5), 646-674. https://doi.org/10.1016/j.cell.2011.02.013.

Hanna, R. N., Cekic, C., Sag, D., Tacke, R., Thomas, G. D., Nowyhed, H., Herrley, E., Rasquinha, N., McArdle, S., Wu, R., Peluso, E., Metzger, D., Ichinose, H., Shaked, I., Chodaczek, G., Biswas, S. K., & Hedrick, C. C. (2015). Patrolling monocytes control tumor metastasis to the lung. *Science*, *350*(6263), 985-990. https://doi.org/10.1126/science.aac9407.

Headley, M. B., Bins, A., Nip, A., Roberts, E. W., Looney, M. R., Gerard, A., & Krummel, M. F. (2016). Visualization of immediate immune responses to pioneer metastatic cells in the lung. *Nature*, *531*(7595), 513-517. https://doi.org/10.1038/ nature16985.

Kondo, T., Nakazawa, H., Ito, F., Hashimoto, Y., Osaka, Y., Futatsuyama, K., Toma, H., & Tanabe, K. (2006). Favorable prognosis of renal cell carcinoma with increased expression of chemokines associated with a Th1-type immune response. *Cancer Sci*, *97*(8), 780-786. https://doi.org/10.1111/j.1349-7006.2006.00231.x.

Kusmartsev, S., Nefedova, Y., Yoder, D., & Gabrilovich, D. I. (2004). Antigen-specific inhibition of CD8+ T cell response by immature myeloid cells in cancer is mediated by reactive oxygen species. *J Immunol*, *172*(2), 989-999. https://doi.org/10.4049/jimmunol.172.2.989.

Kusuda, T., Shigemasa, K., Arihiro, K., Fujii, T., Nagai, N., & Ohama, K. (2005). Relative expression levels of Th1 and Th2 cytokine mRNA are independent prognostic factors in patients with ovarian cancer. *Oncol Rep*, *13*(6), 1153-1158. https://www.ncbi.nlm.nih.gov/pubmed/15870936.

Kyewski, B., & Klein, L. (2006). A central role for central tolerance. *Annu Rev Immunol*, *24*, 571-606. https://doi.org/10.1146/annurev.immunol.23.021704.115601.

Ma, Y., Adjemian, S., Mattarollo, S. R., Yamazaki, T., Aymeric, L., Yang, H., Portela Catani, J. P., Hannani, D., Duret, H., Steegh, K., Martins, I., Schlemmer, F., Michaud, M., Kepp, O., Sukkurwala, A. Q., Menger, L., Vacchelli, E., Droin, N., Galluzzi, L., Krzysiek, R., Gordon, S., Taylor, P. R., Van Endert, P., Solary, E., Smyth, M. J., Zitvogel, L., & Kroemer, G. (2013). Anticancer chemotherapy-induced intratumoral recruitment and differentiation of antigen-presenting cells. *Immunity*, *38*(4), 729-741. https://doi.org/10.1016/j.immuni.2013.03.003.

Mantovani, A., Allavena, P., Sica, A., & Balkwill, F. (2008). Cancer-related inflammation. *Nature*, *454*(7203), 436-444. https://doi.org/10.1038/nature07205.

Mariathasan, S., Turley, S. J., Nickles, D., Castiglioni, A., Yuen, K., Wang, Y., Kadel, E. E., III, Koeppen, H., Astarita, J. L., Cubas, R., Jhunjhunwala, S., Banchereau, R., Yang, Y., Guan, Y., Chalouni, C., Ziai, J., Senbabaoglu, Y., Santoro, S., Sheinson, D., Hung, J., Giltnane, J. M., Pierce, A. A., Mesh, K., Lianoglou, S., Riegler, J., Carano, R. A. D., Eriksson, P., Hoglund, M., Somarriba, L., Halligan, D. L., van der Heijden, M. S., Loriot, Y., Rosenberg, J. E., Fong, L., Mellman, I., Chen, D. S., Green, M., Derleth, C., Fine, G. D., Hegde, P. S., Bourgon, R., & Powles, T. (2018). TGFbeta attenuates tumour response to PD-L1 blockade by contributing to exclusion of T cells. *Nature*, *554*(7693), 544-548. https://doi.org/10.1038/nature25501.

Matsushita, H., Vesely, M. D., Koboldt, D. C., Rickert, C. G., Uppaluri, R., Magrini, V. J., Arthur, C. D., White, J. M., Chen, Y. S., Shea, L. K., Hundal, J., Wendl, M. C., Demeter, R., Wylie, T., Allison, J. P., Smyth, M. J., Old, L. J., Mardis, E. R., & Schreiber, R. D. (2012). Cancer exome analysis reveals a T-cell-dependent mechanism of cancer immunoediting. *Nature*, *482*(7385), 400-404. https://doi.org/10.1038/nature 10755.

Moretta, A., Bottino, C., Vitale, M., Pende, D., Cantoni, C., Mingari, M. C., Biassoni, R., & Moretta, L. (2001). Activating receptors and coreceptors involved in human natural killer cell-mediated cytolysis. *Annu Rev Immunol*, *19*, 197-223. https://doi.org/10. 1146/annurev.immunol.19.1.197.

Nestle, F. O. (2000). Dendritic cell vaccination for cancer therapy. *Oncogene*, *19*(56), 6673-6679. https://doi.org/10.1038/sj.onc.1204095.

Odum, N. (2019). Anti-regulatory T cells are natural regulatory effector T cells. *Cell Stress*, *3*(10), 310-311. https://doi.org/10.15698/cst2019.10.199.

Ott, P. A., Hu, Z., Keskin, D. B., Shukla, S. A., Sun, J., Bozym, D. J., Zhang, W., Luoma, A., Giobbie-Hurder, A., Peter, L., Chen, C., Olive, O., Carter, T. A., Li, S., Lieb, D. J., Eisenhaure, T., Gjini, E., Stevens, J., Lane, W. J., Javeri, I., Nellaiappan, K., Salazar, A. M., Daley, H., Seaman, M., Buchbinder, E. I., Yoon, C. H., Harden, M., Lennon, N., Gabriel, S., Rodig, S. J., Barouch, D. H., Aster, J. C., Getz, G., Wucherpfennig, K., Neuberg, D., Ritz, J., Lander, E. S., Fritsch, E. F., Hacohen, N., & Wu, C. J. (2017). An immunogenic personal neoantigen vaccine for patients with melanoma. *Nature*, *547*(7662), 217-221. https://doi.org/10.1038/nature22991.

Pardoll, D. M., & Topalian, S. L. (1998). The role of CD4+ T cell responses in antitumor immunity. *Curr Opin Immunol*, *10*(5), 588-594. https://doi.org/10.1016/s0952-7915 (98)80228-8.

Pelanda, R., & Torres, R. M. (2012). Central B-cell tolerance: where selection begins. *Cold Spring Harb Perspect Biol*, *4*(4), a007146. https://doi.org/10.1101/cshperspect.a007146.

Rizvi, N. A., Hellmann, M. D., Snyder, A., Kvistborg, P., Makarov, V., Havel, J. J., Lee, W., Yuan, J., Wong, P., Ho, T. S., Miller, M. L., Rekhtman, N., Moreira, A. L., Ibrahim, F., Bruggeman, C., Gasmi, B., Zappasodi, R., Maeda, Y., Sander, C., Garon, E. B., Merghoub, T., Wolchok, J. D., Schumacher, T. N., & Chan, T. A. (2015). Cancer immunology. Mutational landscape determines sensitivity to PD-1 blockade in non-small cell lung cancer. *Science*, *348*(6230), 124-128. https://doi.org/10.1126/science.aaa1348.

Roberts, E. W., Broz, M. L., Binnewies, M., Headley, M. B., Nelson, A. E., Wolf, D. M., Kaisho, T., Bogunovic, D., Bhardwaj, N., & Krummel, M. F. (2016). Critical role for CD103(+)/CD141(+) Dendritic cells bearing CCR7 for tumor antigen trafficking and priming of T cell immunity in melanoma. *Cancer Cell*, *30*(2), 324-336. https://doi.org/10.1016/j.ccell.2016.06.003.

Romagnani, S. (2006). Immunological tolerance and autoimmunity. *Intern Emerg Med*, *1*(3), 187-196. https://doi.org/10.1007/BF02934736.

Sahin, U., Derhovanessian, E., Miller, M., Kloke, B. P., Simon, P., Lower, M., Bukur, V., Tadmor, A. D., Luxemburger, U., Schrors, B., Omokoko, T., Vormehr, M., Albrecht, C., Paruzynski, A., Kuhn, A. N., Buck, J., Heesch, S., Schreeb, K. H., Muller, F., Ortseifer, I., Vogler, I., Godehardt, E., Attig, S., Rae, R., Breitkreuz, A., Tolliver, C., Suchan, M., Martic, G., Hohberger, A., Sorn, P., Diekmann, J., Ciesla, J., Waksmann, O., Bruck, A. K., Witt, M., Zillgen, M., Rothermel, A., Kasemann, B., Langer, D., Bolte, S., Diken, M., Kreiter, S., Nemecek, R., Gebhardt, C., Grabbe, S., Holler, C., Utikal, J., Huber, C., Loquai, C., & Tureci, O. (2017). Personalized RNA mutanome vaccines mobilize poly-specific therapeutic immunity against cancer. *Nature*, *547*(7662), 222-226. https://doi.org/10.1038/nature23003.

Sato, E., Olson, S. H., Ahn, J., Bundy, B., Nishikawa, H., Qian, F., Jungbluth, A. A., Frosina, D., Gnjatic, S., Ambrosone, C., Kepner, J., Odunsi, T., Ritter, G., Lele, S., Chen, Y. T., Ohtani, H., Old, L. J., & Odunsi, K. (2005). Intraepithelial CD8+ tumor-infiltrating lymphocytes and a high CD8+/regulatory T cell ratio are associated with favorable prognosis in ovarian cancer. *Proc Natl Acad Sci U S A*, *102*(51), 18538-18543. https://doi.org/10.1073/pnas.0509182102.

Shankaran, V., Ikeda, H., Bruce, A. T., White, J. M., Swanson, P. E., Old, L. J., & Schreiber, R. D. (2018). Pillars article: IFNgamma and lymphocytes prevent primary tumour development and shape tumour immunogenicity. *Nature*. 2001. 410: 1107-1111. *J Immunol*, *201*(3), 827-831. https://www.ncbi.nlm.nih.gov/pubmed/30038035.

Sharma, P., Hu-Lieskovan, S., Wargo, J. A., & Ribas, A. (2017). Primary, adaptive, and acquired resistance to cancer immunotherapy. *Cell*, *168*(4), 707-723. https://doi.org/10.1016/j.cell.2017.01.017.

Sharma, P., Shen, Y., Wen, S., Yamada, S., Jungbluth, A. A., Gnjatic, S., Bajorin, D. F., Reuter, V. E., Herr, H., Old, L. J., & Sato, E. (2007). CD8 tumor-infiltrating lymphocytes are predictive of survival in muscle-invasive urothelial carcinoma. *Proc Natl Acad Sci U S A*, *104*(10), 3967-3972. https://doi.org/10.1073/pnas.0611618104.

Smyth, M. J., Dunn, G. P., & Schreiber, R. D. (2006). Cancer immunosurveillance and immunoediting: the roles of immunity in suppressing tumor development and shaping tumor immunogenicity. *Adv Immunol*, *90*, 1-50. https://doi.org/10.1016/S0065-2776(06)90001-7.

Soucek, L., Lawlor, E. R., Soto, D., Shchors, K., Swigart, L. B., & Evan, G. I. (2007). Mast cells are required for angiogenesis and macroscopic expansion of Myc-induced pancreatic islet tumors. *Nat Med*, *13*(10), 1211-1218. https://doi.org/10.1038/nm1649.

Sparmann, A., & Bar-Sagi, D. (2004). Ras-induced interleukin-8 expression plays a critical role in tumor growth and angiogenesis. *Cancer Cell*, *6*(5), 447-458. https://doi.org/10.1016/j.ccr.2004.09.028.

Speiser, D. E., Ho, P. C., & Verdeil, G. (2016). Regulatory circuits of T cell function in cancer. *Nat Rev Immunol*, *16*(10), 599-611. https://doi.org/10.1038/nri.2016.80.

Swann, J. B., Vesely, M. D., Silva, A., Sharkey, J., Akira, S., Schreiber, R. D., & Smyth, M. J. (2008). Demonstration of inflammation-induced cancer and cancer immunoediting during primary tumorigenesis. *Proc Natl Acad Sci U S A*, *105*(2), 652-656. https://doi.org/10.1073/pnas.0708594105.

Takahashi, H., Ogata, H., Nishigaki, R., Broide, D. H., & Karin, M. (2010). Tobacco smoke promotes lung tumorigenesis by triggering IKKbeta- and JNK1-dependent inflammation. *Cancer Cell*, *17*(1), 89-97. https://doi.org/10.1016/j.ccr.2009.12.008.

Tian, T., Olson, S., Whitacre, J. M., & Harding, A. (2011). The origins of cancer robustness and evolvability. *Integr Biol (Camb)*, *3*(1), 17-30. https://doi.org/10.1039/c0ib00046a.

Tran Janco, J. M., Lamichhane, P., Karyampudi, L., & Knutson, K. L. (2015). Tumor-infiltrating dendritic cells in cancer pathogenesis. *J Immunol*, *194*(7), 2985-2991. https://doi.org/10.4049/jimmunol.1403134.

Turchinovich, G., Ganter, S., Bärenwaldt, A., & Finke, D. (2018). NKp46 calibrates tumoricidal potential of type 1 innate lymphocytes by regulating TRAIL expression. *The Journal of Immunology*, *200*(11), 3762-3768.

Vakkila, J., & Lotze, M. T. (2004). Inflammation and necrosis promote tumour growth. *Nat Rev Immunol*, *4*(8), 641-648. https://doi.org/10.1038/nri1415.

von Kobbe, C. (2019). Targeting senescent cells: approaches, opportunities, challenges. *Aging (Albany NY)*, *11*(24), 12844-12861. https://doi.org/10.18632/aging.102557.

Wing, J. B., Tanaka, A., & Sakaguchi, S. (2019). Human FOXP3(+) Regulatory T cell heterogeneity and function in autoimmunity and cancer. *Immunity*, *50*(2), 302-316. https://doi.org/10.1016/j.immuni.2019.01.020.

Woo, S. R., Corrales, L., & Gajewski, T. F. (2015). Innate immune recognition of cancer. *Annu Rev Immunol*, *33*, 445-474. https://doi.org/10.1146/annurev-immunol-032414-112043.

Yang, H., Bi, Y., Han, F., Lu, Y., Wang, J., Zhang, Z., & Liu, G. (2015). Myeloid-derived suppressor cells in immunity and autoimmunity. *Expert Rev Clin Immunol*, *11*(8), 911-919. https://doi.org/10.1586/1744666X.2015.1052794.

Yarchoan, M., Johnson, B. A., 3rd, Lutz, E. R., Laheru, D. A., & Jaffee, E. M. (2017). Targeting neoantigens to augment antitumour immunity. *Nat Rev Cancer*, *17*(9), 569. https://doi.org/10.1038/nrc.2017.74.

Zahran, A. M., Hetta, H. F., Zahran, Z. A. M., Rashad, A., Rayan, A., Mohamed, D. O., Elhameed, Z. A. A., Khallaf, S. M., Batiha, G. E., Waheed, Y., Muhammad, K., & Nafady-Hego, H. (2021). Prognostic role of monocytic myeloid-derived suppressor cells in advanced non-small-cell lung cancer: relation to different hematologic indices. *J Immunol Res*, *2021*, 3241150. https://doi.org/10.1155/2021/3241150.

Zeh, H. J., 3rd, Perry-Lalley, D., Dudley, M. E., Rosenberg, S. A., & Yang, J. C. (1999). High avidity CTLs for two self-antigens demonstrate superior *in vitro* and *in vivo* antitumor efficacy. *J Immunol*, *162*(2), 989-994. https://www.ncbi.nlm.nih.gov/pubmed/9916724.

Zhou, Y., Shao, N., Aierken, N., Xie, C., Ye, R., Qian, X., Hu, Z., Zhang, J., & Lin, Y. (2017). Prognostic value of tumor-infiltrating Foxp3+ regulatory T cells in patients with breast cancer: a meta-analysis. *J Cancer*, *8*(19), 4098-4105. https://doi.org/10.7150/jca.21030.

Zitvogel, L., Apetoh, L., Ghiringhelli, F., & Kroemer, G. (2008). Immunological aspects of cancer chemotherapy. *Nat Rev Immunol*, *8*(1), 59-73. https://doi.org/10.1038/nri2216.

Zong, W. X., & Thompson, C. B. (2006). Necrotic death as a cell fate. *Genes Dev*, *20*(1), 1-15. https://doi.org/10.1101/gad.1376506.

Chapter 4

Genetics, Autoimmunity, and Cancer

Sevgi Durna Daştan[1], PhD
and İnanç Baral[2,*], DVM, PhD
[1]Division of Molecular Biology,
Department of Biology, Faculty of Science,
Sivas Cumhuriyet University, Sivas, Turkey
[2]Division of Veterinary Genetics,
Department of Zootechnics and Animal Nutrition,
Faculty of Veterinary Medicine,
Sivas Cumhuriyet University, Sivas, Turkey

Abstract

The majority of people consider cancer to be a single disease, but it is actually a collection of more than 1000 distinct abnormalities in cell and tissue function. However, all cancers have one trait in common: they are all diseases characterized by unregulated cell division. Under normal circumstances, the body regulates the generation of new cells quite precisely. Specific DNA abnormalities in cancer cells cause disruptions in cell communication and growth regulation that are typical in healthy cells. Cancer cells that have evaded these restrictions can become invasive and move to other regions of the body. At the molecular level, cancer is primarily a hereditary disease. It is crucial to understand the fundamental genetic alterations that occur at the somatic level when cancer progresses. The genetics of cancer at the germline layer is still one of the most intriguing and fascinating areas of cancer research, and it is becoming even more so as DNA sequencing technology improves. This has allowed researchers to identify the genetic underpinnings of previously unknown inherited diseases. Newer technologies have also

* Corresponding Author's Email: ibaral@cumhuriyet.edu.tr.

In: Autoimmunity and Cancer
Editors: Soner Şahin and Kenan Demir
ISBN: 978-1-68507-937-6

made it economically feasible to test patients for the presence of common and hereditary cancer susceptibilities. As a result, cancer genetics has become a significant part of the volume of work in clinical genetics programs. This chapter focuses on cancer and autoimmune-related genetic and genomic components.

Keywords: autoimmunity, cancer, genetics, genomics, medicine

Introduction

The pros and challenges of incorporating genomics into conventional healthcare have been widely debated across the world (Collins and Guttmacher, 2001; Scheuner et al. 2008). There are reported examples of successful genetic risk assessment adoption in cancer care (Grimsey et al. 2010; Harris and Lötter, 2012; Jacobs, 2014). However, even when a risk assessment has been made, health professionals may not always feel competent in estimating risk, or be unclear about whose job it is, or do not always recommend patients to genetic counseling (Metcalfe et al. 2010; Meyer et al. 2010; Lanceley et al. 2012). There is still a lot to understand about how genetic diversity affects cancer risk (Jacobs, 2014). Most of the hereditary cancer genes found so far have significant penetration and confer a strong proclivity for cancer development. Because such genes are more difficult to find, there are fewer low-penetrance cancer genes recognized. Genes that change cancer risk in alternative ways are significantly difficult to identify, yet they may cause a large number of carcinogenesis collectively. The activation of proto-oncogenes and the loss of function of tumor suppressor genes cause each of the roughly hundred forms of cancer. Although cancer genomes are complicated, there are certain distinct mutational patterns that may be identified. Several cancer genes are present in abundance in some forms of cancer but are uncommon in others. Other cancer genes, on the other hand, are much more common. Recent investigation of individual cancer genomes has revealed that many mutations originate at extremely low frequency during carcinogenesis as a result of clonal selection. These findings suggest that there are a variety of combinations of cancer genes that can work together to promote tumor development (Azarnezhad and Mehdipour, 2017).

Cancer is a hereditary disease caused mostly by somatic mutations in tumor suppressor and oncogenes (e.g., K-ras and EGFR) (Kim and Jablons, 2017; Hanahan and Weinberg, 2000; 2011). Cancer, on the other hand, is significantly complicated and diverse. Many other pathways, including epigenetics, immunological functions, and environmental variables, contribute to cancer genesis, evolution, metastasis, and acquisition of resistance to treatment in addition to genetic abnormalities. Furthermore, cancer is not a static disease; its attributes fluctuate as it adapts to various settings and habitats within the human body. As a result, identifying a specific target to treat and cure cancer is difficult (Kim and Jablons, 2017; Hanahan and Weinberg, 2000; 2011).

Genetic and epigenetic changes are the causes of human cancer. Numerous discoveries amassed over the last few years reveal that genetic and epigenetic modifications are not confined to protein-coding genes. Mechanisms that control cell proliferation, communication, and differentiation are essential for the precise orchestration of the cellular communities that make up our organs, systems, and ultimately bodies. While the list of cell actions that determine whether a cell is normal or carcinogenic appears lengthy, these seemingly independent traits are really governed by seven interacting processes in a domino-like fashion. And it is in these processes that highly specific molecules occur. Cells are prompted to divide by signal molecules. The signal molecule has an effect on the cell by initiating the first of several stages in the cell's communication route. The signal molecule interacts with a receptor molecule on the cell surface or in the cytoplasm, which is the second component of this route. The second type of molecule that regulates cell activity is the receptor. A molecule known as a signal transducer falls into the third group. This molecule gets the information the cell receives when the signal molecule connects to the receptor and generates another one inside the cell that keeps the information flowing. Transcription factors make up the fourth group of compounds. These variables control which genes are employed in the cell and, as a result, how cells appear and behave. Apoptotic proteins, which are included in the fifth group, instruct injured cells to commit suicide by apoptosis. Molecules that directly affect cellular division pathways fall into the sixth group. Proteins that repair DNA damage are the seventh and final type of molecule. All seven of these molecular groups operate normally in healthy cells. However, any of these categories does not operate normally in cancerous cells. Because all of the information for creating all of the regulatory molecules in all seven categories is encoded in the DNA sequences of particular genes, it means that these genes function normally in normal cells but not in cancerous cells. To put it another way, normal cells contain genes that encode normal proteins, but cancer cells have mutated versions of those same genes that encode aberrant proteins. Genetic coding is the process of transferring genetic information to a protein in order to establish its function. As a result, groups of incorrectly functioning genes are at the center of cancer's cellular process (Bozzone, 2007; Kim and Jablons, 2017; Mehdipour, 2017; Roy and Datta, 2019).

Another important characteristic is the understanding of the role of the immune system in eliminating emerging cancerous lesions and micro-metastases (Roy and Datta, 2019; Hanahan, 2011). The regular functioning of the immune system assumes that its cells are continually monitoring cells and tissues, and that this surveillance of the immune system should eradicate the great majority of early neoplastic lesions and metastatic growths. Maybe the cancerous developments that make it past the immune system's scrutiny are immune to the immune system's efforts. There is, however, evidence to support and refute this hypothesis. It is well recognized that immune-compromised people are more likely to develop certain malignancies. Nevertheless, practically all these cancers are caused by viruses (Roy and Datta, 2019; Vajdic and Leeuwen, 2009). As a result, the immune system's involvement in such circumstances may be to remove virus-infected cells, albeit it is difficult to generalize this role to the overwhelming majority of malignancies. These findings suggest that, at least in some experimental models, the immune system has a role to play in cancer eradication. In several types of human cancer, antitumor immunological responses have also been observed (Nam and Murthy, 2004; Thomas-Tikhonenko, 2010). Finely tuned clinical observational studies establishing the relationship with statistical significance, as well as a greater molecular knowledge of cancers and the toxic millieu created by inflammation, all contributed to persuading scientists and clinicians of the reality of this link (Thomas-Tikhonenko, 2010; Sepulveda and Lynch, 2010). According to existing models, prolonged inflammation generates a milieu that promotes neoplastic progression (Coussens and Werb, 2002; Thomas-Tikhonenko, 2010; Sepulveda and Lynch, 2010). There is a clear-cut difference between the normal cellular microenvironment and the inflammatory states. In the case of an inflammatory environment, the striking increase in stimulated immune system cells and excessive amounts of inflammatory mediators is evident. Among others, eicosanoids, cytokines, chemokines, and nontoxicnon-toxic free radicals stemming from the reactive oxygen and nitrogen species (ROS and RNS, respectively) are more pronounced. Aforementioned inflammatory factors primarily regulate the course of immune response; however, they are known to partake in the activation of different mechanisms, namely, stimulation of mesenchymal and epithelial cells that is leading to tissue regeneration and healing. In such a case, there is an inverse correlation between cellular proliferation and apoptosis, where apoptosis is being inhibited. It should be noted that angiogenesis is also enhanced for the stated regeneration. Finally in the inflammatory milieu, physiological protections of the organism are overwhelmed by the constant stress caused by the oxidative stressors, which particularly leads to striking damaging of cellular subunits, such as proteins, lipids, and even the nuclear DNA. This all adds up to a more favorable environment for the formation of a changed neoplastic cell (Thomas-Tikhonenko, 2010; Sepulveda and Lynch, 2010).

The Theory of the Cancer Genetics

When somatic cells in the body divide, new cells are produced. Each has a complete set of chromosomes. During cell division, anything might go wrong, and chromosomes can become damaged, lost, or abandoned. When these events occur, cells that arise may contain excess chromosomes, chromosomes that have missing sections, chromosomes that break and then reattach the fragments wrongly, or even chromosomes that are missing totally. To correctly balance the activity of genes, cells must have complete normal chromosomes present in the correct quantities. Due to chromosomal abnormalities (Bozzone, 2007), uncontrolled cell division and cancer can emerge when this finely managed scenario breaks down. Most human tumors are caused by germline or somatic cell abnormalities. These flaws might be chromosomal, such as chromosomal dislocations, or specific gene mutations. Individual proteins produced from defective genes have significant metabolic implications as a result of such abnormalities. Furthermore, genes are typically arranged as metabolic circuits, and incorrect transcription of a gene can have cascading effects on a circuit (Roy and Datta, 2019).

However, definitive cells in the body have a system in place to prevent telomere shortening. These are the cells that develop into gametes (eggs or sperm). These germ cells produce the enzyme telomerase, which repairs the telomeres lost during replication, bypassing the cellular aging mechanism. The only other cells in the human body that may synthesize telomerase and so become immortal are cancer cells. Cells in 90% of human cancers generate telomerase. As a result, even if they are damaged or aberrant, these cells ignore the signals that instruct them to die. These cells subsequently continue to multiply and, more than likely, gather more genetic abnormalities, making them even more aggressive. This genetic disorder may prove lethal in the end (Bozzone, 2007).

One of the hypotheses that has emerged from research into the genetics of cancer is that a sequence of isolated events might drive a cell toward malignancy. There is a final straw where chromosomal, telomere, and gene errors and faults avalanche and the pace of fault accumulation accelerates. Although not evident in all cancers, general genetic instability raises the chances of many cancers developing into comprehensive, aggressive, and invasive tumors. In most cases, the instability is caused by a mutation or chromosomal flaw, which leads to other mutations and abnormalities. Cancer development is undeniably influenced by genetic instability (Bozzone 2007).

Cancer researchers distinguish three types of cancer: sporadic, familial, and hereditary. Hereditary factors do not appear to play a role in the development of sporadic tumors. There is no family-related history of the particular cancer, and there is no reason to believe that the genetic component of the disease is anything more than a several mutations that happened in a cell and eventually resulted in a tumor. Familial neoplasms occur when there are a few incidences of the disease in a family, but there is no discernible pattern. It is improbable that cancer will be passed down through generations in cases of family cancer. There is likely to be a pattern of inherited and environmental variables that impact the differential risk of acquiring cancer. Cancer susceptibility can be passed down from one generation to the next, rather than merely from one cell to the next. Inherited cancers are uncommon, making up just 5 to 10% of all malignancies. Still, studies of these malignancies are significant, as they have demonstrated that genes play a definite role in cancer formation. Likewise, knowledge of genes involved in genetically determined malignancies has led to new perspectives on non-hereditary and more prevalent cancers (Bozzone, 2007; Roy and Datta, 2019).

Defects in tumor suppressor genes or proto-oncogenes, as well as chromosomal issues that impact the normal function of suppressor genes or proto-oncogenes, can increase the risk of cancer. Whether errors are novel or acquired from parents, these genetic abnormalities can lead to tumor growth. Investigations and research on factors in human tumors show that carcinogenesis is caused by the aggregation of many genetic flaws, which reinforces the cascading nature of oncogenesis (Bozzone, 2007; Roy and Datta, 2019).

The Oncogenes

Given that certain normal genes can malfunction and turn cells into cancerous states, it is crucial to examine how these genes, also known as proto-oncogenes, behave in typical situations. After all, proto-oncogenes are not like timed bombs in cells, ready to explode. Indeed, proto-oncogenes all code for proteins that are required for cell proliferation, survival, or differentiation in some way. Some proto-oncogene-encoded proteins, for example, are growth factors and are involved in cell communication pathways, while others become receptor proteins for such growth factors. Some are intracellular signal molecules that convey information obtained at the cell surface, where receptors attach to growth factor molecules, to places inside the cell and its nucleus. Some proteins even bind directly to DNA to alter gene expression, regulating specific genes to influence the creation of specific proteins. These kinds of protein work together to control cell division in a complicated mechanism (Bozzone, 2007). Because the proteins expressed by specific proto-oncogenes may govern cell division, it stands to reason that if some or all of these genes are mutated, the protein molecules they encode might become defective, causing cell proliferation to remain in an "always active state." To put it another way, proto-oncogenes can be converted into oncogenes, which can cause cancer if they are present in cells (Bozzone, 2007).

Proto-oncogenes change into oncogenes in all situations due to a change in gene structure, location, or function, resulting in excessive protein synthesis or the development of a hyperactive, uncontrolled protein. An oncogene can become a proto-oncogene by undergoing particular genetic modifications. For starters, a mutation in which one of the four bases of DNA's genetic code is changed to a different base might result in the creation of a new protein. A point mutation is defined as a change in one base of the DNA code. The oncogene "ras" is a representation of an oncogene that arises from a single alteration in the gene's DNA sequence. In the second group, genes can be amplified in some cases. This implies that they become duplicates and implant them into the cell's chromosomes. Consequently, a cell may have too many copies of a proto-oncogene, resulting in excessive protein production and oncogenic activity despite the normal gene structure. Among others, a proto-oncogene that turns oncogenic when amplified is the oncogene "N-myc." In the third group, chromosomes can be broken and their components rearranged. If a proto-oncogene is transferred to a new site on the chromosome, it may become uncontrolled and trapped in the "on" position, leading to oncogenic behavior. The gene "c-myc" is oncogenic due to its translocation on the chromosome. Some of these genes are identified in tumor viruses as oncogenes, but the majority of them are proto-oncogenes that turn oncogenic without entering a virus. Proto-oncogenes encode proteins that regulate cell growth or survival. To become an oncogene, some sort of modification or shift in gene structure, location, or function is required for all proto-oncogenes (Bozzone 2007).

Well-over 100 oncogenes have been found, all of which are derived from normal genes involved in cell growth and survival. To begin with, cells require growth hormones to promote cell division. When oncogenesis is active, it encodes a growth factor that is produced on a constant basis. As a result, cells with an operational oncogene emit the same growth factor that causes their own proliferation, in other words, they encourage their own cell division. Subsequently, to continue the communication channel, growth factors must attach to cell surface receptors. An aberrant form of a growth factor receptor is encoded by the oncogene "erb-B." Even when no growth factor is available, this defective receptor acts as if it is bound all the time. Next, when growth factors and receptors attach to each other, the communication channel is continued by molecules inside the cell. Oncogenes known as "src" and "ras" create aberrant intracellular signal molecules that activate other cascades. The pathway's signal will eventually reach the chromosomes, causing changes in gene expression. The oncogenes "c-myc" and "c-fos" generate transcription factors, which are DNA-binding molecules that control gene activity. These transcription factors, including "c-myc" and "c-fos," overstimulate gene expression and cause excessive proliferation. Lastly, cells have to choose between dividing to generate new cells and dying. The oncogene "bcl-1" produces a protein that prevents cells from committing suicide. Damaged cells that should die fail to do so while "bcl-1" is active and instead divide, resulting in a population of faulty cells. Proto-oncogenes are important regulators of cell growth. Cell division is overstimulated when they transform into oncogenes and act abnormally (Bozzone 2007).

MicroRNAs as Oncogenes

MiRNAs that are significantly elevated in human malignancies are thought to play an oncogenic role. MiR-155 was the first miRNA to be postulated to have an oncogenic role after its increase was discovered in human B-cell lymphomas together with a host noncoding RNA called the B-cell integration cluster on chromosome 21q23 (Eis et al. 2005; Lee and Croce, 2017). MiR-21 was the first to disclose specific miRNA expression. MiR-21 is the most widely elevated miRNA in practically all malignant tumors, including hematological and consistent tumors (Krichevsky and Gabriely, 2009; Lee and Croce, 2017). In the non-coding gene C13orf25 at 13q31.3, a single cistronic miR-17-92 collection containing six miRNAs is situated at 800 base pairs (Olive et al. 2013). Lymphomas typically amplify this location (Lee and Croce, 2017).

Tumor Suppressors

Tumor suppressor genes that have been mutated or damaged are unable to limit cell proliferation, whereas oncogene activity often drives cells to continue cell division even when it is inappropriate. Tumor suppressor genes encode proteins that determine whether cells survive and, if they do, whether they replicate. Only a few dozen genes in each human cell encode tumor suppressors, despite the fact that each cell has more than 30,000 genes. Even if only one of these tumor suppressor genes is malfunctioning, it can have major health repercussions. Tumor suppressor genes are known as "gatekeeper genes" because their absence allows for uncontrolled cell growth. There are also "caretaker genes" that are covered in the repairmen of DNA and chromosomal sorting during cell division (Bozzone, 2007). Caretaker genes are necessary for genomic integrity, but they have little effect on cell growth. Tumor suppressor genes affect cells in a number of different ways. Tumor suppressor genes encode proteins that fall into one of four functional groups. To begin with, there are proteins within the cell that prevent cells from progressing through a specific stage of the cell cycle of growth and division. Second, certain proteins serve as receptors for hormones or chemical signals that instruct cells not to divide. Third, some proteins prevent cell division when DNA is broken or when chromosomes are aberrant. Fourth, if DNA or chromosomal damage is too severe to repair, some proteins will cause apoptosis, or "cell death." Tumor suppressor genes produce proteins that evaluate whether cells should be permitted to proliferate and/or survive in all instances (Bozzone 2007). The suppressor p53, which is transcripted by the p53 gene, is by far the most significant. In 50% of all human cancers, including hereditary and noninherited types, this tumor suppressor is altered or deleted. When DNA is badly damaged, the control system, which contains p53, requires cells to cease proliferating or die through apoptosis. In addition to random mutations or cellular mishaps, there are several events and chemicals that impact the p53 protein. Although the tumor suppressor function of the p53 protein is vital, it is only one of the reasons why it is important in cells. Many issues, such as DNA damage, hypoxia, nucleotide imbalance, and disruption of the mitotic spindle, activate p53 genes as part of an overall response pathway to cellular stress. The defensive actions of the cell against various threats are governed by the p53 protein. The p53 protein, along with a few other components, can determine how much damage has been done to DNA and chromosomes. p53 is a transcription factor, which is a type of molecule that controls whether other genes are activated or not. Genes influence the creation of other proteins when they are active. No proteins are produced when genes are switched off, and therefore dormant. When DNA is broken, p53 controls the genes responsible for mending it, regulating cell division, and guiding apoptosis. If the damage is not too severe, p53 stops the cell's growth and division cycle and guides repair. P53 triggers apoptosis because there is too much injury (Bozzone, 2007).

Another tumor suppressor gene, for example, produces a protein that can halt the cell division process. Although altered tumor suppressor genes have been linked to numerous forms of inherited tumors, they are also seen in non-hereditary tumors. Several tumor suppressors are also critical in the progression of several tumors. As a result, the protein it encodes is missing, which typically suppresses cell growth, and a tumor ultimately develops. It is worth noting that normal proto-oncogene protein products promote cell division, whereas normal tumor suppressor protein products prevent cell division (Bozzone, 2007). In many circumstances, an activating protein and an inhibiting protein are found at the same stage in the same route. The tumor suppressor gene "NF-1" is altered in diverse incarnations of leukemia and nervous system malignancies, for example. Normally, the normal action of the "NF-1" gene suppresses the function of the protein produced by the proto-oncogene "ras." When the "NF-1" protein is faulty, it does not prevent the "ras" protein from activating cell division, resulting in uncontrolled cell proliferation. The delicate balance between cell division activators and inhibitors can be challenging at times. "TGF-β" is a chemical signal released by normal cells that prevents cell division in a variety of cells (Bozzone, 2007). As a result, the receptor becomes inactive and cell division proceeds. Other steps in the regulatory cascade can go awry even when the TGF-β signal connects to a normal receptor. TGF-β inhibits cell division under normal conditions by interacting with another protein named p15. The p15 protein is absent in various malignancies, and consequently, the signal to terminate cell division is not effectively passed on. An intricate agreement between activating chemicals encoded by proto-oncogenes and inhibitory agents from tumor suppressors determines whether cells should live and proliferate (Bozzone, 2007).

MicroRNAs as Tumor Suppressors

When loss of activity of a miRNA is related to malignancy of a normal cell, it can behave as a suppressor, much like a protein-coding gene. According to Lee and Croce (2017), the function of a miRNA can be lost due to chromosomal mutation, epigenetic silencing, and/or changes in miR processing. The 30-kb deletion region between the LEU2 gene from the 13q14.2 region, the most documented chromosomal abnormality, produced two miRNAs, reported as miR-15a and miR16-1 (Calin et al. 2002; 2004; 2005; Lee and Croce, 2017). Because the miR-15a/miR16-1 cluster was shown to target the anti-apoptotic protein BCL-2, the miR-15a/16-1 cluster was postulated to have a suppressing role. As a result, in individuals with chromosomal deletions or, less commonly, mutations, low levels of miR15a/miR-16-1 may promote BCL-2 protein production (Calin et al. 2002; 2004; 2005; Lee and Croce, 2017). In addition, miR-29b-1/miR-29a of the miR-29 family, were discovered on chromosome 7q32, a frequently deleted location in different cancer types (Garzon et al. 2008; 2009; Lee and Croce, 2017). The downregulated miR-29 family was also shown to be inversely linked with upregulated oncogenic products, notably "BCL-2" and "MCL-1" (Xu et al. 2014; Lee and Croce, 2017), strongly implying a tumor suppressor role (Lee and Croce, 2017).

Biomarkers in Cancers

Because late discovery typically leads to a poor prognosis due to metastasis to other organs, early detection of the malignant phenotype is one of the most important variables in cancer diagnosis that determines favorable outcomes of cancer treatment choices. Global profiling of total miRNAs is a time-consuming and expensive procedure that should not be performed on each patient sample. Identification of a small number of miRNAs may be done quickly. A solid understanding of precise and cheap biomarkers for each kind of human cancer is crucial in this regard. A microRNA signature is the recommended course of action. The discovery of miRNA signatures in diverse forms of human cancer encouraged many researchers to dig deep to identify the most important miRNAs, even after taking into account the genetic and historical background of different specimens. If possible, such miRNAs might be used as diagnostic and prognostic biomarkers. MiR-15/16 clusters, for example, have been discovered to be regularly eliminated and downregulated (Calin et al. 2004; Lee and Croce, 2017). When miRNA profiles from 166 human bladder tumor samples were compared with miRNA profiles from 11 normal bladder samples, only three out of 15 miRNAs were determined to represent the miRNA signature linked with tumor aggressiveness. These three miRNA signatures have the potential to be valuable prognostic indicators. Although miRNA signatures obtained from extensive profiling of a variety of patient samples can be effective diagnostic and prognostic indicators, there are still significant differences in profiling methods (Lee and Croce, 2017). The majority of miRNA profiling was done on RNA samples taken directly from patients' cancer tissue retrieved through biopsies. Alternatively, circulating RNAs, or RNA extracts from plasma and serum, have been proposed as a noninvasive, low-cost, and quick cancer diagnostic technique (Tsang and Lo, 2007; Lee and Croce, 2017). Proliferation, apoptosis, invasion, metastasis, angiogenesis, and maintenance have all been found to be influenced by miRNAs in human malignancies. Furthermore, specific miRNA expression patterns are linked to carcinogenesis and progression. High-throughput characterization of miRNA expression in a range of human cancer patient samples revealed a distinct signature of unregulated miRNAs in malignancies. The discovery of definitive miRNA signatures can be used to develop diagnostic and prognostic tools, as well as therapeutics (Lee and Croce, 2017).

Tumor Immunology

The connection between carcinogenesis and immunity begins at the onset of the disease. Regular immune cells are thought to target aberrant cells for death as part of normal immune surveillance. However, cancer cells appear to elude destruction in a variety of ways. The absence of co-stimulatory signal generation by the cancer cell, as well as its inherently low immunogenicity, might result in immune tolerance of the malignant cell (Murphy, 2011; Yandle, 2014; Jacobs et al. 2014). Immune editing, which involves the continuing killing of aberrant cells recognized by the immune system and the survival of cancer cells expressing antigens that are poorly recognized by the immune system, may also contribute to cancer escape from immune control. A crucial number of live cancer cells without antigens capable of eliciting a substantial immune response is eventually achieved, allowing the tumor to proliferate unabated (Schreiber et al. 2011; Yandle, 2014; Jacobs et al. 2014).

Different types of immune cells can be shown in various regions of the tumor and surrounding tissue, and among them are cells that are hypothesized to inhibit immune responses in tumors (Murphy, 2011; Yandle, 2014; Jacobs et al. 2014). Cancerous cells also appear to regulate their immunological surroundings by releasing pro-inflammatory and other cytokines, keeping immune responses aimed at cancer cells suppressed. Immune cell subgroups appear to play a role in guaranteeing the survival of cancer cells and the spread of metastases (Pollard, 2004). Cancerous cells, immune cells, and extracellular matrix components interact in ways that might lead to tumor suppression or development. The dynamic and intricate interactions between cancer cells and their immediate surroundings are considered to have a role in their abnormal behavior (Bissell and Radiski, 2001; Lu et al. 2012). Finally, these factors add to the complicated character of cancer biology (Yandle, 2014; Jacobs et al. 2014).

Conclusion

There are various reasons why the characterization of cancer types remains incomplete despite increasing research in the field. Among the many postulated reasons, some of them are more prevalent. To name a few, the following can be stated: (1) unclear genetic patterns present in "gatekeeper genes" and their associated pathways lead to obscure mapping of dominant traits; (2) the lack of convincing data to represent each clinical phase of a given malignancy in a population; and (3) genetic heterogeneity of patients diagnosed with cancer that leads to conflicting clinical patterns. Cancer genes have been discovered in all the most common kinds of cancer, despite these roadblocks. The expanded use of sequencing methods on cancers holds the prospect of revealing a substantial number of new cancer genes in the future. Circulating tumor DNA and cells are two potential molecular indicators for cancer diagnosis in the early stages (Murtaza et al. 2013; Bianchi et al. 2014; Kim and Jablons, 2017; Kim, 2017). Genetic or proteomic abnormalities of specific cells or tissues can be analyzed in a large number of cells or tissues using microarray technology (Shim and Lee, 2017; Kim, 2017). Many conserved gene expression profiles connected to novel therapeutic targets or predicting prognosis in terms of survival or recurrence-free survival in various malignancies have been uncovered using these methods, which outperform conventional staging systems. Microarray technology is also commonly employed in other investigations, such as identifying SNP linked to cancer risk, variations, expression profiling, and cancer genome profiling (Shim and Lee, 2017; Kim, 2017). Furthermore, pedigree-based evaluation is the key for cancers and clinical discoveries, as it allows scientists and clinicians to discover the most suitable target genes, the most appropriate personalized management and, if needed, their relatives who carry the cancer risk, and the rational mentoring for target-based diagnosis (Azarnezhad and Mehdipour, 2017; Mehdipour, 2017). To progress into the present era of "personalized" or "precision" medicine (PM), which may be described as a medical care choice and response based on a patient's genetic, epigenetic, histopathological, or any other patient data, a novel conceptual framework of cancer therapy was required.

References

Azarnezhad, A., and Mehdipour, P., (2017). Cancer genetics at a glance: The comprehensive insights. In P. Mehdipour (Ed.) *Cancer Genetics and Psychotherapy.* (pp. 79-390). Springer International Publishing AG.

Bianchi, D. W., Parker, R. L., Wentworth, J., Madankumar, R., Saffer, C., Das, A. F., Craig, J. A., Chudova, D. I., Devers, P. L., Jones, K. W., Oliver, K., Rava, R. P., Sehnert, A. J., and Care Study Group. (2014). DNA sequencing versus standard prenatal aneuploidy screening. *The New England Journal of Medicine*, 27; 370(9), 799-808.

Bissell, M. J., and Radiski, D. (2001). Putting tumours in context. *Nature Reviews Cancer*, 1, 46-54.

Bozzone, D. M. (2007). *Biology of Cancer: Cancer Genetics.* Infobase publishing, New York. ISBN 0-7910-8818-9.

Calin, G. A., Dumitru, C. D., Shimizu, M., Bichi, R., Zupo, S., Noch, E., Aldler, H., Rattan, S., Keating, M., Rai, K., Rassenti, L., Kipps, T., Negrini, M., Bullrich, F., and Croce, C. M. (2002). Frequent deletions and down-regulation of micro- RNA genes miR15 and miR16 at 13q14 in chronic lymphocytic leukemia. *Proceedings of the National Academy of Sciences of the United States of America*, 99, 15524-15529.

Calin, G. A., Ferracin, M., Cimmino, A., Di Leva, G., Shimizu, M., Wojcik, S. E., Iorio, M. V., Visone, R., Sever, N. I., Fabbri, M., Iuliano, R., Palumbo, T., Pichiorri, F., Roldo, C., Garzon, R., Sevignani, C., Rassenti, L., Alder, H., Volinia, S., Liu, C. G., Kipps, T. J., Negrini, M., and Croce, C. M. (2005). A MicroRNA signature associated with prognosis and progression in chronic lymphocytic leukemia. *The New England Journal of Medicine*, 353, 1793-1801.

Calin, G. A., Liu, C. G., Sevignani, C., Ferracin, M., Felli, N., Dumitru, C. D., Shimizu, M., Cimmino, A., Zupo, S., Dono, M., Dell'Aquila, M. L., Alder, H., Rassenti, L., Kipps, T. J., Bullrich, F., Negrini, M., and Croce, C. M. (2004). MicroRNA profiling reveals distinct signatures in B cell chronic lymphocytic leukemias. *Proceedings of the National Academy of Sciences of the United States of America*, 101, 11755-11760.

Collins, F. and Guttmacher, A. (2001). Genetics moves into the medical mainstream. *JAMA The Journal of the American Medical Association*, 286, 2322-2324.

Coussens, L. M., and Werb, Z. (2002). Inflammation and cancer. *Nature*, 420, 860-867.

Eis, P. S., Tam, W., Sun, L., Chadburn, A., Li, Z., Gomez, M. F., Lund, E., and Dahlberg, J. E. (2005). Accumulation of miR-155 and BIC RNA in human B cell lymphomas. *Proceedings of the National Academy of Sciences of the United States of America*, 102, 3627-3636.

Garzon, R., Garofalo, M., Martelli, M. P., Briesewitz, R., Wang, L., Fernandez-Cymering, C., Volinia, S., Liu, C. G., Schnittger, S., Haferlach, T., Liso, A., Diverio, D., Mancini, M., Meloni, G., Foa, R., Martelli, M. F., Mecucci, C., Croce, C. M., and Falini, B. (2008). Distinctive microRNA signature of acute myeloid leukemia bearing cytoplasmic mutated nucleophosmin. *Proceedings of the National Academy of Sciences of the United States of America*, 105, 3945-3950.

Garzon, R., Heaphy, C. E., Havelange, V., Fabbri, M., Volinia, S., Tsao, T., Zanesi, N., Kornblau, S. M., Marcucci, G., Calin, G. A., Andreeff, M., and Croce, C. M. (2009). MicroRNA 29b functions in acute myeloid leukemia. *Blood*, 114, 5331-5341.

Grimsey, E., Howlett, D., Allan, S., et al. (2010). Implementation and progress review of a nurse-led family history risk assessment clinic. *European Journal of Cancer*, 8, 241.

Hanahan, D., and Weinberg, R. A. (2000). The hallmarks of cancer. *Cell,* 7; 100(1), 57-70.

Hanahan, D., and Weinberg, R. A. (2011). Hallmarks of cancer: the next generation. *Cell,* 4; 144(5), 646-674.

Harris, K., and Lötter, B. (2012). Focus on patients with a family history of cancer. *Cancer Nursing Practice*, 11, 14-19.

Jacobs, C. (2014). Putting cancer genetics into context. pp. 3-8. In C. Jacobs, P. Webb and L. Robinson (Eds.) *Genetics for Health Professionals in Cancer Care; From Principles to Practice* (pp. 3-8). Oxford University Press.

Jacobs, C., Webb, P., and Robinson, L. (2014). *Genetics for Health Professionals in Cancer Care: From Principles to Practice*. Oxford University Press. ISBN 978–0–19–967 284–4.

Kim, J. (2017). *Cancer Genetics and Genomics for Personalized Medicine*. Taylor and Francis Group, Pan Stanford Publishing Pte. Ltd. ISBN 978-1-315-36476-6 (eBook).

Kim, J. and Jablons, D. (2017). Personalized medicine for cancer: Introduction and overview of the book. In J. Kim (Eds.) *Cancer Genetics and Genomics for Personalized Medicine* (pp. 1-15). Taylor and Francis Group, Pan Stanford Publishing Pte. Ltd.

Krichevsky, A. M., and Gabriely, G. (2009). miR-21: a small multi-faceted RNA. *Journal of Cellular and Molecular Medicine*, 13, 39-5332.

Lanceley, A, Eagle, Z., Ogden, G., et al. (2012). Family history and women with ovarian cancer: is it asked and does it matter? An observational study. *International Journal of Gynecological Cancer*, 22, 254-259.

Lee, T. J., and Croce, C. M. (2017). MicroRNAs in human cancers. In J. Kim (Eds.) *Cancer Genetics and Genomics for Personalized Medicine* (pp. 239-265). Taylor and Francis Group, Pan Stanford Publishing Pte. Ltd.

Lu, P., Weaver, V., and Werb, Z. (2012). The extra-cellular matrix: a dynamic niche in cancer progression. *Journal of Cell Biology*, 196, 395-406.

Mehdipour, P. (2017). *Cancer Genetics and Psychotherapy*. Springer International Publishing AG. ISBN 978-3-319-64550-6 (eBook).

Meyer, L. A., Anderson, M. E., Lacour, R. A., et al. (2010). Evaluating women with ovarian cancer for BRCA1 and BRCA2 mutations: missed opportunities. *Journal of Obstetrics and Gynaecology*, 115, 945-952.

Murphy, K. (2011). *Janeway's Immunobiology*, 8th edn. New York: Garland Science.

Murtaza, M., Dawson, S. J., Tsui, D. W., Gale, D., Forshew, T., Piskorz, A. M., Parkinson, C., Chin, S. F., Kingsbury, Z., Wong, A. S., Marass, F., Humphray, S., Hadfield, J., Bentley, D., Chin, T. M., Brenton, J. D., Caldas, C., Rosenfeld, N. (2013). Noninvasive analysis of acquired resistance to cancer therapy by sequencing of plasma DNA. *Nature,* 2; 497(7447), 108-112.

Nam, J. H., and Murthy, S. (2004) *Chronic Inflammation and Cancer in Various Organ Systems*. Springer Basel AG, Birkhauser Verlag Basel, Basel.

Olive, V., Li, Q., and He, L. (2013). Mir-17-92: a polycistronic oncomir with pleiotropic functions. *Immunological Reviews,* 253, 158-166.

Phillips J, Murray P, Kirk P 2001. *Biology of Disease*, 2nd edn. Oxford: Blackwell Science.

Pollard, J. (2004). Tumour-educated macrophages promote tumour progression and metastasis. *Nature Reviews Cancer*, 4, 71-78.

Roy, M., and Datta, A. (2019). *Cancer Genetics and Therapeutics.* Springer Nature Singapore Pte. Ltd. ISBN 978-981-13-9471-3.

Scheuner, M., Sieverding, P., Shekelle, P. (2008). Delivery of genomic medicine for common chronic adult diseases: a systematic review. *JAMA The Journal of the American Medical Association*, 299, 1320-1334.

Schreiber, R. D., Old, L. J., and Smyth, M. J. (2011). Cancer immunoediting: integrating immunity's roles in cancer suppression and promotion. *Science*, 331, 1565-1570.

Sepulveda, A. R., and Lynch, J. P. (2010). Genetic instability and chronic inflammation in gastrointestinal cancers. pg: 351-398. In A. Thomas-Tikhonenko (Ed.) *Cancer Genome and Tumor Microenvironment* (pp. 351-398). Springer New York Dordrecht Heidelberg London. e-ISBN 978-1-4419-0711-0.

Shim, J. J., and Lee, J. S. (2017). Genome- based personalized Medicine in liver cancer. In J. Kim (Eds.) *Cancer Genetics and Genomics for Personalized Medicine* (pp. 39-53). Taylor and Francis Group, Pan Stanford Publishing Pte. Ltd.

Thomas-Tikhonenko, A. (2010). *Cancer Genome and Tumor Microenvironment*. Springer New York Dordrecht Heidelberg London. e-ISBN 978-1-4419-0711-0.

Tsang, J. C., and Lo, Y. M. (2007). Circulating nucleic acids in plasma/serum. *Pathology*, 39, 197-207.

Vajdic, C. M., and van Leeuwen, M. T. (2009). Cancer incidence and risk factors after solid organ transplantation. *International Journal of Cancer*, 125, 1747-1754.

Xu, L., Xu, Y., Jing, Z., Wang, X., Zha, X., Zeng, C., Chen, S., Yang, L., Luo, G., Li, B., and Li, Y. (2014). Altered expression pattern of miR-29a, miR-29b and the target genes in myeloid leukemia. *Experimental Hematology and Oncology*, 3, 17-3619-3-17.

Yandle, A. (2014). Cancer biology. In C. Jacobs, P. Webb and L. Robinson (Eds.) *Genetics for Health Professionals in Cancer Care: From Principles to Practice* (pp. 36-46). Oxford University Press.

Chapter 5

Effects of p53 and Other Antioncogenes on Cancer

Gözde Öztan*, PhD

Department of Medicine,
Istanbul University, Istanbul, Turkey

Abstract

The proliferation and differentiation of all cells are controlled by two types of genes, oncogenes and anti-oncogenes. Oncogenes stimulate cell growth, whereas anti-oncogenes inhibit it. Oncogenes and anti-oncogenes are crucial to the complex step-by-step process that leads to cancer.

Both Rb and p53 play a role in tumor suppression. When cancers develop, they become inactive and their reactivation is the reason most cancer therapies work. Rb and p53 are both genetically inactivated, so cells lose their antitumor properties irreparably. It is widely known that $p16^{INK4A}$ and $p14^{ARF}$ play a critical role in cell cycle arrest, cellular senescence, and cancer. PTEN plays an important role in cell growth, proliferation, and survival because it functions as a down-regulator of the PI3K/Akt/mTOR pathway. In addition, it is involved in the control of DNA damage response and modeling of tumor immune micro-environments. APC is a tumor suppressor gene that is involved in the Wnt signaling pathway associated with APC mutations and CRC carcinogenesis.

In this chapter, the effects of the p53 gene and other anti-oncogenes in various cancer diseases are stated, and the most important tumor suppressor genes are classified. The relationship between the

* Corresponding Author's Email: gozdeoztan@yahoo.com.

In: Autoimmunity and Cancer
Editors: Soner Şahin and Kenan Demir
ISBN: 978-1-68507-937-6

biochemical processes that control cell division, the proteins that control the growth mechanism, the genes and mechanisms responsible for limiting growth when necessary, and the formation and development of cancer has been revealed at the molecular level.

Keywords: antioncogen, cancer, genes, tumor suppressor

Introduction

Oncogenes and Antioncogenes (Tumor Suppressor Genes)

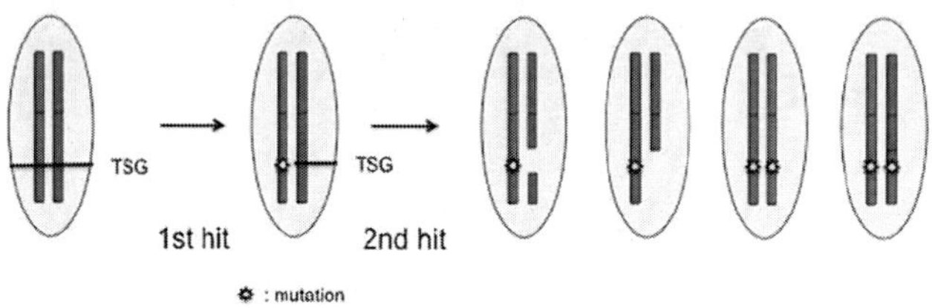

Figure 1a. Knudson's two hit model.

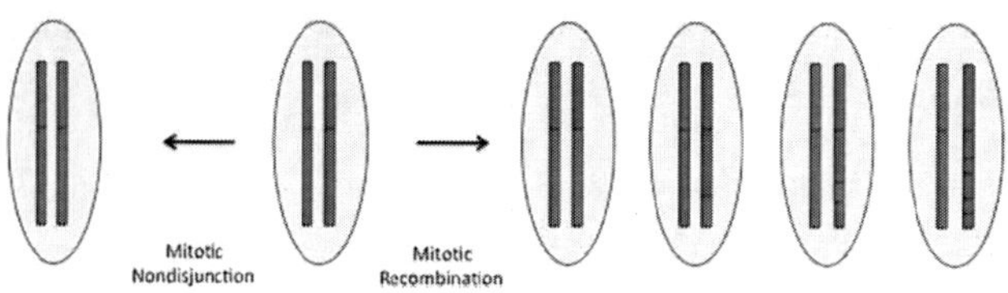

Figure 1b. Mechanism of acquired uniparental disomy (copy neutral LOH).

Figure 1a. A two-hit model of inactivation using Knudson's tumor suppressor gene. First hits are typically rare mutations, while second hits are usually caused by gross chromosomal mechanisms. Sporadic tumors acquire these two hits somatically. *Figure 1b.* A copyneutral LOH (cnLOH) can result from mitotic nondisjunction or mitotic recombination. As a result of incomplete segregation during mitosis, there may be monosomic or trisomic cells as a result of the number of chromosomes. CnLOH occurs when all chromosomes are duplicated or deleted in a non-disjunction mitotic cycle. There may also be a single or multiple mitotic recombination event during mitosis, resulting in segmental cnLOH (Mizoguchi et al., 2011).

The world's most serious disease is cancer. During the cancer development process, five steps occur: initiating, advancement, malignancy, progression, and metastasis. Cancers can be caused by various factors: some reduce tumor development, and some promote it. Oncogenes and tumor suppressors work together to induce cancer (Zhang et al., 2007).

The proto-oncogenes are cancer-causing genes that act dominantly. Activation of one copy of the gene is sufficient to generate tumor growth. Contrary to this, the second major type of cancer gene, tumor suppressor genes, acts in a recessive manner at the cellular level. Tumor growth requires inactivation of both copies. Tumor cells fusioned with normal cells provide evidence for recessive mechanisms in tumorigenesis (Cornelisse & Devilee, 1997).

According to Knudson's two-hit hypothesis, tumor suppressor genes can be inactivated by two genetic events. Both genetic hits in the disease are acquired at the somatic level, rather than inherited. First-hit chromosomal mutations normally result in a second hit, resulting from recombination followed by mitotic recombination or non-disjunctional chromosomal loss, respectively. A loss of heterozygosity (LOH) test can be performed using PCR-based assays or fluorescence *in situ* hybridization. PCR-based tests frequently use polymorphic markers to detect LOH. LOH analysis can be performed with SNP arrays, which allow the simultaneous detection of allelic imbalances and copy number changes. The copy number profile of LOH was copy neutral even after mitotic recombination and non-disjunction occurred in glioblastoma (Figure 1) (Mizoguchi et al., 2011).

TP53 (Tumor Protein p53)

Cancerous cells grow uncontrollably and abnormally in the body. The gene that encodes the protein is TP53, which is also called the genome guardian and was identified as involved in the regulation of the cell cycle and tumor suppression. Different events such as heat shock, hypoxia, DNA damage, and oncogene overexpression activate p53. This protein plays a crucial role as a regulator, which controls many diverse biological responses and prevents mutations in the genome. Murine double minute 2 gene expression (mdm2), caused by more than 50% of human cancer mutations, has been found to play an important role in the development of cancer. MDM2 regulates p53 gene expression via an autoregulatory feedback loop. As an E3 ubiquitin ligase, murine double minute 2 plays a crucial role in the ubiquitination and degradation of the p53 gene. Numerous drugs and compounds have been developed to reactivate the p53 gene by blocking the interaction between P53 and MDM2, as well as inhibiting the ubiquitination of p53 by E3. Clinical trials of compounds have been conducted in tumors caused by hematologic malignancies (Gupta et al., 2019).

The tumor suppressor p53 regulates multiple cellular functions. The survival-death axis mediated by p53 includes transient or permanent inhibition of cell proliferation or induction of cell death pathways in response to genotoxic stress. TP53 mutations are common in many types of human cancers due to the biological properties of TP53. TP53 inactivation often occurs during tumor development and progression. Tumor cells expressing wild-type p53 will be more susceptible to elimination by cytotoxic treatments than those expressing mutant p53 without wtp53 activities, because p53's potency in suppressing tumor growth is well known. TP53 mutations are rare in some cancer entities, which supports the idea that wtp53 activity is not always beneficial for tumor prevention. An interesting example is the etiology of glioblastoma multiforme, the most common and malignant form of adult brain cancer (Kim et al., 2009).

On chromosome 17, the short arm of TP53 is located. The gene consists of 11 exons and 19,200 base pairs in length. Two promoters are found in the TP53 sequence. p53 or its half-formed isoform Δ40p53 is produced by transcription from the first promoter, but transcription from the internal promoter gives rise to p53 or its truncated isoforms Δ133p53 and Δ160p53. Also, TP53 transcripts are subjected to alternative splicing, which can result in dozens of different isoforms of the gene. There are some of these truncated proteins that function similarly to their full-length counterparts, while others are antagonistic. P53 contains five domains: an N-terminal transcriptional activation domain (TAD), a proline rich domain (PR), a central DNA binding domain (DBD), an oligomerization domain (OD), and a regulatory domain (REG). Because DBD binds p53 to the regulatory motifs of its target genes, the majority of p53 mutations occur in this domain (Curylova et al., 2022).

The transcription factor p53, which plays an essential role in maintaining genetic stability, has been studied a lot. p63 and p73, two highly related proteins, are members of the same family of genes. A large proportion of human cancers are characterized by the loss of p53, which serves as a crucial pathway to prevent cancer formation. Approximately 60% of cancer cases are caused by mutations in the p53 gene. Cancers containing a WTp53 gene are inactivated by cell signaling along the p53 pathway, as well as upstream or downstream of it (Machado-Silva et al., 2010).

There are now nine distinct isoforms instead of the originally proposed three due to alternate promoters, initiation sites, and splicing sites. Intron 9 is alternatively spliced into p53α, p53β, and p53γ, the last two lacking an oligomerization domain (Figure 2) (Machado-Silva et al., 2010).

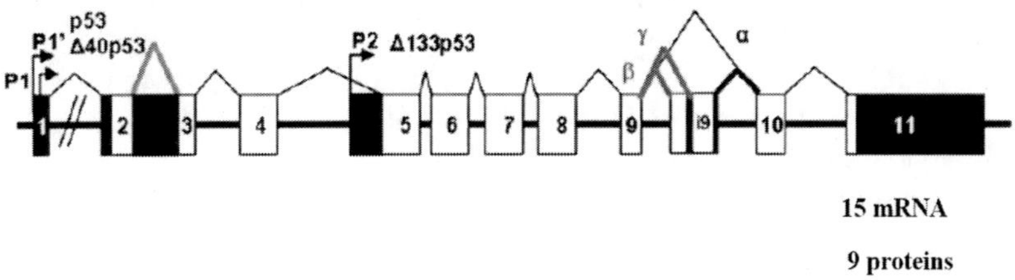

Figure 2a. Structure of the human p53 gene.

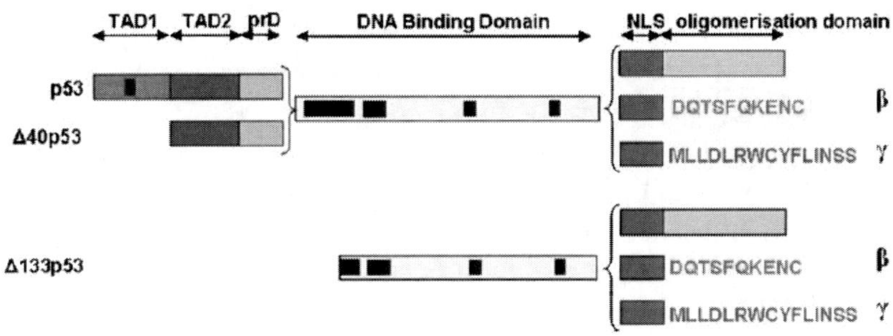

Figure 2b. p53 protein isoforms.

Figure 2a. Schematic diagram of the p53 gene. Various types of alternative splicing (α, β, γ) are available, as are alternative promoters (P1, P1', P2).
Figure 2b. p53 protein: The transactivation domains found on p53, p53β and p53γ encoded by promoters P1 or P1' are conserved. As the name implies, Δ133p53 is encoded by promoter P2. They contain a truncated amino acid sequence and lack the entire transactivation domain. ATG-133 is the starting point for translation. Alternative promoters for ATG-40 lead to amino-truncated Δ40p53 proteins when expressed from the P1 or P1' promoters. Despite losing the conserved N-terminal transactivation domain, the Δ40p53 protein still contains some transactivation domain (Machado-Silva et al., 2010).

The p53 gene and the p53 protein are believed to be responsible for the inactivation of human cancers. These two molecules act together to protect a cell from genotoxic stress, which radiotherapy and chemotherapy can produce. These changes may contribute greatly to resistance to tumor treatment. Among tumor suppressor genes, p53 is unique due to its specific characteristics; 80% of its mutations result in missense mutations that cause heterogeneous proteins. Mutant p53 proteins probably possess an oncogenic function, which allows them to facilitate cellular transformation. Furthermore, the ability of p53 to independently activate both apoptosis and antiproliferation in some mutants suggests that the relationship between p53 inactivation and cancer is more complex than previously thought (Soussi & Lozano, 2005).

PTEN (Phosphatase and Tensin Homolog)

PTEN controls cell proliferation, migration, and death by suppressing tumor growth. It was initially discovered that PTEN is located at 10q23, which is a frequently mutated or deleted site in cancer. PTEN loss or mutations have been detected in many different types of cancers, and heterozygous PTEN mice are highly susceptible to many types of tumors, supporting the hypothesis that PTEN plays an important tumor suppressor role in a wide variety of cancers. As a phosphatase that functions on both lipid and protein substrates, PTEN is a protein phosphatase with a broad spectrum of activity. As a tumor suppressor, PTEN utilizes its lipid substrates to function. When entering the cell membrane, PTEN converts phosphatidylinositol-3,4,5-trisphosphate (PIP3) into phosphatidylinositol-4,5-bisphosphate (PIP2), which facilitates 3-kinesis of phosphoinositide and downstream activation of AKT (Kavela et al., 2013).

When PIP3 stimulates the recruitment of AKTs to the membrane, other kinases that also rely on PIP3 activate it. The cancer pathway contains a number of components that have been described as causal factors. Human cancers that are affected by mutations, deletions, or silencing of promoter methylation have loss of PTEN activity. The number of cancer predisposition syndromes are linked to gene mutations in PTEN. Human tumors have recently been found to contain a number of mutations encoding the PI3KCA gene. Cancers of the breast, ovary, pancreas, esophagus, and other organs activate PI3K and AKT. Cancer is usually triggered by tissue-specific deletions of PTEN. Furthermore, the lack of PTEN promotes cancer in combination with p53 deficiency. An activated AKT transgenic line has not seen tumor development in breast or prostate tissue and has not been found to be compatible with the absence of p53. In transgenic mice that express PTEN targets, the researchers found that cyclin D1 and p53 are not expressed as these AKT-independent targets. Although AKT does enable PTEN tumorigenesis, it also enforces and accelerates it when it is expressed along with other oncogenes (Blanco-Aparicio et al., 2007).

In homeostasis, the phosphate groups are removed from PIP3 and PIP2 is converted to inactive PIP3. The findings also indicated that PTEN plays a fundamental antioncogenic role, including maintaining chromosomal stability and preserving the function of the DNA repair protein RAD51 through positive regulation. It was described that PTEN forms homodimers to acquire the lipid phosphatase configuration. In contrast, mutant PTEN units lack the catalytic function observed in wild-type PTEN units and, therefore, establish an inactive state by a dominant-negative mechanism. As a result, mechanisms that interfere with dimerization may prevent its proper activity and lead to oncogenesis. In any case, the active conformation of PTEN can be restored by eliminating phosphorylation residues. The PTEN family of proteins, as well as PTEN-L, a variant that is 173 amino acids longer, is secreted into the extracellular environment, exerting its tumor-defeating effects directly in recipient cells (Figure 3) (Gkountakos et al., 2019).

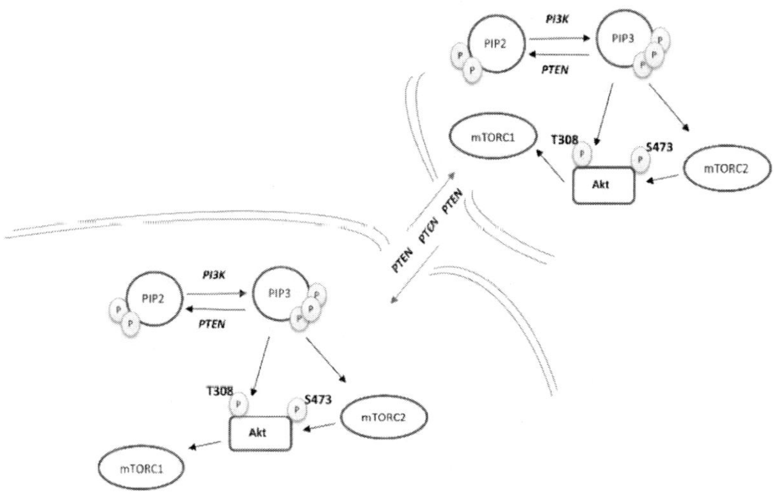

Figure 3. A tumor suppressor created by PTEN that can leave the cell and enter the recipient cell in a paracrine manner, exerting its effects on the target cell. mTORC1, mTOR complex 1; mTORC2, mTOR complex 2; PIP2, phosphatidylinositol 4,5-bisphosphate; PIP3, phosphatidylinositol 3,4,5-trisphosphate, PI3K, phosphoinositide 3-kinase (Gkountakos et al., 2019).

Although loss of PTEN increases insulin sensitivity, these metabolic effects are thought to explain the tumor suppressing effects of the protein. It is recognized that metabolic signals such as the activation of hexokinase and phosphofructokinase, as well as de novo lipogenesis, are several of the factors that promote tumor growth. Several metabolic enzymes, in particular glycolytic genes, are oncogenes or can suppress tumor growth when manipulated. Tumorigenesis appears to be strongly correlated with the expression of metabolic isoform-specific genes. There is growing evidence that lipogenic and other lipid-metabolizing genes contribute to tumorigenesis, but more research is needed (Chen et al., 2018).

p14ARF (Alternative Reading Frame)

In response to oncogenic stress, p14ARF (ARF) is up-regulated. There is widespread expression of ARF and surprisingly low levels of expression. In the absence of oncogenic stress, ARF inhibits the E3 ligase activity of MDM2 toward p53, causing apoptosis, cell cycle arrest, and cell senescence. 40% of cancers lose ARF, which is an obstacle to transformation. Recent studies suggested that ARF plays a noncanonical role in the detection of inflammation and inducing pro-inflammatory genes independent of p53. ARF also promotes the conjugation of small ubiquitin-like modifiers to various proteins independently of p53. SUMOylation is an analogous post-translational modification process involving enzymes E1 (SAE1/2), E2 (UBC9) and E3. SUMOylation influences protein activity, stability, and localization. Infections and inflammatory stimuli are typically used to initiate conjugation of SUMO2 and SUMO3. ARF has been found to not serve as a SUMO E3 ligase but rather promotes SUMOylation of p53, MDM2, NPM1, and Werner's helicase interactions (Alagu et al., 2018).

On chromosome 9p21, CDKN2A (INK4A/ARF) is a cancer suppressor gene that encodes two tumor suppressor genes, p16INK4A and p14ARF, which regulate the stability of P53. The most common form of brain tumor is malignant glioma, which is also the most deadly. Sixty-eight to eighty percent of malignant gliomas lack P14ARF tumor suppressor activity as a result of somatic alterations at the INK4A/ARF locus. In part, P14ARF's tumor suppressive properties are due to its ability to sequester HDM2 and prevent its degradation. Although P14ARF loss was found to be associated with TP53 loss in some tumors, this suggests that the protein has other tumor suppressor functions that do not depend on P53. Tumor suppressor p53 is known to be negatively regulated by p19Arf, which binds and inactivates Mdm2. Upon activation of P14ARF, the transcription factor P53 is stabilized, leading to the expression of important P53 target genes, which may lead to apoptosis or arrest of the cell cycle. There is generally acceptance that P14ARF inhibits tumor growth through P53 and that HDM2 amplification and P14ARF loss are alternative methods to inactivate this pathway (Zerrouqi et al., 2012).

P14ARF in humans is only 49% similar to murine p19ARF and is a little smaller at 5 kDa. Both p19ARF and p14ARF exhibit a similar structure despite the large size differences and the divergence of the sequence. MDM2 is directly accessed by M19ARF and M14ARF. In addition, MDM2 binds to p53, causing its degradation through ubiquitin. MDM2 is transactivated by p53, which produces a negative feedback loop between MDM2 and p53. Based on the cellular context, ARF inhibits the degradation of MDM2-mediated p53, stabilizing and activating p53, which then induces cell cycle arrest or apoptosis. Human cancers are often associated with the locus of the INK4a / ARF gene. In many human cancers, p16Ink4a is a tumor suppressor that is frequently deleted, mutated, and hypermethylated exclusively targeting p16Ink4a (Weber et al., 2002).

CDKN2A ($P16^{INK4A}$) (INK4 Family Member p16)

$P16^{INK4a}$ is a tumor suppressor protein also inactivated by cancer. It is encoded by each of the two tumor suppressor genes: multiple tumor suppressor 1 (MTS1) and cyclin-dependent kinase inhibitor 2A (CDKN2A) (Figure 4) (Zhao et al., 2016).

The 8.5 kb gene encodes $p16^{INK4a}$. Two introns and three exons are found in it. $P16^{INK4a}$ is a 16 kDa protein with 156 amino acids and is a negative cell cycle regulator. Exon 1β, which has its own promoter, complicates the simple tandem arrangement. A distinct protein is obtained from the RNA derived from exons 2 and 3 since the RNA is translated by a new reading frame. In other words, both mRNAs encode different proteins, $p16^{INK4a}$ and ARF, although their exons 2 and 3 are shared. The formation of the p16INK4a-CDK4 or $p16^{INK4a}$-CDK6 complex is inhibited by binding the $p16^{INK4a}$ protein to these proteins specifically and, through this, an allosteric conformational change is induced within the proteins. The retinoblastoma protein (Rb) persists in its hypophosphorylated and growth suppressing state due to the lack of this complex formation. Therefore, the repressive complex Rb/E2F induces G1 phase cell cycle arrest (Zhao et al., 2016).

During carcinogenesis, gene silencing often occurs in the context of altered cell cycle regulation. Many cancers are associated with deletion of the CDKN2A gene, which encodes $p16^{INK4a}$. $p16^{INK4a}$ regulates the CDK 4/6 complex, as well as cyclin D, which are critical in the regulation of the cell cycle and senescence. Multiple genetic and epigenetic defects in CDKN2A are associated with increased tumorigenesis and metastasis, as well as poor prognoses and recurrence of cancer (Zhao et al., 2016).

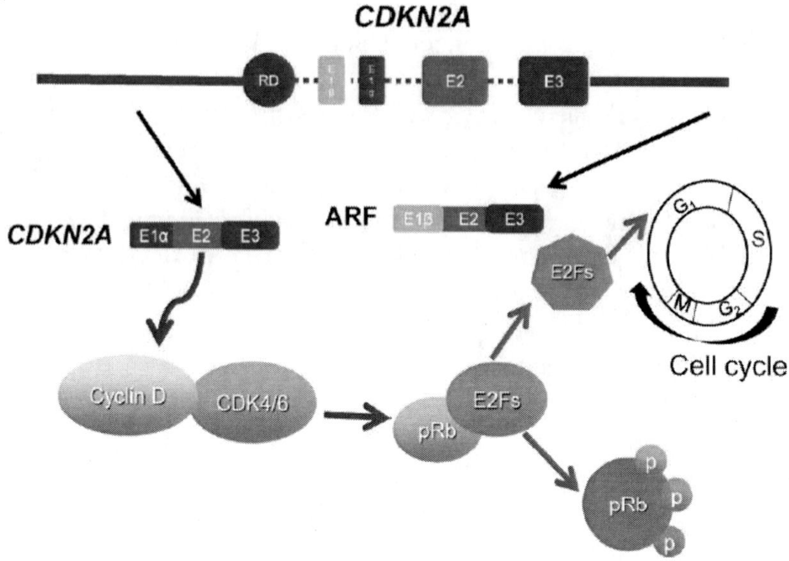

Figure 4. An illustration of the INK4a/ARF locus and the function of p16^{INK4a} can be found in this diagram. Cell cycle proteins move from phase G1 to phase S when p16^{INK4a} binds to cyclin D and CDK4/6 complexes, inhibiting transcription factor E2F1 (Zhao et al., 2016).

Tumor suppressive mechanisms, such as cellular senescence or DNA damage-induced growth arrest, are often associated with the induction of p16^{Ink4a}. In mice lacking both copies of p16Ink4a, tumorigenesis is highly exacerbated, despite the fact that p16Ink4a acts as a strong tumor suppressor. Tumors derived from mutations affecting p16^{Ink4a} often have loss-of-function mutations, which are common prerequisites to tumorigenesis. However, mutations in RB or CDK4 / 6, do not interfere with the activity of p16Ink4a. Furthermore, overexpression of p16Ink4a has been found in cancers of the endometrium, colorectal, and basal cell types with high levels of aggression. Kohli et al. formed murine sarcomas by overexpressing the RAS oncogene while simultaneously inhibiting p53 activity. This method was used to examine the effects of specific treatments. ABT-263 and ABT-737, which had previously been shown to eliminate murine sarcoma cells expressing p16^{Ink4a}, proved ineffective in eliminating senescent cells expressing p16Ink4a + when overexpressed by p16Ink4a. Suicide activation of sarcoma cells overexpressing p16^{Ink4a} both in vitro and in vivo resulted in sarcoma cells overexpressing 3MR, when the entire p16^{Ink4a} promoter was activated (Kohli et al., 2018).

RB (Retinoblastoma)

As part of a cellular process, tumor suppressors, such as retinoblastoma (RB), suppress the G1-S transition by integrating extracellular and intracellular signals. p107 and p130 play a role in mediating cellular responses to signals by controlling how E2F transcription factors function and target genes are expressed during cell cycle progression. RB family members are inhibited by cyclin-dependent kinases (CDK) upon exposure to growth factors. Cytostatic conditions inhibit cyclin-CDK complexes by inhibiting members of the p16INK4a and p21CIP1 family. Cancer has mutations that target the RB pathway almost universally, although different components are selectively affected in different types of cancer. In general, methylating the INK4a promoter or amplification of CDK genes inhibits three members of the RB family simultaneously and leads to uncontrolled proliferation. The RB gene is rarely mutated in human cancers, in contrast to p107 and p130, which are uncommon mutations in these cancers. Furthermore, the RB gene is seldom mutated in other types of cancer, such as retinoblastoma and osteosarcoma (Viatour & Sage, 2011).

Each member of the RB family has many structural similarities (Figure 5A). In the small pocket region, which is made up of two A domains and a flexible spacer region, highly homologous sequences tend to accumulate. Oncoproteins, such as E1A and TAg, can interact with a pocket on pRB. Despite their highly unrelated origins, each of the viral proteins possesses a unique peptide motif called LXCXE required to interact with the proteins of the RB family (Henley & Dick, 2012).

A large pocket forms when combined with the C-terminal domain (Figure 5A). A large pocket is formed by combining the small pocket and the C-terminal domain. This is the smallest growth suppressor found in RB family proteins. The interaction between proteins of the RB family and E2Fs is essential for proliferation control. However, p107 and p130 share more sequence similarities than pRB or pRB2 with each other, despite their shared pocket domain structure. The central tumor suppressor pRB, despite recognition as the central member of this family of cancer suppressors and divergence in sequence similarities, shows few differences in the structural characteristics of p107 and p130. The local pRB coupling site is used exclusively by E2F1, and the short peptide region of the C-terminus is occupied by CDK or protein phosphatase 1, two characteristics that are unique to pRB (Figure 5B) (Henley & Dick, 2012).

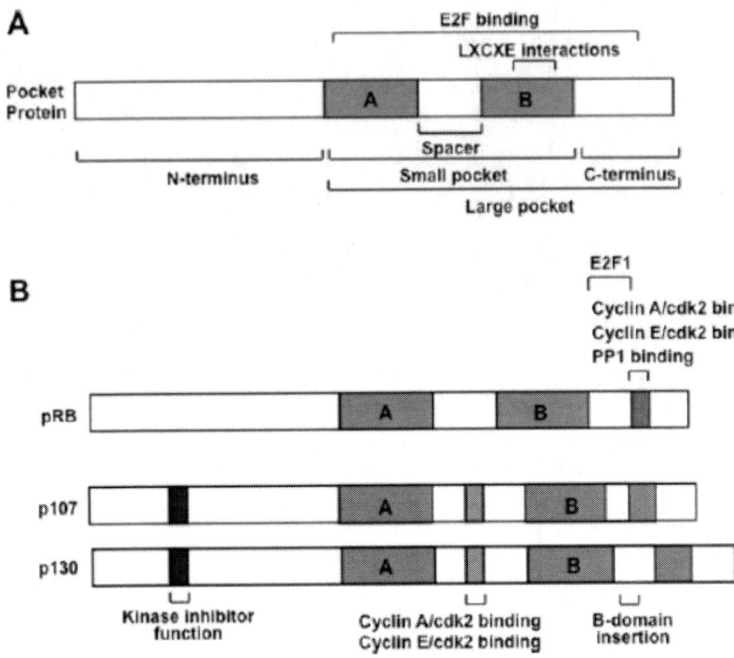

Figure 5. As shown in this figure, there are three open reading frames: pRB, P107, and P130. A) The pocket domain appears to be the defining feature of proteins in the RB family. In this figure, it is indicated as the 'small pocket' (which is named after the LXCXE motif) that is possible for binding to viral oncoproteins such as TAg from the simian virus. B) Comparison of the structures of the open reading frames of pocket proteins. Additional features of these proteins include an inhibitory site for kinases, a binding site for cyclin, and the insertion of a sequence into the B-domain of the pocket (Henley & Dick, 2012).

Almost all human cancers involve mutations of the Ras oncogene pathway or inactivation of the RB pathway. Cancer cells harboring Ras mutations almost always express wild-type Prb. Compared to wild-type cells, pRB-deficient tumor cells are much less susceptible to the cancer-causing potential of H-RasV12, while activated Ras inhibits pRB-deficient tumor cells from proliferating. The proliferation and anchorage-independent growth of Ras-transformed murine cells and human tumor cells with Ras pathway mutations are also inhibited by the loss of pRB. There is a distinct difference between fibroblasts lacking other members of the pRB family (p107 and p130) and those lacking $pRB^{-/-}$ 3T3 cells. Ras mutant tumor cells express increased amounts of p107 as a result of loss of pRB. However, expression of both p107 and pRB does not inhibit proliferation in these tumor cells (Williams et al., 2006).

APC (Adenomatous Polyposis Coli)

Due to its dysregulated structure and function, Adenomatous polyposis coli was identified as a tumor suppressor gene in colorectal carcinomas (CRCs). On chromosome 5q21-q22, APC is located in a gene assembly of 8535 nucleotides and consists of 21 exons. This gene codes for a 310-kDa protein that contains 2843 amino acids. Mutations in the APC gene cause familial adenomatous polyposis (FAP), an important cause of CRC. Most sporadic colorectal tumors contain somatic mutations of APC, and between 30% and 40% of tumors have loss of heterozygosity on chromosome 5q (Zhang & Shay, 2017).

Asef, PP2A, IQGAP1, and KAP3 bind to a conserved domain, the armadillo repeat, of the IQ-motif. Cell migration and adhesion are often stimulated by these interactions. By aiding in the degradation of β-catenin through proteosomal mechanisms, the 15 and 20 residue repeat domains and SAMP repeats are essential for working against the canonical Wnt signaling pathway. A component of the cytoskeleton, EB1 is known to play a crucial role in microtubule fixation, kinetochore activity, and chromosomal separation. Cell movement, cell adhesion, cell proliferation, cell differentiation, and chromosome segregation are all regulated by APC through its interaction with a variety of proteins (Figure 6A and 6B) (Zhang & Shay, 2017).

Almost all intestinal tumors exhibit a combination of both APC alleles at early stages of their development, which is in line with Knudson's two-hit hypothesis. According to Knudson's hypothesis, the two hits are independent mutation events, which are the cause of loss of tumour suppressor function. MYC and cyclin D1, the first two targets identified downstream of the APC/β-catenin pathway, are clearly involved in tumor proliferation, apoptosis, and cell cycle progression. The expression of MYC and cyclin D1 is likely to alter intestinal epithelial regeneration by increasing overall proliferation if expression patterns change. Several studies have shown that colorectal tumors contain an increased number of cycling cells. Matrilysin, CD44, Myc itself and urokinase-type plasminogen activator receptors are WNT target genes whose products play a major role in tumour promotion rather than initiation (Fodde et al., 2001).

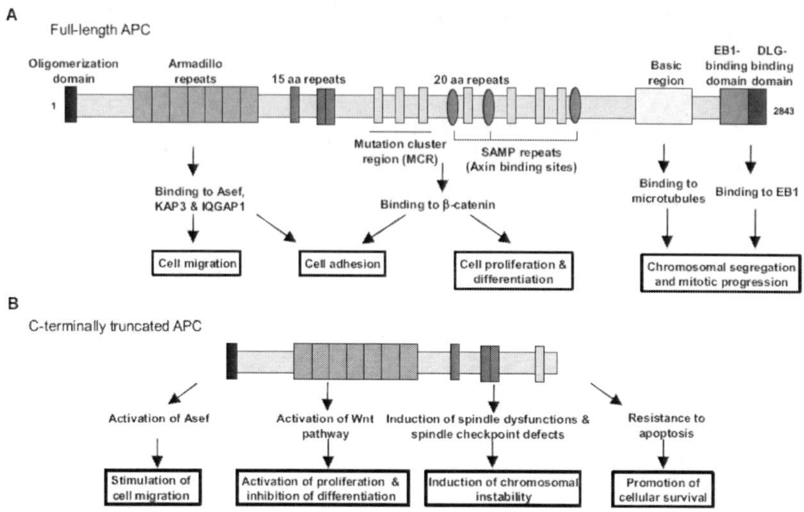

Figure 6. Structures and functions of full-size and truncated APC. A) Multiple APC domains bind to β-catenin, repeats bind to axin, and domains bind to EB1. Furthermore, APC participates in the processes of migration, proliferation, differentiation, adhesion, and chromosomal segregation in the cell. B) As a result, chromosomally unstable cells are caused by truncated proteins lacking domains required to interact with microtubules, EB1 and β-catenin, leading to instability of chromosome structure, stimulation of proliferation, and inhibition of differentiation. Cellular survival is promoted by truncated APC due to its dominant properties that promote cell migration and proliferation (Zhang & Shay, 2017).

Conclusion

Carcinogenesis refers to uncontrolled cell growth after activation of oncogenes and/or deactivation of antioncogenes (tumor suppressor genes). Based on studies, it has been determined that defective antioncogenes and hyperactive oncogenes are major contributors to cell proliferation and apoptosis during cancer development by means of somatic mutations and deletions.

The TP53 gene encodes the tumor suppressor p53 protein. Most sporadic cancers are caused by TP53 mutations, and TP53 responds to a number of cellular stresses. Normal cells contain a low level of p53 due to the mouse double minute 2 homolog (MDM2), which binds to p53. p53 and MDM2 are stabilized and activated by post-translational cellular stress. In most human cancers, mutations occur that abolish the function of the p53 tumor suppressor. It is hypothesized that molecular understanding of the action of p53 due to its potent tumor suppressor activity will provide treatments that limit tumorigenesis and can identify key molecular targets for therapeutic intervention (Lee & Muller, 2010). CDKN2A encodes two distinct proteins, separated by translating the common second exon into alternative reading frames. The $p16^{INK4a}$ protein encoded by this gene inhibits CDK4 and CDK6 from phosphorylating the retinoblastoma protein. In contrast, the CDKN2A β-transcript, p14ARF, triggers an apoptotic response manifested by a low level of p21CIP1 and MDM2, which stops cell division in both the G1 and G2/M phases (Stott et al., 1998).

The available evidence suggests that p14ARF exerts its tumor suppressor activity by controlling signaling pathways that have profound effects on gene expression and cell growth. Mdm2 inhibition triggers the accumulation of p53 through p14ARF, which triggers RB hypophosphorylation and cell cycle arrest through p53 transcription. p14ARF is a tumor suppressor gene involved in p53-dependent or independent cell growth control, and evidence suggests that this gene is modified by molecules involved in the RB signaling pathway, which may mediate its antiproliferative properties (Leduc et al., 2006). PTEN functions as a negative regulator of the PI3K/AKT pathway. Inactivation of PTEN mutations or loss of heterozygosity results in hyperactivation of AKT signaling and an increased risk of developing cancer. PTEN is among the most commonly mutated tumor suppressor genes in sporadic cancer (Manning & Toker, 2017). There is evidence that PTEN is regulated through a variety of mechanisms, including transcriptional regulation or post-translational regulation. The peroxisome proliferator activated receptor gamma (PPAR-γ), Early growth response protein 1 (EGR-1) and p53 at the transcriptional level regulate the expression of PTEN, while the ubiquitination and phosphorylation of PTEN at the post-translational level control it (Kavela et al., 2013).

The two-hit hypothesis applies in spontaneous cases of sporadic non-hereditary colorectal cancer, which occurs when adenomatous polyps occur and then tumors develop. The loss of both copies of the adenomatous polyposis coli (APC) gene in adenomas can lead to epithelial cells undergoing uncontrolled cell division. 80% of adenomas were found to have an APC gene mutation (Strate & Syngal, 2005).

The Wnt interface is controlled by the APC gene. Activation of the Wnt pathway increases cell proliferation. Wnt-binding proteins bind to Wnt receptors on cell surfaces. As a consequence, they activate proteins that block the APCaxinGSK (glycogen synthase kinase-3) complex. In this complex, a phosphorylation reaction occurs, leading to ubiquinization of the β-catenin protein and its degradation. Therefore, the Wnt interface becomes inactive with a decrease in β-catenin levels in the cell and active with a rise in levels. Transcription factors interact with β-catenin in the nucleus. Therefore, it correlates with active reading of many genes, resulting in cell proliferation. Mutation of both APC alleles leads to an inability to control the Wnt pathway, so cell division is caused to remain uncontrolled (Sachse et al., 2002).

Tumor suppressor genes and oncogenes often carry out their cellular functions together. Thus, a comprehensive elucidation of the relationships between tumor suppressor genes and oncogenes may help shed light on their roles in cancer development. In this chapter, the aim is to guide the pathogenesis of cancer by revealing the properties and mechanisms of other effective anti-oncogenes (p16INK4A, p14ARF, Rb, PTEN, APC) associated with cancer, especially the p53 gene.

In conclusion, the roles of oncogenes and antioncogenes in the proliferation and differentiation of cells cannot be overstated. Cancer cells often express these genes differently due to mutations, deletions, rearrangements, inactivation, and overexpression of specific genes. The development of tumors can cause some of these changes. Recovery of the normal function of these genes may be effective in the treatment of cancer.

References

Alagu, J., Itahana, Y., Sim, F., Chao, S. H., Bi, X., Itahana, K. (2018). Tumor suppressor p14ARF enhances IFN-γ-activated immune response by inhibiting PIAS1 via SUMOylation. *The Journal of Immunology.* 201(2), 451-464. https://doi.org/10.4049/jimmunol.1800327.

Blanco-Aparicio, C., Renner, O., Leal, J. F. M., Carnero, A. (2007). PTEN, more than the AKT pathway. *Carcinogenesis.* 28(7), 1379-86. https://doi.org/10.1093/carcin/bgm052 .

Chen, C. Y., Chen, J., He, L., Stiles, B. L. (2018). PTEN: Tumor suppressor and metabolic regulator. *Frontiers in Endocrinology.* 9,338. https://doi.org/10.3389/fendo.2018.00338.

Cornelisse, C. J., & Devilee, P. (1997). Facts in cancer genetics. *Patient Education and Counseling.* 32(1-2), 9-17. https://doi.org/10.1016/S0738-3991(97)00059-1.

Curylova, L., Ramos, H., Saraiva, L., & Skoda, J. (2022). Noncanonical roles of p53 in cancer stemness and their implications in sarcomas. *Cancer Letters.* 525,131-145.

Fodde, R., Smits, R., Clevers, H. (2001). APC, signal transduction and genetic instability in colorectal cancer. *Nature Reviews Cancer.* 1(1):55-67. https://doi.org/10.1038/35094067.

Gkountakos, A., Sartori, G., Falcone, I., Piro, G., Ciuffreda, L., Carbone, C., Tortora, G., Scarpa, A., Bria, E., Milella, M., Rosell, R., Corbo, V., Pilotto, S. (2019). PTEN in lung cancer: dealing with the problem, building on new knowledge and turning the game around. *Cancers.* 11(8),1141. https://doi.org/10.3390/cancers11081141.

Gupta, A., Shah, K., Oza, M. J., Behl, T. (2019). Reactivation of p53 gene by MDM2 inhibitors: A novel therapy for cancer treatment. *Biomedicine&Pharmacotherapy.* 109,484-492. https://doi.org/10.1016/j.biopha.2018.10.155.

Henley, S. A., & Dick, F. A. (2012). The retinoblastoma family of proteins and their regulatory functions in the mammalian cell division cycle. *Cell Division.* 7(1), 10. https://doi.org/10.1186/1747-1028-7-10.

Kavela, S., Shinde, S. R., Ratheesh, R., Viswakalyan, K., Bashyam, M. D., Gowrishankar, S., Vamsy, M., Pattnaik, S., Rao, S., Sastry, R.A., Srinivasulu, M., Chen, J., Maddika, S. (2013). PNUTS functions as a proto-oncogene by sequestering PTEN. *Cancer Res.* 73(1), 205–214. https://doi.org/10.1158/0008-5472.CAN-12-1394.

Kim, E., Giese, A., & Deppert, W. (2009). Wild-type p53 in cancer cells: When a guardian turns into a blackguard. *Biochemical Pharmacology,* 77(1), 11-20. https://doi.org/10.1016/j.bcp.2008.08.030.

Kohli, J., Campisi, J., & Demaria M. (2018). A novel suicide gene therapy for the treatment of p16Ink4a overexpressing tumors. *Oncotarget.* 9(7),7274-7281. https://doi.org/10.18632/oncotarget.23752.

Leduc, C., Claverie, P., Eymin, B., Col, E., Khochbin, S., Brambilla, E., Gazzeri, S. (2006). p14ARF promotes RB accumulation through inhibition of its Tip60-dependent acetylation. *Oncogene.* 25:4147 4154. https://doi.org/10.1038/sj.onc.1209446.

Lee, E. Y., & Muller, W. J. (2010). Oncogenes and tumor suppressor genes. *Cold Spring Harbor Perspectives in Biology.* 2(10): a003236. https://doi.org/10.1101/cshperspect.a003236.

Machado-Silva, A., Perrier, S., & Bourdon, J. C. (2010). p53 family members in cancer diagnosis and treatment. *Seminars in Cancer Biology.* 20(1),57-62.

Manning, B. D., & Toker, A. (2017). AKT/PKB signaling: navigating the network. *Cell.* 169(3):381-405. https://doi.org/10.1016/j.cell.2017.04.001.

Mizoguchi, M., Kuga, D., Guan, Y., Hata, N., Nakamizo, A., Yoshimoto, K., & Sasaki, T. (2011). Loss of heterozygosity analysis in malignant gliomas. *Brain Tumor Pathol.* 28(3),191-6. https://doi.org/10.1007/s10014-011-0038-0.

Sachse, C., Smith, G., Wilkie, M. J. V., Barrett, J. H., Waxman, R., Sullivan, F., Forman, D., Bishop, D. T., Wolf, C. R. (2002). A pharmacogenetic study to investigate the role of dietary carcinogens in the etiology of colorectal cancer. *Carcinogenesis.* 23(11): 1839-49.

Soussi, T., & Lozano, G. (2005). p53 mutation heterogeneity in cancer. *Biochemical and Biophysical Research Communications,* 331(3), 834-42. https://doi.org/10.1016/j.bbrc.2005.03.190.

Stott, F. J., Bates, S., James, M. C., McConnell, B. B., Starborg, M., Brookes, S., Palmero, I., Ryan, K., Hara, E., Vousden, K. H., Peters, G. (1998). The alternative product from the human CDKN2A locus, p14(ARF), participates in a regulatory feedback loop with p53 and MDM2. *The EMBO Journal.* 17(17), 5001-14. https://doi.org/10.1093/emboj/17.17.5001.

Strate, L. L., & Syngal, S. (2005). Hereditary colorectal cancer syndromes. *Cancer Causes & Control.* 16(3):201-13. https://doi.org/10.1007/s10552-004-3488-4.

Viatour, P., & Sage, J. (2011). Newly identified aspects of tumor suppression by RB. *Disease Models & Mechanisms.* 4, 581-585. https://doi.org/10.1242/dmm.008060.

Weber, H. O., Samuel, T., Rauch, P., Funk, J. O. (2002). Human p14ARF-mediated cell cycle arrest strictly depends on intact p53 signaling pathways. *Oncogene.* 21,3207-3212. https://doi.org/10.1038/sj/onc/1205429.

Williams, J. P., Stewart, T., Li, B., Mulloy, R., Dimova, D., Classon, M. (2006). The retinoblastoma protein is required for Ras-induced oncogenic transformation. *Molecular and Cellular Biology.* 26(4), 1170-82. https://doi.org/10.1128/MCB.26.4.1170-1182.2006.

Zerrouqi, A., Pyrzynska, B., Febbraio, M., Brat, D. J., Van Meir, E. G. (2012). P14ARF inhibits human glioblastoma-induced angiogenesis by upregulating the expression of TIMP3. *The Journal of Clinical Investigation.* 122(4), 1283-95. https://doi.org/10.1172/JCI38596.

Zhang, B., Pan, X., Cobb, G. P., & Anderson, T. A. (2007). microRNAs as oncogenes and tumor suppressors. *Developmental Biology.* 302(1), 1-12. https://doi.org/10.1016/j.ydbio.2006.08.028.

Zhang, L., & Shay, J. W. (2017). Multiple roles of APC and its therapeutic implications in colorectal cancer. *JNCI J Natl Cancer Inst.* 109(8), djw332. https://doi.org/10.1093/jnci/djw332.

Zhao, R., Choi, B. Y., Lee, M. H., Bode, A. M., Dong, Z. (2016). Implications of genetic and epigenetic alterations of CDKN2A (p16INK4a) in cancer. *EBioMedicine.* 8, 30–39. https://doi.org/10.1016/j.ebiom.2016.04.017.

Chapter 6

Effects of p53 on Autoimmunity

Asli Kireçtepe Aydin*, **PhD**
Department of Medical Biology,
Nişantaşı University, Istanbul, Turkey

Abstract

The p53 protein, the product of the tumor suppressor gene *TP53*, plays a central role in the suppression of tumorigenesis by regulation of cell cycle arrest, DNA damage repair, senescence, and apoptosis. It performs these functions by interacting with p21, cyclin G, Bcl-2-like protein 4 (Bax), growth arrest and DNA damage-inducible 45a (Gadd45a), and p53 upregulated modulator of apoptosis (PUMA). Recent studies indicated that p53 is also involved in immune responses, and p53 dysfunction causes the development of autoimmune disorders in humans and murine. p53 performs its function by suppressing the production of the pro-inflammatory cytokine, controlling the activation of T cells, and regulating the balance of Th17 and Treg cells, as well as inducing apoptosis. Although the transcription factor p53 is an essential protein for cancer suppression, it also plays a role in immune responses and the development of autoimmunity. Therefore, it is suggested that therapeutics targeted to p53 and the proteins involved in the p53 pathway could be useful for the treatment of autoimmune diseases.

Keywords: p53, autoimmune diseases, autoimmunity, cancer

---

* Corresponding Author's Email: akirectepe@gmail.com.

In: Autoimmunity and Cancer
Editors: Soner Şahin and Kenan Demir
ISBN: 978-1-68507-937-6

Introduction

TP53, a tumor suppressor gene, is located at 17p13.1 covering a region of approximately 19.15 kb and contains 11 exons. The p53 protein, the product of the *TP53* gene, was first identified in cells transformed with simian virus 40 (SV) as an oncogene (Lane & Crawford, 1979). In 1989, it was understood that the previously defined p53 protein was mutant and wild-type (wt) p53 has tumor suppressor function (Finlay et al., 1989). p53, which is a tumor suppressor protein and also a transcription factor, plays a role in cell cycle arrest, DNA damage repair, senescence, and apoptosis. Many *TP53* mutations are commonly seen in many types of cancer and are associated with poor prognoses (Kastenhuber & Lowe, 2017; Li et al., 2019).

The p53 protein consists of two transcription activation domains at the N-terminus, followed by a proline-rich domain, a DNA-binding domain at the central region, and nuclear localization signals, an oligomerization domain at the C-terminus. Each domain has its own function, and the mutation hotspot is generally located in the sequences of the gene that encodes the DNA binding domain (Kastenhuber & Lowe, 2017; Li et al., 2019). Under non-stressed conditions, p53 expression is present at very low levels, which is regulated by the E3 ubiquitin-protein ligase Mdm2. p53 is activated by cellular stresses that cause DNA damage or oncogene dysregulation, such as ultraviolet radiation, chemicals, oxidative stress, inflammation, and response through different pathways. p53 performs its functions, regulating the transcription of genes of interest, either by interacting with other proteins or directly with DNA (Pflaum et al., 2014). p21, cyclin G, Bcl-2-like protein 4 (Bax), growth arrest and DNA damage-inducible 45a (Gadd45a), and p53 upregulated modulator of apoptosis (PUMA) are the well-known proteins associated with p53. They play a role in cell cycle arrest, DNA repair, apoptosis, and all of them function together to suppress tumorigenesis (Harms & Chen, 2006; Lowe et al., 2017). Furthermore, p53 can activate genes involved in antiviral immunity, such as IFN regulatory factor 5 (IRF5), IRF9, protein kinase RNA-activated (PKR), Toll-like receptor 3 (TLR3), and ISG15. Although transcription factor p53 is an essential protein for cancer suppression by regulating cell cycle arrest, DNA repair, senescence, and apoptosis by activating cellular stress, it also plays a role in immune responses and the development of autoimmunity (Muñoz-Fontela et al., 2016).

p53 in Autoimmunity

Autoimmune diseases, which are clinically heterogeneous chronic disorders, are the result of an abnormal immune response against the cells and tissues of their own body. It is characterized by self-reactive T and B cells and the production of antibodies targeting self-antigens. 3-5% of the population are reported to suffer from more than 80 different autoimmune diseases and women are more affected than men (Wang et al., 2015). The etiology of many autoimmune diseases is not clear yet; however, many studies emphasize the combination of the roles of genetic and environmental factors in the pathogeneses of the diseases. Previous studies revealed that the tumor suppressor p53 is associated with autoimmune diseases by affecting the expression of immune response genes, cytokine production, and the expression of MHC and co-inhibitory molecules (Eggenhuizen et al., 2020).

Repression of interleukin 6 (IL-6) by wt p53 and dysregulation of IL-6 expression level by p53 mutations in neoplastic cells were shown by two studies in the 1990s (Santhanam et al., 1991; Margulies & Sehgal, 1993). These studies can be considered as the first evidence that p53 plays a role in autoimmunity, because IL-6 is involved in the pathogenesis of autoimmune disorders such as rheumatoid arthritis (RA), systemic lupus erythematosus (SLE), and diabetes mellitus. Subsequently, many studies focused on investigating the effect of p53 on RA, associated with increased IL-6 levels. Firestein et al., (1997) detected a *TP53* mutation in synovial cells of RA patients and showed the effects of suppression of p53 in cell culture studies based on DNA breaks and apoptotic morphology seen in synovial tissues of RA patients in previous studies. On the other hand, the mutation in p53 has not been detected in skin samples from the same patients and osteoarthritis synovial samples (Firestein et al., 1997). It was shown that synovial cells with *TP53* mutations were clustered specific regions of synovial tissues and increased IL-6 expression levels were observed in these regions. Furthermore, it was suggested that *TP53*-mutated cells can activate neighboring cells by increasing pro-inflammatory cytokines (Yamanishi et al., 2002a). Several variations of *TP53*, such as P151, R213, N239, G245, R248, R280, and R282, have been identified in RA and are generally located in the DNA-binding domain, which is also a mutation hot spot for cancer cases. These mutations can cause loss of transcriptional function, gain of function, and dominant negative effects (Han et al., 2001; Sun & Cheung, 2002; Zhang et al., 2020). The common variation P72R, which causes conformational changes in p53 and thus affects protein function, such as binding to specific transcriptional genes, apoptosis, and DNA repair, was not found to be associated with RA (Lee et al., 2001; Macchioni et al., 2007; Moodley et al., 2010; Lee et al., 2012). Furthermore, several studies have investigated the association between P72R variation and SLE in different populations (Lee et al., 2005; Sanchez et al., 2006; Piotrowski et al., 2008; Onel et al., 2009). A meta-analysis of six studies emphasizes that the association between P72R and SLE may differ by ethnicity and the variation of P72R could increase the susceptibility to SLE in Asia but not in Europe (Lee et al., 2012). The ratio of homozygote arginine at codon 72 in the p53 gene in Hashimoto's thyroiditis was found to be higher than healthy controls, so it is suggested that this variation could be a biomarker of the disease (Chen et al., 2008).

An increase in the level of expression of the p53 protein has been reported in synovial tissues of RA patients, and this can be explained by the production of mutant p53 or the production of wt p53 resulting from DNA damage (Firestein et al., 1997; Tak et al., 1999; Tak et al., 2000; Salvador et al., 2005; Takatori et al., 2014). Additionally, the level of p53 protein was found to be higher in pediatric patients with RA and SLE compared to healthy controls (El-Sayed et al., 2003). A higher level of p53 has been reported in SLE patients with active phase than in SLE patients with inactive phase and healthy controls (El-Sayed et al., 2003; Miret et al., 2003). As the known regulatory role of p53 in inflammation, it is suggested that increasing p53 expression or function can be affected in many autoimmune or autoinflammatory disorders (Yamanishi et al., 2002b, Takatori et al., 2014). Despite the increased level of p53 expression in synovial tissues of RA, a lower level of p53 was reported in peripheral mononuclear cell (PBMC) samples obtained from patients with RA compared to healthy controls (Maas et al., 2005; Park et al., 2013). Mass et al., showed that cell death in gamma radiation-exposed RA PBMCs was lower compared to healthy PBMC, which could be caused by the dysregulation of the p53-regulated apoptosis mechanism (Maas et al., 2005). Increased expression levels of p53 have also been reported in different autoimmune diseases such as Sjögren's syndrome and Hashimoto's thyroiditis (Tapinos et al., 2001; Mariette et al., 2002; Okayasu et al., 1998).

Autoantibodies against antigen and DNA are a common feature of many autoimmune diseases. The relationship between autoimmune diseases and anti-p53 antibodies, which are found in many types of cancer, was first indicated by Kovacs et al., (Kovacs et al., 1997). Thereafter, many studies showed increased anti-p53 antibodies in different autoimmune diseases, such as SLE, autoimmune thyroid disease, systemic sclerosis, autoimmune hepatitis, dermatomyositis/polymyositis and rarely in RA and Sjögren's syndrome (Kuhn et al., 1999; Herkel et al., 2001; Chauhan et al., 2004; Fenton et al., 2000; Hara et al., 2008; Mimura et al., 2007; Herkel et al., 2002; Mariette et al., 1999). p53 autoantibodies were also shown in pediatric patients with SLE and juvenile rheumatoid arthritis (JRA) (El-Sayed et al., 2003). Contrary to these results, an absence of anti-p53 antibodies was reported in Chinese patients with RA and SLE, and it was suggested that this was caused by ethnic differences (Shiau et al., 2002; Chauhan et al., 2004). p53 autoantibodies of sera obtained from patients with autoimmune diseases react to p53 carboxy-terminal in contrast to sera from cancer patients and mostly against to the DNA-binding domain of p53 which recognizes damaged DNA. Therefore, p53 autoantibodies could mimic damaged DNA and could cause apoptosis defects in SLE by blocking the activity of p53 (Herkel et al., 2001; Herkel et al., 2004; Herkel & Cohen, 2007).

There are several studies that showed the relationship between p53 and the development of autoimmune and inflammatory disorders in animal models. Collagen-induced arthritis (CIA) or antigen-induced arthritis (AIA) were developed in $p53^{-/-}$ mice with increased severity of arthritis (Yamanishi et al., 2002b; Simelyte et al., 2005; Leech et al., 2008). Additionally, mice with p53 deficiency have more risk to develop experimental autoimmune encephalomyelitis and streptozotocin (STZ)-induced diabetes compared to mice with wt p53 (Okuda et al., 2003; Zheng et al., 2005). Yamanishi et al., showed a decreased apoptosis rate and significantly increased expression levels of pro-inflammatory cytokines IL-6 and IL-1β in mice with CIA mouse model with $p53^{-/-}$ (Yamanishi et al., 2002b). Similarly, Leech et al., have reported a decreased apoptosis rate in the synovium and an increased T cell proliferation and release of interferon γ (IFN-γ) in AIA mouse model with $p53^{-/-}$ (Leech et al., 2008). Expression levels of IL-1β, IL-6, and IL-12 were higher in macrophages from STZ-induced diabetes mice with $p53^{-/-}$. Macrophages with $p53^{-/-}$ also showed higher immunity to lipopolysaccharide (LPS) and IFN-γ compared to $p53^{+/+}$ mice. In addition, the finding of increased levels of proinflammatory cytokines and signal transducer and activator of transcription-1 (STAT-1) in $p53^{-/-}$ STZ-induced diabetes mice suggests that p53 can prevent autoimmune disorders by inhibiting the expression of STAT-1, which plays a role in cytokine production (Zheng et al., 2005).

Activation of T cells and regulation of Th17 and Treg cell balance is controlled by p53 through interaction with STAT in CD4+ T cells isolated from $p53^{-/-}$ mice. Differentiation of Th17 cells, which are the effector cells in autoimmunity, is repressed by binding of p53 to STAT-3. On the other hand, differentiation of regulatory T cells (Tregs), which play a role in autoimmunity by suppression of the proliferation of T cells, was stimulated by binding of p53 to STAT-5 (Kawashima et al., 2013; Park et al., 2013). Additionally, it was shown that p53 regulates the differentiation of Tregs by activating Foxp3 transcription (Jung et al., 2010). Many studies have shown that dysfunction of p53-related proteins can cause immune system disorders as well as dysfunctions of p53. Deficiency of p21 and Gadd45a, which are the well-known p53 target proteins, were found to be related with lupus-like syndromes in $p21^{-/-}$ and $Gadd45^{-/-}$ mice, due to lack of repression of T cell activation (Santiago-Raber et al., 2001; Salvador et al., 2002).

Conclusion

Previous studies in humans and murine have shown that p53, which is a well-known tumor suppressor, plays an important role in the pathogenesis of autoimmune disorders and tumorigeneses. Although the mechanism of p53 in immune responses and autoimmune diseases is not yet clear, p53 dysfunction was shown to cause the development of autoimmune diseases by affecting the production of the pro-inflammatory cytokine, controlling activating T cells, and regulating Th17 and Treg cell balance. In addition to the direct role of p53 in autoimmunity, p53-related proteins are also involved in the pathogenesis of autoimmune diseases. As a result of several studies on p53 in autoimmunity, it is suggested that the use of p53 targeted therapeutics might be effective for the treatment of autoimmune diseases.

References

Chauhan, R., Handa, R., Das, T. P., & Pati, U. (2004). Over-expression of TATA binding protein (TBP) and p53 and autoantibodies to these antigens are features of systemic sclerosis, systemic lupus erythematosus and overlap syndromes. *Clin Exp Immunol*, 136(3): 574-84. https://doi.org/10.1111/j.1365-2249.2004.02463.x.

Chen, R. H., Chang, C. T., Wang, T. Y., Huang, W. L., Tsai, C. H., & Tsai, F. J. (2008). p53 codon 72 proline/arginine polymorphism and autoimmune thyroid diseases. *J Clin Lab Anal*, 22(5): 321-6. https://doi.org/10.1002/jcla.20249.

El-Sayed, Z. A., Farag, D. H., & Eissa, S. (2003). Tumor suppressor protein p53 and anti-p53 autoantibodies in pediatric rheumatological diseases. *Pediatr Allergy Immunol*, 14(3): 229-33. https://doi.org/10.1034/j.1399-3038.2003.00033.x.

Eggenhuizen, P. J., Ng, B. H., & Ooi, J. D. (2020). Treg enhancing therapies to treat autoimmune diseases. *International Journal of Molecular Sciences*, 21(19): 7015. https://doi.org/10.3390/ijms21197015.

Fenton, C. L., Patel, A., Tuttle, R. M., & Francis, G. L. (2000). Autoantibodies to p53 in sera of patients with autoimmune thyroid disease. *Ann Clin Lab Sci*, 30(2): 179-83.

Finlay, C. A., Hinds, P. W., & Levine, A. J. (1989). The p53 proto-oncogene can act as a suppressor of transformation. *Cell*, 57(7): 1083-93. https://doi.org/10.1016/0092-8674(89)90045-7.

Firestein, G. S., Echeverri, F., Yeo, M., Zvaifler, N. J., & Green, D. R. (1997). Somatic mutations in the p53 tumor suppressor gene in rheumatoid arthritis synovium. *Proc Natl Acad Sci USA*, 94(20): 10895-900. https://doi.org/10.1073/pnas.94.20.10895.

Han, Z., Boyle, D. L., Shi, Y., Green, D. R., & Firestein, G. S. (1999). Dominant-negative p53 mutations in rheumatoid arthritis. *Arthritis Rheum,* 42(6):1088-92. https://doi.org/10.1002/1529-0131(199906)42:6<1088::AID-ANR4>3.0.CO;2-E.

Hara, T., Ogawa, F., Muroi, E., Komura, K., Takenaka, M., Hasegawa, M., Fujimoto, M., & Sato, S. (2008). Anti-p53 autoantibody in systemic sclerosis: association with limited cutaneous systemic sclerosis. *J Rheumatol*, 35(3): 451-7.

Harms, K. L., & Chen, X. (2006). The functional domains in p53 family proteins exhibit both common and distinct properties. *Cell Death Differ*, 13(6): 890-7. https://doi.org/10.1038/sj.cdd.4401904.

Herkel, J., Mimran, A., Erez, N., Kam, N., Lohse, A. W., Märker-Hermann, E., Rotter, V., & Cohen, I. R. (2001). Autoimmunity to the p53 protein is a feature of systemic lupus erythematosus (SLE) related to anti-DNA antibodies. *J Autoimmun*, 17(1): 63-9. https://doi.org/10.1006/jaut.2001.0518.

Herkel, J., Modrow, J. P., Bamberger, S., Kanzler, S., Rotter, V., Cohen, I. R., & Lohse, A. W. (2002). Prevalence of autoantibodies to the p53 protein in autoimmune hepatitis. *Autoimmunity*. 35(8): 493-6. https://doi.org/10.1080/0891693021000054075.

Herkel, J., & Cohen I. R. (2007). p53 Autoantibodies. In Y. Shoenfeld, M. E. Gershwin, P. L. Meroni (Eds.), *Autoantibodies (*2nd Ed.). (pp. 271-276). Elsevier. https://doi.org/10.1016/B978-044452763-9/50040-8.

Herkel, J., Kam, N., Erez, N., Mimran, A., Heifetz, A., Eisenstein, M., Rotter, V., & Cohen, I. R. (2004). Monoclonal antibody to a DNA-binding domain of p53 mimics charge structure of DNA: anti-idiotypes to the anti-p53 antibody are anti-DNA. *Eur J Immunol*, 34(12): 3623-32. https://doi.org/10.1002/eji.200425371.

Jung, D. J., Jin, D. H., Hong, S. W., Kim, J. E., Shin, J. S., Kim, D., Cho, B. J., Hwang, Y. I., Kang, J. S., & Lee, W. J. (2010). Foxp3 expression in p53-dependent DNA damage responses. *The Journal of Biological Chemistry*, 285(11): 7995-8002. https://doi.org/10.1074/jbc.M109.047985.

Kastenhuber, E. R., & Lowe, S. W. (2017). Putting p53 in context. *Cell*, 170(6): 1062-1078. https://doi.org/10.1016/j.cell.2017.08.028.

Kawashima, H., Takatori, H., Suzuki, K., Iwata, A., Yokota, M., Suto, A., Minamino, T., Hirose, K., & Nakajima, H. (2013). Tumor suppressor p53 inhibits systemic autoimmune diseases by inducing regulatory T cells. *J Immunol*, 191(7): 3614-23. https://doi.org/10.4049/jimmunol.1300509.

Kovacs, B., Patel, A., Hershey, J. N., Dennis, G. J., Kirschfink, M., & Tsokos, G. C. (1997). Antibodies against p53 in sera from patients with systemic lupus erythematosus and other rheumatic diseases. *Arthritis Rheum.* 40(5): 980-2. https://doi.org/10.1002/art.1780400531.

Kuhn, H. M., Kromminga, A., Flammann, H. T., Frey, M., Layer, P., & Arndt, R. (1999). p53 autoantibodies in patients with autoimmune diseases: a quantitative approach. *Autoimmunity*, 31(4): 229-35. https://doi.org/10.3109/08916939908994068.

Lane, D. P., & Crawford, L. V. (1979). T antigen is bound to a host protein in SV40-transformed cells. *Nature*, 278(5701): 261-3. https://doi.org/10.1038/278261a0.

Lee, Y. H., Bae, S. C., Choi, S. J., Ji, J. D., & Song, G. G. (2012). Associations between the p53 codon 72 polymorphisms and susceptibility to systemic lupus erythematosus and rheumatoid arthritis: a meta-analysis. *Lupus*, 21(4): 430-7. https://doi.org/10.1177/0961203311434941. PMID: 22427364.

Lee, Y. H., Kim, Y. R., Ji, J. D., Sohn, J., & Song, G. G. (2001). p53 codon 72 polymorphism and rheumatoid arthritis. *J Rheumatol*, 28(11): 2392-4.

Lee, Y. H., Rho, Y. H., Choi, S. J., Ji, J. D., & Song, G. G. (2005). The functional p53 codon 72 polymorphism is associated with systemic lupus erythematosus. *Lupus*, 14(10): 842-5. https://doi.org/10.1191/0961203305lu2224oa.

Leech, M., Xue, J. R., Dacumos, A., Hall, P., Santos, L., Yang, Y., Li, M., Kitching, A. R., & Morand, E. F. (2008). The tumour suppressor gene p53 modulates the severity of antigen-induced arthritis and the systemic immune response. *Clin Exp Immunol*, 152(2): 345-53. https://doi.org/10.1111/j.1365-2249.2008.03629.x.

Li, V. D., Li, K. H., & Li, J. T. (2019). *TP53* mutations as potential prognostic markers for specific cancers: analysis of data from the Cancer Genome Atlas and the International Agency for Research on Cancer *TP53* Database. *J Cancer Res Clin Oncol*, 145(3): 625-636. https://doi.org/10.1007/s00432-018-2817-z.

Lowe, J. M., Nguyen, T. A., Grimm, S. A., Gabor, K. A., Peddada, S. D., Li, L., Anderson, C. W., Resnick, M. A., Menendez, D., & Fessler, M. B. (2017). The novel p53 target TNFAIP8 variant 2 is increased in cancer and offsets p53-dependent tumor suppression. *Cell Death Differ*, 24(1): 181-191. https://doi.org/10.1038/cdd.2016.130.

Maas, K., Westfall, M., Pietenpol, J., Olsen, N. J., & Aune, T. (2005). Reduced p53 in peripheral blood mononuclear cells from patients with rheumatoid arthritis is associated with loss of radiation-induced apoptosis. *Arthritis Rheum*, 52(4): 1047-57. https://doi.org/10.1002/art.20931.

Macchioni, P., Nicoli, D., Casali, B., Catanoso, M., Farnetti, E., Boiardi, L., & Salvarani, C. (2007). The codon 72 polymorphic variants of p53 in Italian rheumatoid arthritis patients. *Clin Exp Rheumatol*, 25(3): 416-21.

Margulies, L., & Sehgal, P. B. (1993). Modulation of the human interleukin-6 promoter (IL-6) and transcription factor C/EBP beta (NF-IL6) activity by p53 species. *J Biol Chem*, 268(20): 15096-100.

Mariette, X., Sibilia, J., Delaforge, C., Bengoufa, D., Brouet, J. C., & Soussi, T. (1999). Anti-p53 antibodies are rarely detected in serum of patients with rheumatoid arthritis and Sjögren's syndrome. *J Rheumatol*. 26(8): 1672-5.

Mimura, Y., Yazawa, N., Tamaki, Z., Ashida, R., Jinnin, M., Asano, Y., Tada, Y., Kubo, M., Ihn, H., & Tamaki, K. (2007). Anti-p53 antibodies in patients with dermatomyositis/polymyositis. *Clin Rheumatol*, 26(8): 1328-31. https://doi.org/10.1007/s10067-006-0473-1.

Miret, C., Molina, R., & Filella, X., García-Carrasco, M., Claver, G., Ingelmo, M., Ballesta, A., Font, J. (2003). Relationship of p53 with other oncogenes, cytokines and systemic lupus erythematosus activity. *Tumour Biol*, 24(4): 185-8. https://doi.org/10.1159/000074428. PMID: 14654712.

Moodley, D., Mody, G. M., & Chuturgoon, A. A. (2010). Functional analysis of the p53 codon 72 polymorphism in black South Africans with rheumatoid arthritis - a pilot study. *Clin Rheumatol*, 29(10): 1099-105. https://doi.org/10.1007/s10067-010-1505-4.

Muñoz-Fontela, C., Mandinova, A., Aaronson, S. A., & Lee, S. W. (2016). Emerging roles of p53 and other tumour-suppressor genes in immune regulation. *Nature Reviews. Immunology*, 16(12): 741-750. https://doi.org/10.1038/nri.2016.99.

Okuda, Y., Okuda, M., & Bernard, C. C. (2003). Regulatory role of p53 in experimental autoimmune encephalomyelitis. *J Neuroimmunol*, 135(1-2): 29-37. https://doi.org/10.1016/s0165-5728(02)00428-9.

Onel, K. B., Huo, D., Hastings, D., Fryer-Biggs, J., Crow, M. K., & Onel, K. (2009). Lack of association of the *TP53* Arg72Pro SNP and the MDM2 SNP309 with systemic lupus erythematosus in Caucasian, African American, and Asian children and adults. *Lupus*, 18(1): 61-6. https://doi.org/10.1177/0961203308094558.

Park, J. S., Lim, M. A., Cho, M. L., Ryu, J. G., Moon, Y. M., Jhun, J. Y., Byun, J. K., Kim, E. K., Hwang, S. Y., Ju, J. H., Kwok, S. K., & Kim, H. Y. (2013). p53 controls autoimmune arthritis via STAT-mediated regulation of the Th17 cell/Treg cell balance in mice. *Arthritis Rheum*. 65(4): 949-59. https://doi.org/10.1002/art.37841.

Pflaum, J., Schlosser, S., & Müller, M. (2014). p53 Family and cellular stress responses in cancer. *Frontiers in Oncology*, 4: 285. https://doi.org/10.3389/fonc.2014.00285.

Piotrowski, P., Lianeri, M., Mostowska, M., Wudarski, M., Chwalinska-Sadowska, H., & Jagodzinski, P. P. (2008). Contribution of polymorphism in codon 72 of p53 gene to systemic lupus erythematosus in Poland. *Lupus*, 17(2): 148-51. https://doi.org/10.1177/0961203307084722.

Salvador, G., Sanmarti, R., Garcia-Peiró, A., Rodríguez-Cros, J. R., Muñoz-Gómez, J., & Cañete, J. D. (2005). p53 expression in rheumatoid and psoriatic arthritis synovial tissue and association with joint damage. *Ann Rheum Dis*, 64(2): 183-7. https://doi.org/10.1136/ard.2004.024430.

Sánchez, E., Sabio, J. M., Callejas, J. L., de Ramón, E., de Haro, M., Jiménez-Alonso, J., Ortego-Centeno, N., Sánchez-Román, J., González-Gay, M. A., López-Nevot, M. A., González-Escribano, M. F., & Martín, J. (2006). Study of a functional polymorphism in the p53 gene in systemic lupus erythematosus: lack of replication in a Spanish population. *Lupus*, 15(10): 658-61. https://doi.org/10.1177/0961203306070986.

Santhanam, U., Ray, A., & Sehgal, P. B. (1991). Repression of the interleukin 6 gene promoter by p53 and the retinoblastoma susceptibility gene product. *Proc Natl Acad Sci USA*, 88(17), 7605-9. https://doi.org/10.1073/pnas.88.17.7605.

Shiau, M. Y., Kuo, T. M., Tsay, G. J., Chiou, H. L., Lee, Y. L., & Chang, Y. H. (2002). Absence of anti-p53 antibodies in Chinese patients with rheumatoid arthritis and systemic lupus erythematosus: comment on the concise communication by Kovacs et al., *Arthritis Rheum.* 46(1): 276-7. https://doi.org/10.1002/1529-0131(200201)46:1<276::aid-art10032>3.0.co;2-i.

Simelyte, E., Rosengren, S., Boyle, D. L., Corr, M., Green, D. R., & Firestein, G. S. (2005). Regulation of arthritis by p53: critical role of adaptive immunity. *Arthritis Rheum*, 52(6): 1876-84. https://doi.org/10.1002/art.21099.

Sun, Y., & Cheung, H. S. (2002). p53, proto-oncogene and rheumatoid arthritis. *Semin Arthritis Rheum*, 31(5): 299-310. https://doi.org/10.1053/sarh.2002.31550.

Tak, P. P., Smeets, T. J., Boyle, D. L., Kraan, M. C., Shi, Y., Zhuang, S., Zvaifler, N. J., Breedveld, F. C., & Firestein, G. S. (1999). p53 overexpression in synovial tissue from patients with early and longstanding rheumatoid arthritis compared with patients with reactive arthritis and osteoarthritis. *Arthritis Rheum*, 42(5): 948-53. https://doi.org/10.1002/1529-0131(199905)42:5<948::AID-ANR13>3.0.CO;2-L.

Tak, P. P., Zvaifler, N. J., Green, D. R., & Firestein, G. S. (2000). Rheumatoid arthritis and p53: how oxidative stress might alter the course of inflammatory diseases. *Immunol Today*, 21(2): 78-82. https://doi.org/10.1016/s0167-5699(99)01552-2.

Takatori, H., Kawashima, H., Suzuki, K., & Nakajima, H. (2014). Role of p53 in systemic autoimmune diseases. *Crit Rev Immunol*, 34(6): 509-16. https://doi.org/10.1615/critrevimmunol.2014012193.

Wang, L., Wang, F. S., & Gershwin, M. E. (2015). Human autoimmune diseases: a comprehensive update. *Journal of Internal Medicine*, 278(4): 369-395. https://doi.org/10.1111/joim.12395.

Yamanishi, Y., Boyle, D. L., Pinkoski, M. J., Mahboubi, A., Lin, T., Han, Z., Zvaifler, N. J., Green, D. R., & Firestein, G. S. (2002b). Regulation of joint destruction and inflammation by p53 in collagen-induced arthritis. *Am J Pathol*, 160(1): 123-30. https://doi.org/10.1016/S0002-9440(10)64356-8.

Yamanishi, Y., Boyle, D. L., Rosengren, S., Green, D. R., Zvaifler, N. J., & Firestein, G. S. (2002a). Regional analysis of p53 mutations in rheumatoid arthritis synovium. *Proc Natl Acad Sci USA*, 99(15): 10025-30. https://doi.org/10.1073/pnas.152333199.

Zhang, K. X., Ip, C. K., Chung, S. K., Lei, K. K., Zhang, Y. Q., Liu, L., & Wong, V. K. W. (2020). Drug-resistance in rheumatoid arthritis: the role of p53 gene mutations, ABC family transporters and personal factors. *Curr Opin Pharmacol*, 54: 59-71. https://doi.org/10.1016/j.coph.2020.08.002.

Zheng, S. J., Lamhamedi-Cherradi, S. E., Wang, P., Xu, L., & Chen, Y. H. (2005). Tumor suppressor p53 inhibits autoimmune inflammation and macrophage function. *Diabetes*, 54(5): 1423-8. https://doi.org/10.2337/diabetes.54.5.1423.

Chapter 7

Effects of Ras and Other Proto-Oncogenes on Cancer

Özlem Aldemir*, MD

Department of Infectious Diseases
and Clinical Microbiology,
Sivas Numune Hospital, Sivas, Turkey

Abstract

Cancer, one of the leading causes of death worldwide and causes more than 10 million deaths annually, represents the pathological condition due to changes in critical regulatory genes that control cell growth and survival (Zaimy et al., 2017). Genetic studies on viral oncogenes have obtained data on the development of normal cells and cancer-causing genes. The presence of different genes (called oncogenes) in their genome is responsible for the carcinogenic effect of retroviruses that cause cancer. Molecular genetic studies have shown that normal eukaryotic cells are similar to retroviral oncogenes. These normal cellular genes, which have essential roles in growth regulation, differentiation, and proliferation, are called proto-oncogenes. With mutation of proto-oncogenes, its effect on neoplastic transformation occurs. Proto-oncogenes are activated by various genetic mechanisms and turn into oncogenes. These mechanisms are transduction, insertional mutagenesis, amplification, point mutation, and chromosomal translocation. The genetic alteration brought about by these mechanisms results in a proto-oncogene that is detached from its traditional regulatory agencies. This deregulation of function causes marked proliferation of cells (Torry & Cooper, 1991).

* Corresponding Author's Email: ozlem_gulgec@hotmail.com.

In: Autoimmunity and Cancer
Editors: Soner Şahin and Kenan Demir
ISBN: 978-1-68507-937-6

Keywords: protooncogene, ras, cancer

Introduction

Proto-oncogenes are involved in the regulation of growth, proliferation, differentiation, and apoptosis. Proto-oncogenes control the synthesis of the oncoprotein and encode proteins associated with mitosis regulation. These proteins include growth factors, growth factor receptors, proteins that transmit exogenous signals across the plasma membrane, and nuclear transcription factors. When proto-oncogenes (Erb- B1, Erb-B2, Ras, cis, hst-1, ret, abl, Myc, cyclin D, CDK4, etc.) are mutated, the overproduction of growth factors, uncontrolled stimulation of the pathways between the cell membrane and the nucleus, increased synthesis of transcription factors, results such as the inability to prevent cell division. The products of proto-oncogenes can be found in the plasma membrane, cytoplasm, or nucleus. The nucleic acid sequences of cellular proto-oncogenes and viral oncogenes, and thus the products' proteins, are similar. Viral oncogenes are denoted by v- (v-Fos, v-Myc), and cellular proto-oncogenes are characterized by c- (c-Fos, c-Myc) (Yokus & Ülker, 2012).

Activation Mechanisms of Protooncogenes

Insertion, chromosomal translocation, amplification, point mutation, and transduction are genetic mechanisms that cause activation of proto-oncogenes. Oncogenes formed by mutations or aberrant proto-oncogenes can induce neoplastic transformation (Lynch, 1987; Torry & Cooper, 1991).

1 - *Insertion*: A change occurs in the number and order of nucleotides in the genome when a new pair is introduced between nucleotide pairs in the cell genome. Such a mutation results in a difference in the protein synthesized by the proto-oncogene (Altınbas, 2020).

2 - *Chromosomal translocation* is defined as chromosomal rearrangement involving the exchange of parts between two non-homologous chromosomes (Rowley, 1973). Translocations generally result in two ways. First, the coding region of one gene localizes to the transcriptionally active promoter/enhancer region of another gene under the influence of the promoter, which can lead to overexpression of the transplaced gene. Second, translocations may also form

a fusion or chimeric gene (Nambiar et al., 2008). It is known that chromosomal translocations are more common in hematopoietic and lymphoid tumors among cancers (Mitelman et al., 2007).

Burkitt's lymphoma, a B-cell neoplasm, is the first example of oncogene activation by chromosome translocation. With translocation of t(8;14) in Burkitt's lymphoma, the c-Myc gene located on chromosome 8 is localized to the IgH locus on chromosome 14 so that the c-Myc gene is overstimulated under the influence of the IgH promoter, leading to overexpression of the c-Myc gene (Hecht & Aster, 2000).

One of the cancers recently shown to contain specific chromosomal translocations is prostate cancer, one of the most common epithelial carcinomas. In this carcinoma, translocation of the TMPRSS2 gene with the ETS gene family on chromosome 21 is the most common. The ETS genes encode nuclear transcription factors that regulate cellular growth and differentiation, and the ETS genes are involved in various malignancies. The TMPRSS2 gene is specific for the prostate gland and is androgen sensitive. Therefore, due to translocation, up-regulation of ETS genes by regulatory factors on this gene occurs in response to androgen (Nambiar et al., 2008).

Chronic myelocytic leukemia (CML) was the first neoplasm in which fusion gene formation with chromosomal translocation was described. In this translocation, the c-ABL proto-oncogene on chromosome 9 is transferred to the BCR gene region on chromosome 22. The chromosome 22 variant is known as the Philadelphia chromosome (Ph). Just as Ph disrupts normal signaling pathways in leukemia cells, it also disrupts genome stability. The resulting BCR-ABL gene is overexpressed, leading to increased oncogenic protein synthesis, exhibiting abnormal tyrosine kinase (TK) activity associated with carcinogenesis of CML and acute lymphoblastic leukemia (ALL). Kinase activity provides resistance to cell apoptosis, maintaining proliferation and blocking differentiation (Kang et al., 2016; Zheng, 2013).

Ewing sarcoma is the second most common bone tumor in childhood and adolescence (Grünewald et al., 2018). This small round cell tumor originating from mesenchymal stem cells originating from the primordial bone marrow is characterized by fusion transcription, usually involving the EWS-FLI-1 or EWS-ERG genes (Eaton et al., 2021). FLI-1 and ERG belong to the ETS family of transcription factors, with sequence-specific DNA binding domains. 85% of Ewing sarcoma cases are associated with translocation of t (11;22), 10-15% with t(21;12) translocation. The t(11;22) translocation leads to the formation of the EWS-FLI-1 fusion gene and the chimeric protein expression. In addition, the t(21;12) translocation produces the EWS-ERG fusion protein

(May, Gishizky, et al., 1993; Sorensen et al., 1994; Turc-Carel et al., 1983). Thus, chimeric proteins act as abnormal transcription factors involved in malignant transformation (May, Lessnick, et al., 1993).

3 - *Gene Amplification:* One of the critical events programmed for the development of eukaryotic organisms is gene amplification. In the process of oncogenesis, a segment of DNA is replicated, and sometimes hundreds of new copies of a proto-oncogene contained in that segment are added to the genome. Proto-oncogenes such as Myc, cyclin D1, epidermal growth factor receptor (EGFR), and RAS are amplified in small cell lung cancer, breast, esophagus, cervix, and ovarian cancer. The ERBB2 gene (also known as HER2/neu), an epidermal growth factor receptor, is amplified and evaluated as a poor prognostic indicator.

4 - *Point Mutation:* These are mutations that occur on one or more nucleotides. They appear to be the result of base pair substitutions in DNA or the insertion or removal. These mutated genes cause the synthesis of oncoproteins whose activity and functions are different. For example, point mutations that activate the BRAF gene occur in melanoma, colorectal cancer, hepatocellular carcinoma, and glioma (Croce, 2008).

5 - *Transduction Activation*: When a retrovirus infects a cell, a segment of the cellular DNA sequences enters the viral genome by recombination. The cellular sequence that becomes part of the viral genome replicates with the virus and thus spreads to other cells. Activation in this way is thought to be an effective way in the stimulation of proto-oncogenes and tumor formation.

Effect of Ras and Other Proto-Oncogenes on Cancer

Ras proteins are small GTPases that regulate signaling networks that control cell proliferation and survival. Three members of the Ras gene group that encode a 21 Kd protein have been identified and most extensively studied: the classic Ras proteins Harvey Ras viral oncogene homolog (H-Ras), Kirsten Ras viral oncogene homolog (K-Ras), and neuroblastoma Ras (N-Ras). Mutation in the Ras gene has been detected in more than 30% of all cancers. In addition, it is observed in 90% of lung, colon, and pancreatic cancer (Zinatizadeh et al., 2019).

Ras Activation Mechanism

Small GTPases belonging to the Ras protein family play a critical role in all aspects of cell biology and regulate cell division, differentiation, intracellular protein transport, organization of the cytoskeleton, growth factor signal transduction, and gene expression. With their GTP-bound or GDP-bound forms, Ras family proteins oscillate between the two conformations and affect various proteins in the cell, causing their conformation to change and their phosphorylation, triggering intracellular signal transduction. After Ras hydrolyzes the bound GTP, Guanine Exchange Factors is needed to remove the protein-bound GDP. GEF proteins interact with Ras-GDP and allow GDP to move away from the protein, allowing Ras to bind to GTP with a higher intracellular concentration. The bound GTP is hydrolyzed by the intrinsic GTPase activity of Ras, as well as by the action of GTPase Activating Proteins (GAP) that bind to Ras. The GTP-bound conformation of Ras leads to the fact that molecules located at the lower step of the signal transduction to which this protein binds also undergo conformational changes and participate in signal transduction by phosphorylation. Some mutations that occur activate Ras proteins, prevent the hydrolysis of GTP, and cause abnormal Ras-GTP forms to accumulate in the cell. It is known to trigger uncontrolled cell proliferation in this way.

The Ras family proteins in the GTP-bound conformation activate these proteins by directly binding to effector proteins located in the lower steps of the signaling pathway. Ras effectors are divided into three groups:

1. Effectors in the RAF ("Ras Associated Factor") and MAPK/ERK ("Mitogen-Activated Protein Kinase" and "Extracellular Signal Regulated Kinase") cascade;
2. Effectors in the phosphoinositide-3-kinase (PI3-K) and Ral ("Ras-like" Ras-like protein) cascade;
3. Ras effectors with various functions:
   - RalGDS protein
   - Rgl and Rlf
   - Phospholipase C-epsilon (PLCe)
   - T-cell invasion and metastasis factor-1 (TIAM-1)
   - Ras interaction/interference protein (RIN1)
   - Afadin Protein (AF-6)

- Family of proteins with Ras interaction site (RASSF) (Telkoparan & Tazebay, 2011)

Ras Mediated MAPK Pathway Activation Mechanism

The MAPK pathway includes three major kinases that activate and phosphorylate downstream proteins: MAPK kinase kinase, MAPK kinase, and MAPK. ERK1 and ERK2 are extracellular signal-regulated serine-threonine kinases. Hyperactivation of this pathway, which regulates cellular signaling under normal and pathological conditions, causes cancer development and progression. Among all MAPK signal transduction pathways, the Ras/Raf/ MAPK (MEK)/ERK pathway plays the most critical role and plays an essential role in the formation and progression of tumor cells (Guo et al., 2020).

Ras Mediated PI3K Pathway Activation Mechanism

A phosphoinositide-3 kinase (PI3K) is a plasma membrane-bound enzyme that regulates cellular growth and metabolism. PI3Ks are divided into three classes (I-III), each with different roles in signal transmission. PI3Ks are divided into class I, class IA, IB, and IC. IA-PI3Ks act as a heterodimer consisting of catalytic activity proteins (p110a, p110β, p110δ, p110γ) and a regulatory unit (p85α, p85β, p85γ). IA-PI3Ks are found in many tissue types and are directly activated by cell surface receptors such as the small G protein Ras, G protein-coupled receptors, receptor tyrosine kinases (RTKs). Activated PI3Ks catalyze the phosphorylation of inositol phospholipids in the cell membrane, thereby producing phosphatidylinositol triphosphate (PIP3). PIP3 recruits AKT to the membrane and allows activation of mTOR. PIP3 is also responsible for activating PIP3-dependent kinases (PDK) and protein kinase B (PKB). Protein kinase B is a protein encoded by the Akt1 and Akt2 genes (Miricescu et al., 2021).

Ras Mutations and Cancer Relationship

Since Ras proteins play an active role in the proliferative and change signals of the growing cell, they are very susceptible to acquired somatic functional mutations in all cancers. Studies on some tumors have shown 'hot-spots' in the RAS gene family prone to point mutations. Mutations in exons 12, 13 (segment 1), and 61 (segment 2), known as hot spot codons, cause-specific amino acid changes. Frequent mutations are the change of glycine to valine at codon 12, glycine to cysteine at codon 13, and glutamine to arginine/lysine/leucine at codon 61. By disrupting GTPase activity and leading to the development of resistance to GAPs, these changes lead to the accumulation of mutant Ras proteins remaining in the GTP-bound form in the cell, and the cell begins to be stimulated in an uncontrolled manner. Ras is more associated with cancer than Ras mutation frequency; Confusions in GDP-GTP regulation, loss of GAPs or disturbances in expression and protein activity levels such as persistent receptor tyrosine kinase-mediated activation of GEFs are additional mechanisms of Ras activation in cancer (Aslan Koşar et al., 2011; Hobbs et al., 2016).

Ras/Raf/Mek/Erk (MAPK) Pathway and Cancer

It is known that the MAPK pathway is activated in more than 85% of cancers. This condition is directly caused by genetic changes in receptor tyrosine kinases (RTKs), Ras, BRAF, and their activators or components, or indirectly by factors independent of Ras or RAF. Ras is an oncogene identified in one-third of all cancers. Ras mutations are frequently encountered in pancreatic (90%), thyroid (50%), colon (50%), lung (30%), and melanoma (25%) cancers. Ras mutants encode proteins mutated in human cancers primarily due to a single amino acid change in glycine 12 (G12) and glutamine 61 (Q61). These mutated proteins are GAP-insensitive and constitutively dependent on GTP, causing uncontrolled activation of downstream effectors. Within the members of the Ras gene group, K-Ras is the most frequently mutated, followed by N-Ras and H-Ras in order of frequency. While K-Ras mutations are more common in colorectal, pancreatic, lung, endometrial, cervical, and biliary tract cancers, N-Ras and K-Ras mutations are seen in myelomas, N-Ras, and H-Ras mutations are found in melanomas and bladder cancers, respectively.

BRAF mutations are prevalent in hair cell leukemia, papillary thyroid cancer, melanoma, pilocytic astrocytoma, colorectal cancer, and non-small cell lung cancer and have been identified in approximately 7% of all cancers. In general, BRAF activation occurs with a single point mutation (within the kinase domain of the BRAF protein) that converts valine 600 to glutamic acid and accounts for more than 90% of cases. As a result of this mutation, a structurally active protein is formed by uncontrollably stimulating the MAP kinase cascade, disrupting the functioning of genes related to the regulation of essential cellular functions such as cell proliferation and differentiation. Melanoma and papillary thyroid carcinoma are the most common types of cancer with the BRAF-V600E mutation.

MEK and ERK are overactivated as a result of oncogenic BRAF mutations. Unlike Ras and RAF, MEK and ERK have rare mutations in cancers. Still, their transformations are responsible for some RAF inhibitors (RAFi) resistant cases in current cancer treatments. MEK mutations have been identified mainly in melanoma, ovarian cancer cell lines, and gliomas. Upstream mutations can lead to uncontrolled stimulation of the ERK protein, which causes substrate activation, which is regulated by a series of ERK signals. ERK hyperactivation mediates the development of various types of cancer in these and similar ways. For example, overexpression of ERK can induce modulation of anti-apoptotic molecules such as BCL-2, a drug resistance-associated protein in some types of breast cancer (Liu et al., 2018; Yuan et al., 2020).

PI3K Pathway and Cancer

Phosphatidylinositol-3-kinase (PI3K)/Akt and rapamycin (mTOR) signaling pathways are essential for many events, including proliferation, angiogenesis, metabolism, differentiation, survival. While PIK3 is overexpressed in ovarian and cervical cancers, its mutations have been observed in breast cancer, glioblastoma, and gastric cancer.

The PI3 kinase/Protein kinase B signal transduction pathway is one of the most common pathways in cancers. In this pathway, phosphoinositol-3-phosphate (PIP-3) is activated by phosphorylating membrane phospholipids via PI3K as a result of cell stimulation. This activation activates protein kinase B (Akt). Protein kinase B is encoded by the Akt 1 and Akt 2 genes. Akt1 overexpression was detected in gastric cancer, Akt2 overexpression in ovarian and pancreatic cancer. Although the Akt mutation is rare, somatic mutations in Akt1 have been described in a small percentage of breast, ovarian, and colorectal cancers. Protein kinase B stimulation affects the activities of various proteins within the cell. One is the "mammalian target of rapamycin (m TOR)" protein. The mTOR protein has kinase activity and is inhibited by rapamycin. mTOR activates ribosomal proteins, stimulating the translation of mRNAs.

Rapamycin is used to treat tumors with increased mTOR synthesis (Sekulic' et al., 2000).

There may be an increased synthesis of PI3K in cancer. Located on chromosome 10, PTEN acts as a negative regulator of PI3K/Akt signaling. The PTEN tumor suppressor protein loses function by mutation, leading to permanent activation of the PI3K/Akt pathway. As a result, protein kinase B synthesis is increased. With the effect of these and similar factors, activation of mTOR may occur. The effects of protein kinase B activation on the cell cycle are also crucial in carcinogenesis. The p21 protein exerts a positive and stimulating effect on the cyclin D and cyclin-dependent kinase 4/6 (cdk4/6) complex in the early G1 phase of the cell cycle. Protein kinase B triggers the formation of the stable form of p21 and stimulates the progression of the cell cycle. In addition, it inhibits the protein that stimulates the degradation of protein kinase B p21. One of the cellular functions in which protein kinase B stimulation is directly effective is apoptosis. While protein kinase B exerts an inhibitory effect on caspase 9 with the proapoptotic BAD protein, it also supports the anti-apoptotic response with NFκB stimulation. BAD proteins antagonize the anti-apoptotic functions of the anti-apoptotic BCL2 and BCL-x(L) proteins. Changes in protein kinase B stimulation initiate carcinogenesis by disrupting the apoptosis mechanism (Zinkel et al., 2006).

Epidermal Growth Factor Receptor and Cancer

A large family of cell surface receptors is the receptor tyrosine kinase. RTKs play an essential role in regulating the most basic cellular processes such as cell cycle, migration, and cell metabolism. In addition, they have essential roles in controlling cell proliferation and differentiation. EGFR is a 170 kDa monomeric glycoprotein, one of four structurally similar members of the erythroblastosis oncogene B (ErbB) family of RTK: EGFR (ErbB1, HER1: "human epidermal growth factor receptor"), ErbB2 (HER2), ErbB3 (HER3), ErbB4 (HER4) (Scaltriti & Baselga, 2006).

It is known that EGFR affects normal cellular processes in humans and neoplastic growth processes. Some tumors such as glioblastomas, head and neck, non-small cell lung cancer, pancreatic, colorectal, prostate, breast, and ovarian cancer exhibit increased EGFR activity through increased synthesis of EGF overexpression or mutation of EGFR.

EGF and EGFR are associated with progressive tumor growth and metastasis in several ways:

- Increase tumor cell proliferation and migration through the Ras/Raf/MEK/ERK and PI3K/AKT pathways;
- Localization of EGFR to the nucleus to promote cell proliferation;
- Dysregulation of autophagic activity;
- Stimulation of several matrix metalloproteinases facilitates cancer invasion and metastasis (Rajaram et al., 2017).

ErbB2(HER2/neu) and Cancer

In the ErbB2 oncoprotein activated by gene amplification, tyrosine kinase is constantly active and continuously transmits cleavage signals to the nucleus. Overexpression of the HER2 protein through gene amplification or transcriptional dysregulation occurs in approximately a quarter of breast and ovarian cancers and is associated with a poor prognosis. It has also been detected in subtypes of endometrial, stomach, and esophageal cancers and rarely in oropharynx, lung, and bladder cancer (Moasser, 2007).

Myc and Cancer

The Myc protein is a transcription factor dimerized with MAX to bind DNA and regulate gene expression. Myc expression is tightly regulated in healthy tissue. It has been shown that the Myc gene is expressed more than the average level or to change structurally in different types of cancer. Such changes in the Myc gene have been detected in 70% of cancers. Gene amplification, retroviral promoter insertion, chromosomal translocation, enhanced call signaling, activation of super-enhancers, altered protein degradation, and mutation are among the mechanisms leading to these changes.

Gene amplification is one of the mechanisms that cause changes in the Myc gene most frequently encountered in solid organ tumors. C- Myc amplification is most commonly seen in ovarian, esophageal, breast, and squamous cell lung cancer. The frequency of amplification detected in L-Myc and N-Myc in cancer formation is not as high as that detected in C-Myc. One of the cancers in which amplification of L-Myc has been detected is small cell lung cancer. In contrast, N-Myc overexpression or amplification has been demonstrated in tumors with neuroendocrine features such as retinoblastoma neuroblastoma, medulloblastoma, small cell lung cancer, and neuroendocrine type prostate cancer.

While there is mostly amplification of Myc in epithelial tumors, activation by translocation of Myc has been shown to be more in hematologic malignancies. The first cancer in which translocations are identified was Burkitt's lymphoma. Three different Myc translocations have been identified in Burkitt lymphoma; t(8;14), t(2;8), t(8;22). Diffuse large B-cell lymphoma, low-grade follicular lymphoma, and mantle-cell lymphoma contain Myc translocation. Myc translocation has been demonstrated in 36% of patients with multiple myeloma (Duffy et al., 2021; Schaub et al., 2018; Schick et al., 2017).

Cyclin D1, Cyclin E Protooncogenes, and Cancer

Cyclins form complexes with cyclin-dependent kinase (CDK) and regulate their activities. The formed CDK/Cyclin complexes are regulatory molecules that are important at all stages of the cell cycle. D-type cyclins regulate G1-S-phase progression. As a result of a mutation in which the control of D cyclin release is disrupted, the cell enters the S phase, and as a result, a neoplastic transformation develops. It is known that Cyclin D1 proto-oncogene play a role in the development of various cancers such as parathyroid adenoma, breast, squamous cell lung cancer, and B cell neoplasm (Motokura & Arnold, 1993).

Cyclin E is found in the late G1-S phase. Cyclin E expression is dependent on E2F transcription factors, and its expression is regulated at the transcriptional level. Cyclin E binds to the kinase Cdk2, activates it, and phosphorylates its substrates, called "pocket proteins," providing the initiation of the S-stage. Besides this function, it plays a direct role in initiating DNA replication, controlling genomic stability, and centrosome cycling. Cyclin E is highly expressed in many tumors.

It has been shown that the cyclin E gene is overexpressed in cancer types such as breast, non-small cell lung cancer, colon, leukemia, and lymphoma (Möröy & Geisen, 2004).

Conclusion

Normal development and cell differentiation are regulated and managed by genes. As a result of the activation of proto-oncogenes, their transformation into oncogenes activates critical pathways for carcinogenesis, and cells turn into cancer cells due to uncontrolled proliferation, inhibition of apoptosis, disruption of the natural immune system, and more frequent mutations. Ras GTPases function as molecular controllers for vital cellular activities such as cell proliferation, maturation, differentiation, and survival of normal cells and are tightly and temporally regulated by multiple signalling pathways. Therefore, RAS has been the main focus of the cancer study in the ~40 years since it was first identified as an oncogene.

References

Altınbas, R. (2020). Oncogenes. In E. Bozgeyik (Ed.), *Molecular Biology and Immunology of Cancer* (pp. 29-43). Akademisyen Kitabevi.

Aslan Koşar, P., Çapar, E., & Koşar, A. (2011). Bladder cancer and RAS proto-oncogenes. *The New Journal of Urology*, 7(1), 55-58.

Croce, C. M. (2008). Oncogenes and cancer. *The New England Journal of Medicine*, 358(5), 502-511.

Duffy, M. J., O'Grady, S., Tang, M., & Crown, J. (2021). MYC as a target for cancer treatment. *Cancer Treatment Reviews*, 94, 1-7. https://doi.org/10.1016/j.ctrv.2021.102154.

Eaton, B. R., Claude, L., Indelicato, D. J., Vatner, R., Yeh, B., Schwarz, R., & Laack, N. (2021). Ewing sarcoma. *Pediatric Blood and Cancer*, 68(S2), 1-8. https://doi.org/10.1002/pbc.28355.

Grünewald, T. G. P., Cidre-Aranaz, F., Surdez, D., Tomazou, E. M., de Álava, E., Kovar, H., Sorensen, P. H., Delattre, O., & Dirksen, U. (2018). Ewing sarcoma. *Nature Reviews Disease Primers*, 4(5), 1-22. https://doi.org/10.1038/s41572-018-0003-x.

Guo, Y., Pan, W., Liu, S., Shen, Z., Xu, Y., & Hu, L. (2020). ERK/MAPK signalling pathway and tumorigenesis. *Experimental and Therapeutic Medicine*, 19, 1997-2007. https://doi.org/10.3892/etm.2020.8454.

Hecht, J. L., & Aster, J. C. (2000). Molecular biology of Burkitt's lymphoma. *Journal of Clinical Oncology*, *18*(21), 3707-3721. https://doi.org/10.1200/JCO.2000.18.21.3707.

Hobbs, G. A., Der, C. J., & Rossman, K. L. (2016). RAS isoforms and mutations in cancer at a glance. *Journal of Cell Science*, 129(7), 1287-1292. https://doi.org/10.1242/jcs.182873.

Kang, Z. J., Liu, Y. F., Xu, L. Z., Long, Z. J., Huang, D., Yang, Y., Liu, B., Feng, J. X., Pan, Y. J., Yan, J. S., & Liu, Q. (2016). The Philadelphia chromosome in leukemogenesis. *Chinese Journal of Cancer*, 35(1), 1-15. https://doi.org/10.1186/s40880-016-0108-0.

Liu, F., Yang, X., Geng, M., & Huang, M. (2018). Targeting ERK, an Achilles' Heel of the MAPK pathway, in cancer therapy. *Acta Pharmaceutica Sinica B,* 8(4), 552-562. https://doi.org/10.1016/j.apsb.2018.01.008.

Lynch, D. H. (1987). Oncogenes and cancer. *American Journal of Reproductive Immunology and Microbiology*, 15(1), 24-28). https://doi.org/10.1111/j.1600-0897.1987.tb00145.x.

May, W. A., Gishizky, M. L., Lessnick, S. L., Lunsford, L. B., Lewis, B. C., Delattre, O., Zucman, J., Thomas, G., & Denny, C. T. (1993). Ewing sarcoma 11;22 translocation produces a chimeric transcription factor that requires the DNA-binding domain encoded by FLI1 for transformation. *Proceedings of the National Academy of Sciences of the United States of America*, 90(12), 5752-5756. https://doi.org/10.1073/pnas.90.12.5752.

May, W. A., Lessnick, S. L., Braun, B. S., Klemsz, M., Lewis, B. C., Lunsford, L. B., Hromas, R., & Denny, C. T. (1993). The Ewing's sarcoma EWS/FLI-1 fusion gene encodes a more potent transcriptional activator and is a more powerful transforming gene than FLI-1. *Molecular and Cellular Biology*, 13(12), 7393-7398. https://doi.org/10.1128/mcb.13.12.7393.

Miricescu, D., Totan, A., Stanescu-Spinu, I. I., Badoiu, S. C., Stefani, C., & Greabu, M. (2021). PI3K/AKT/mTOR signaling pathway in breast cancer: From molecular landscape to clinical aspects. *International Journal of Molecular Sciences*, 22(1), 1-24. https://doi.org/10.3390/ijms22010173.

Mitelman, F., Johansson, B., & Mertens, F. (2007). The impact of translocations and gene fusions on cancer causation. *Nature Reviews Cancer*, 7(4), 233-245. https://doi.org/10.1038/nrc2091.

Moasser, M. M. (2007). The oncogene HER2: Its signaling and transforming functions and its role in human cancer pathogenesis. *Oncogene*, 26(45), 6469-6487. https://doi.org/10.1038/sj.onc.1210477.

Möröy, T., & Geisen, C. (2004). Cyclin E. *International Journal of Biochemistry and Cell Biology*, 36(8), 1424-1439. https://doi.org/10.1016/j.biocel.2003.12.005.

Motokura, T., & Arnold, A. (1993). Cyclin D and oncogenesis. *Current Opinion in Genetics and Development*, 3(1), 5-10. https://doi.org/10.1016/S0959-437X(05)80334-X.

Nambiar, M., Kari, V., & Raghavan, S. C. (2008). Chromosomal translocations in cancer. *Biochimica et Biophysica Acta - Reviews on Cancer*, 1786(2), 139-152. https://doi.org/10.1016/j.bbcan.2008.07.005.

Rajaram, P., Chandra, P., Ticku, S., Pallavi, B., Rudresh, K., & Mansabdar, P. (2017). Epidermal growth factor receptor: Role in human cancer. *Indian Journal of Dental Research*, 28(6), 687-694. https://doi.org/10.4103/ijdr.IJDR_534_16.

Rowley, J. D. (1973). Chromosomal patterns in myelocytic leukemia. *New England Journal of Medicine*, 289(4), 220-221. https://doi.org/10.1056/nejm197307262890422.

Scaltriti, M., & Baselga, J. (2006). The epidermal growth factor receptor pathway: A model for targeted therapy. *Clinical Cancer Research*, 12(18), 5268-5272. https://doi.org/10.1158/1078-0432.CCR-05-1554.

Schaub, F. X., Dhankani, V., Berger, A. C., Trivedi, M., Richardson, A. B., Shaw, R., Zhao, W., Zhang, X., Ventura, A., Liu, Y., Ayer, D. E., Hurlin, P. J., Cherniack, A. D., Eisenman, R. N., Bernard, B., Grandori, C., Caesar-Johnson, S. J., Demchok, J. A., Felau, I., … Mariamidze, A. (2018). Pan-cancer alterations of the MYC oncogene and its proximal network across the cancer genome atlas. *Cell Systems*, 6(3), 282-300. https://doi.org/10.1016/j.cels.2018.03.003.

Schick, M., Habringer, S., Nilsson, J. A., & Keller, U. (2017). Pathogenesis and therapeutic targeting of aberrant MYC expression in haematological cancers. *British Journal of Haematology*, 179(5), 724-738. https://doi.org/10.1111/bjh.14917.

Sekulic, A., Hudson, C. C., Homme, J. L., Yin, P., Otterness, D. M., Karnitz, L. M., & Abraham, R. T. (2000). A direct linkage between the phosphoinositide 3-Kinase-AKT signaling pathway and the mammalian target of rapamycin in mitogen-stimulated and transformed cells. *Cancer Research,* 60(13), 3504-13.

Sorensen, P. H. B., Lessnick, S. L., Lopez-Terrada, D., Liu, X. F., Triche, T. J., & Denny, C. T. (1994). A second ewing's sarcoma translocation, t(21;22), fuses the EWS gene to another ETS-family transcription factor, ERG. *Nature Genetics*, 6(2), 146-151. https://doi.org/10.1038/ng0294-146.

Telkoparan, P., & Tazebay, U. H. (2011). Ras family of proteins: cellular function, molecular control, and its role in oncogenesis. *Turkish Journal of Biochemistry - Turk J Biochem*, 36(4), 367-373.

Torry, D. S., & Cooper, G. M. (1991). Proto-oncogenes in development and cancer. *American Journal of Reproductive Immunology*, 25(3), 129-132. https://doi.org/10.1111/j.1600-0897.1991.tb01080.x.

Turc-Carel, C., Philip, I., Berger, M. P., Philip, T., & Lenoir, G. (1983). [Chromosomal translocation (11; 22) in cell lines of Ewing's sarcoma]. *Comptes Rendus Des Seances de l'Academie Des Sciences. Serie III, Sciences de La Vie*, 296(23), 1101-1103.

Yokus, B., & Ülker, D. Ü. (2012). Cancer biochemistry. *Dicle Üniv Vet Fak Derg*, 1(2), 7-18. http://www.dicle.edu.tr/bolum/Muh/veteriner/dergi/.

Yuan, J., Dong, X., Yap, J., & Hu, J. (2020). The MAPK and AMPK signalings: Interplay and implication in targeted cancer therapy. *Journal of Hematology and Oncology*, 13(1), 1-19. https://doi.org/10.1186/s13045-020-00949-4.

Zaimy, M. A., Saffarzadeh, N., Mohammadi, A., Pourghadamyari, H., Izadi, P., Sarli, A., Moghaddam, L. K., Paschepari, S. R., Azizi, H., Torkamandi, S., & Tavakkoly-Bazzaz, J. (2017). New methods in the diagnosis of cancer and gene therapy of cancer based on nanoparticles. *Cancer Gene Therapy*, 24(6), 233-243. https://doi.org/10.1038/cgt.2017.16.

Zheng, J. (2013). Oncogenic chromosomal translocations and human cancer (Review). *Oncology Reports*, 30(5), 2011-2019. https://doi.org/10.3892/or.2013.2677.

Zinatizadeh, M. R., Momeni, S. A., Zarandi, P. K., Chalbatani, G. M., Dana, H., Mirzaei, H. R., Akbari, M. E., & Miri, S. R. (2019). The role and function of Ras-association domain family in cancer: a review. *Genes and Diseases*, 6(4), 378-384. https://doi.org/10.1016/j.gendis.2019.07.008.

Zinkel, S., Gross, A., & Yang, E. (2006). BCL2 family in DNA damage and cell cycle control. *Cell Death and Differentiation*, 13(8), 1351-1359. https://doi.org/10.1038/sj.cdd.4401987.

Chapter 8

Effects of Ras and Other Proto-Oncogenes on Autoimmunity

Mehtap Şahin*
Health Sciences Institute,
Physiology Doctorate Programme,
Sivas Cumhuriyet University, Sivas, Turkey

Abstract

Control and regulation of cell growth, development, and reproductive functions are provided by proteins encoded by proto-oncogene and tumor suppressor genes. Ras proteins are essential as a complement to cellular networks that control signaling pathways that regulate cell movement, cytoskeleton regulation, adhesion, differentiation, survival, and growth regulation. The relationship between autoimmune diseases and Ras and proto-oncogenes has gained importance in recent years.

Keywords: autoimmunity, protooncogene, Ras

Introduction

Changes in critical regulatory genes (a proto-oncogene) that control cell proliferation, differentiation, and survival cause various cancers. The first information on the molecular basis of carcinogenesis emerged with studies on retroviruses. As little as 10-20% of human cancers are caused by viruses (80-

---

* Corresponding Author's Email: 20189142002@cumhuriyet.edu.tr.

In: Autoimmunity and Cancer
Editors: Soner Şahin and Kenan Demir
ISBN: 978-1-68507-937-6

90% are caused by other causes such as radiation, chemical carcinogens, and errors during DNA replication). Studies on viral oncogenes have enabled the identification of oncogenes that cause nonviral cancers. The control and regulation of cells' growth, development, and reproductive functions are made by proteins encoded by proto-oncogene and tumor suppressor genes. As a result of genetic changes, proto-oncogenes turn into cellular oncogenes (c-onc), and eventually cancer develops. The effects of the use of immunosuppressive drugs due to congenital or acquired immunodeficiency on the cellular and humoral immune response play an essential role in the development and progression of cancers. Proto-oncogenes are essential genes in the genomes and are meticulously protected.

Proto-oncogenes require four factors to control the synthesis of the oncoprotein:

- Growth factors
- Growth factor receptors
- Signal transfer factors
- Nuclear transcription factors

If proto-oncogenes come under the control of oncoviruses such as retroviruses, they are overstimulated. This overstimulation causes them to undergo transcription and translation, and causes the synthesis of oncoproteins and the uncontrolled and unlimited reproduction of cells with the effect of oncoproteins.

Ras Proteins

Ras proteins play an important role in cellular networks that control signaling pathways that regulate cell movement, cytoskeleton regulation, adhesion, differentiation, survival, and growth (Murugan et al., 2019). For more than 60 years, studies on Ras and Ras genes have been ongoing. In these studies, they were defined as retroviral oncogenes. Harvey and Kirstein were identified as the cellular part of rat sarcoma oncogenes. These Ras proteins are GTPase and consist mainly of 3 Ras proto-oncogenes; Harvey rat sarcoma virus oncogene (HRAS), Kirsten rat sarcoma virus oncogene (KRAS), Neuroblastoma rat oncogene (NRAS) (Murugan et al., 2019). Studies conducted in the process have shown that mutations in human Ras genes are associated with cancer development and tumorigenesis (Riller & Rieux-Laucat, 2021). These Ras mutations are responsible for approximately 30% of all human cancers. (Riller & Rieux-Laucat, 2021). HRAS and NRAS, small series of the GTPase family, encode two isoforms of KRAS (KRASA and KRASB). This GTPase family controls the activation of RAF-MEK-ERK, which is a protein that forms RAS / mitogen-activated protein kinase (MAPK). Extracellular matrix receptors, cytokine receptors, G-protein coupled receptors, and growth factor binding receptor tyrosine kinases (RTKs) are affected by GTPase activation. As a result of these interactions, phosphorylated ERK1/2 regulates many vital functions of the cell. For example, regulation of growth, apoptosis, and differentiation. In recent years, diseases originating from RAS-related pathways have been termed "RASopathies." Hematopoietic and nonhemetopoietic cancers, neurofibromatosis type 1, Noonan syndrome, Costello syndrome, cardio-faciocutaneous syndrome, Legius syndrome can be given as examples of Rasopathies (Riller & Rieux-Laucat, 2021). Many of the biological functions of the Ras superfamily depend on the cytoplasmic edge of the cell membrane, where specific signals are received and transmitted further. Ras superfamily members function as lipid scavengers and have membrane-associated structural features. They are oriented in one direction in the regulatory GTPase cycle. Similar to the alpha subunits of the heterotrimeric G protein, Ras family proteins are controlled in the "off" or "on" position, respectively, as a double switch to which GDP or GTP binds (Simanshu et al., 2017). Ras signaling pathway activation has been reported in T lymphocytes to be related to the development of autoimmunity and especially lupus-like disease. T lymphocytes interact with their environment via T cell receptors (TCR). TCR signals are required for the development, differentiation, and activation of T lymphocytes. Regular functioning of the Ras signaling system is necessary for the development of T lymphocytes, normal immune responses, and the maintenance of immune tolerance (Mor et al., 2007). Ras dysfunction leads to immunodeficiency and autoimmunity. Mature T lymphocytes are divided into two main subgroups, Th1 and Th2, into groups such as Th17. Systemic lupus erythematosus (SLE), an autoimmune disease, is particularly associated with the Th2 response, and IL-4 is important in this response. As cells grow and age, they face apoptosis and are cleared by professional or nonprofessional phagocytes (Erwig & Henson, 2007). A disruption in apoptosis, the physiological process of programmed cell death, can lead to degenerative and autoimmune disorders and cancer (Khan et al., 2014; Goldar et al., 2015). This process was first brought up by Carl Vogt in 1842 and later by Lockshin and Williams in 1965 (Khan et al.,

2014). Only 5% of the thymocytes transform into mature T lymphocytes, the rest undergo negative selection, and self-reactive and potentially autoimmune T lymphocytes are cleared. Many apoptotic cells are released under growth, aging, and pregnancy conditions. Caspases carry out apoptosis and play an important role in tissue hemostasis. The disruption of apoptosis is an important step in tumorigenesis. Whether a cell will live or die is often determined by the family of pro-and anti-apoptotic regulators, Bcl-2. Bcl-2 overexpression, myc translocations, and p53 mutations in lymphoid malignancies, deletion in chromosome 7 and 6q in human follicular lymphoma, BCL-6 gene mutations play an important role in oncogenesis (Cory et al., 2003). Insufficient removal of dead cells from the body activates the immune system. As a result of innate and adaptive immune activation, autoimmune diseases such as severe anemia, chronic arthritis, and SLE occur (Nagata et al., 2010). In another study, the importance of the Bcl-2 family was studied in Rheumatoid Arthritis (RA), an autoimmune rheumatic disease that mainly affects the joints and can also cause extra-articular involvement. Autoimmune diseases occur with the contribution of genetic predisposition and environmental factors and can result in tissue and organ damage due to immune dysfunction. Many signaling pathways activate T and B lymphocytes in autoimmune diseases. One of them is the GTP-binding protein Ras family. As a result of inhibition of Ras activation, T lymphocyte activation is suppressed. This has been demonstrated in the MRL/LPR mouse model using S-trans-farnesylthiosalycylic acid (FTS), a Ras inhibitor, and in the experimental antiphospholipid antibody (APS) and SLE model (Centre et al., 2001).

Ras-associated autoimmune leucoproliferative disease (RALD) is a rare immune disorder syndrome due to NRAS or KRAS mutations in hematopoietic cells characterized by lymphadenopathy splenomegaly hyper-gammaglobulinemia, autoimmunity, and monocytosis. RAID patients have an increased risk of malignancy and can be confused with other autoimmune rheumatic diseases such as SLE (Papa et al., 2021). Primary immune-deficiencies that affect lymphocyte development can lead to severe infection and susceptibility to tumorigenesis. Many systems in the human body control autoreactive T lymphocytes, such as clonal deletion in primary lymphoid organs, receptor editing, anergy, suppression of effector lymphocytes by regulatory lymphocytes, and programmed cell death. This issue has gained even more importance with the discovery of FAS (Apo-1/CD95) and the FAS ligand, which are known as "death receptors" that specifically trigger apoptosis (Meynier & Rieux-Laucat, 2019). FAS is the sixth member of a tumor necrosis factor receptor superfamily (TNFRSF6). FAS mutations lead to autoimmune lymphoproliferative syndrome (ALPS), a tumoral syndrome (Meynier & Rieux-Laucat, 2019; Takagi et al., 2013). In recent years, RAS-associated autoimmune lymphoproliferative disease (RALD), similar to ALPS disease, has been reported (Meynier & Rieux-Laucat, 2019). In 1983, the effects of the interaction between activated RAS and Myc on oncogenicity came to the fore. Myc is directly involved in angiogenesis, inflammation, and immunosuppression. Interleukin-23 (IL-23) and CCL9 have been implicated in Myc-related carcinogenesis. IL-23 is also a cytokine involved in many autoimmune-autoinflammatory diseases. Myc-associated tumor development is associated with immunosuppression (Kortlever et al., 2017). PD-L1, an immunosuppressor protein, has been up-regulated in many types of cancer and allows the person with cancer to avoid the immune system. The Ras signaling pathway stimulates PD-L1 upregulation on PD-L1 mRNA by modulation of tristetra protein (TTP) (AU-rich protein) in tumor cells (Coelho et al., 2017). In addition, the RAs-Ros-p38 signaling pathway controls TTP activity. H-Ras activation is associated with non-obese diabetes and diabetic retinopathy and abnormal vascular development (Fernández-Medarde & Santos, 2011). Blocking the Ras signaling pathway will also block the intracellular G protein pathway (Mott & Owen, 2019). Exosome "rasosomes" have come to the fore in targeted cancer therapy for Ras signaling pathway blockade (Sexton et al., 2019; Marín-ramos et al., 2019). This blocking may also work in autoimmune signal blocking. The relationship between the mitogen-activated protein kinase (MAPK) pathway and the Ras pathway has been demonstrated (Nussinov, 2019). The MAPK pathway is essential in many autoimmune diseases (Rieux-Laucat, 2017). In SLE, an autoimmune disease, auto-antibodies against self-antigens are produced due to excessive B lymphocyte proliferation. Increased proto-oncogene expression has been reported in SLE. Increased c-myc and N-ras proto-oncogene expression have been demonstrated in NZB and BXSB rats (Klinman et al., 1986). The Ras signaling pathway is associated with many metabolic lipids, nucleotide, and glycolytic pathways. In addition to these metabolic pathways, the interaction between cancer cells and the immune system is essential for cancer biology. Cancer cells must survive and multiply without being immunized by immune effector cells. The Ras signaling pathway reduces MHC class I expression in cancer cells, thus preventing the destruction of these cells by cytotoxic T cells. Immune checkpoints such as PD-L1 (CD274) prevent immune system reactivity and autoimmunity. In addition, KRAS increases IL-6-related chronic inflammation. IL-6-related chronic inflammation is essential in many rheumatic diseases, especially rheumatoid arthritis (RA). The pro-inflammatory microenvironment is essential for cancer cells. KRAS signaling stimulates the expression of another pro-inflammatory cytokine, the IL-17 receptor (Gimple & Wang, 2019).

The immune system elements associated with Ras and other proto-oncogenes are summarized in Table 1.

Table 1. Immune system elements associated with Ras and other proto-oncogenes

T lymphocytes
B lymphocytes
Neutrophils
Macrophages
IL-6
IL-17
IL-23
IL-8
MAPK pathway
PI3K pathway

IL; interleukin, MAPK; mitogen-activated protein kinase.

Furthermore, the ras signal acts through the MAPK and PI3K pathways and IL-8 in the continuation of vascularization and inflammation. KRAS signaling increases the production of inflammatory chemokines, allowing the migration of neutrophils and macrophages to the site of inflammation (Gimple & Wang, 2019; Downward, 2003; Weber & Carroll, 2021; Molina & Adjei, 2006; Hamarsheh et al., 2020). Ras signal is associated with integrins, E-cadherin, N-cadherin, semaphorins, plexins (Weber & Carroll, 2021). The Ras pathway is essential in cancer immunity and autoimmunity and other autoimmune diseases, thanks to many different pathways, interleukins, and chemokines with which it interacts.

Conclusion

Both the onset and progression of cancer are associated with many factors such as environmental, genetic, infection (viral), and lifestyle. Transformation of proto-oncogenes into oncogenes and inactivation of tumor suppressor genes lead to activation of critical pathways for carcinogenesis. Chronic inflammation after tissue damage contributes to cancer induction by causing cells to transform and proliferate vigorously. Many other autoimmune disorders and diseases are also associated with chronic inflammation. Although many different mechanisms are known that cause T and B lymphocytes, which play a role in most autoimmune diseases, the GTP-binding protein Ras family has also been demonstrated. However, it is known that KRAS increases IL-6-related inflammation and stimulates IL-17 expression. Considering that T and B lymphocytes, IL6 and IL-17 cytokines play an essential role in autoimmune diseases such as rheumatoid arthritis, spondyloarthritis, and SLE, we think that Ras proteins and proto-oncogenes should also be investigated in terms of these diseases. Unfortunately, there are hardly any studies in this field in the literature.

References

Centre, S. M., Hashomer, T., & Faculty, S. (2001). *Anti-Ras Therapy.Pdf.* 570–577.

Coelho, M. A., de Carné Trécesson, S., Rana, S., Zecchin, D., Moore, C., Molina-Arcas, M., East, P., Spencer-Dene, B., Nye, E., Barnouin, K., Snijders, A. P., Lai, W. S., Blackshear, P. J., & Downward, J. (2017). Oncogenic RAS signaling promotes tumor immunoresistance by stabilizing PD-L1 mRNA. *Immunity*, *47*(6), 1083-1099.e6. https://doi.org/10.1016/j.immuni.2017.11.016.

Cory, S., Huang, D. C. S., & Adams, J. M. (2003). The Bcl-2 family: Roles in cell survival and oncogenesis. *Oncogene*, *22*(53), 8590–8607. https://doi.org/10.1038/sj.onc.1207102.

Downward, J. (2003). *Targeting RAS Signalling*. *3*(January). https://doi.org/10.1038/nrc969.

Erwig, L. P., & Henson, P. M. (2007). Immunological consequences of apoptotic cell phagocytosis. *American Journal of Pathology*, *171*(1), 2–8. https://doi.org/10.2353/ajpath.2007.070135.

Fernández-Medarde, A., & Santos, E. (2011). Ras in cancer and developmental diseases. *Genes and Cancer*, *2*(3), 344–358. https://doi.org/10.1177/1947601911411084.

Gimple, R. C., & Wang, X. (2019). RAS: Striking at the Core of the Oncogenic Circuitry. *Frontiers in Oncology*, *9*(September), 1–16. https://doi.org/10.3389/fonc.2019.00965.

Goldar, S., Khaniani, M. S., Derakhshan, S. M., & Baradaran, B. (2015). Molecular mechanisms of apoptosis and roles in cancer development and treatment. *Asian Pacific Journal of Cancer Prevention*, *16*(6), 2129–2144. https://doi.org/10.7314/APJCP.2015.16.6.2129.

Hamarsheh, S., Groß, O., Brummer, T., & Zeiser, R. (2020). Immune modulatory effects of oncogenic KRAS in cancer. *Nature Communications*, *11*(1). https://doi.org/10.1038/s41467-020-19288-6.

Khan, K. H., Blanco-Codesido, M., & Molife, L. R. (2014). Cancer therapeutics: Targeting the apoptotic pathway. *Critical Reviews in Oncology/Hematology*, *90*(3), 200–219. https://doi.org/10.1016/j.critrevonc.2013.12.012.

Klinman, B. Y. D. M., Mushinski, J. F., Honda, M., Ishigatsubo, Y., Mountz, J. D., & Raveche, E. S. (1986). Expression in autoimmune and normal peripheral and Alfred D. Steinberg. *Journal of Experimental Medicin*e 163(May), 1292–1307.

Kortlever, R. M., Sodir, N. M., Wilson, C. H., Burkhart, D. L., Pellegrinet, L., Brown Swigart, L., Littlewood, T. D., & Evan, G. I. (2017). Myc cooperates with Ras by programming inflammation and immune suppression. *Cell*, *171*(6), 1301-1315.e14. https://doi.org/10.1016/j.cell.2017.11.013.

Marín-Ramos, N. I., Ortega-gutiérrez, S., & López-rodríguez, M. L. (2019). Seminars in cancer biology blocking Ras inhibition as an antitumor strategy. *Seminars in Cancer Biology*, *54*(December 2017), 91–100. https://doi.org/10.1016/j.semcancer.2018.01.017.

Meynier, S., & Rieux-Laucat, F. (2019). FAS and RAS related Apoptosis defects: From autoimmunity to leukemia. *Immunological Reviews*, *287*(1), 50–61. https://doi.org/10.1111/imr.12720.

Molina, J. R., & Adjei, A. A. (2006). The Ras/Raf/MAPK pathway. *Journal of Thoracic Oncology*, *1*(1), 7–9. https://doi.org/10.1016/s1556-0864(15)31506-9.

Mor, A., Philips, M. R., & Pillinger, M. H. (2007). The role of Ras signaling in lupus T lymphocytes: Biology and pathogenesis. *Clinical Immunology*, *125*(3), 215–223. https://doi.org/10.1016/j.clim.2007.08.008.

Mott, H. R., & Owen, D. (2019). Seminars in cancer biology bioblockades join the assault on small G protein signalling. *Seminars in Cancer Biology*, *54*(December 2017), 149–161. https://doi.org/10.1016/j.semcancer.2018.01.001.

Murugan, A. K., Grieco, M., & Tsuchida, N. (2019). RAS mutations in human cancers: Roles in precision medicine. *Seminars in Cancer Biology*, *59*(June), 23–35. https://doi.org/10.1016/j.semcancer.2019.06.007.

Nagata, S., Hanayama, R., & Kawane, K. (2010). Autoimmunity and the clearance of dead cells. *Cell*, *140*(5), 619–630. https://doi.org/10.1016/j.cell.2010.02.014.

Nussinov, R. (2019). Seminars in cancer biology oncogenic KRas mobility in the membrane and signaling response. *Seminars in Cancer Biology*, *54*(December 2017), 109–113. https://doi.org/10.1016/j.semcancer.2018.02.009.

Papa, R., Rusmini, M., Schena, F., Traggiai, E., Coccia, M. C., Caorsi, R., Arrigo, S., Pasetti, F., Signa, S., Barone, P., Santamaria, G., Spirito, G., Sanges, R., Vozzi, D., Cavalli, A., Gustincich, S., Ravelli, A., Gattorno, M., Ceccherini, I., & Volpi, S. (2021). Type I interferon activation in RAS-associated autoimmune leukoproliferative disease (RALD). *Clinical Immunology*, *231*(August), 1–5. https://doi.org/10.1016/j.clim.2021.108837.

Rieux-Laucat, F. (2017). What's up in the ALPS. *Current Opinion in Immunology*, *49*, 79–86. https://doi.org/10.1016/j.coi.2017.10.001.

Riller, Q., & Rieux-Laucat, F. (2021). RASopathies: From germline mutations to somatic and multigenic diseases. *Biomedical Journal*, *44*(4), 422–432. https://doi.org/10.1016/j.bj.2021.06.004.

Sexton, R. E., Mpilla, G., Kim, S., Philip, P. A., & Azmi, A. S. (2019). Seminars in cancer biology Ras and exosome signaling. *Seminars in Cancer Biology*, *54*(April 2018), 131–137. https://doi.org/10.1016/j.semcancer.2019.02.004.

Simanshu, D. K., Nissley, D. V., & McCormick, F. (2017). RAS proteins and their regulators in human disease. *Cell*, *170*(1), 17–33. https://doi.org/10.1016/j.cell.2017.06.009.

Takagi, M., Piao, J., Lin, L., Kawaguchi, H., Imai, C., Ogawa, A., Watanabe, A., Akiyama, K., Kobayashi, C., Mori, M., Ko, K., Sugimoto, M., & Mizutani, S. (2013). Autoimmunity and persistent RAS-mutated clones long after the spontaneous regression of JMML. *Leukemia*, *27*(9), 1926–1928. https://doi.org/10.1038/leu.2013.82.

Weber, S. M., & Carroll, S. L. (2021). The role of R-Ras proteins in normal and pathologic migration and morphologic change. *American Journal of Pathology*, *191*(9), 1499–1510. https://doi.org/10.1016/j.ajpath.2021.05.008.

Chapter 9

Cancer in Autoimmune Diseases

Ela Delikgoz Soykut*, MD
Health Sciences University,
Samsun Training and Research Hospital, Samsun, Turkey

Abstract

The unregulated inflammatory process leads to the development of two devastating conditions, cancer and autoimmune diseases. Cancer arises as a result of uncontrolled growth due to many mutations and changes in the metabolic balance of the tumor cell and its surroundings. Autoimmune diseases are chronic inflammatory disorders characterized by immune-mediated self-tissue destruction due to loss of self-tolerance. Although the exact mechanism is not yet clearly understood, it is known that autoimmune diseases are associated with a high risk of malignancy. Similar inflammatory conditions are involved in the development of cancer and autoimmune diseases. In this article, it is aimed to discuss the relationship between the most common autoimmune diseases and malignancies and to mention the increasing types of cancer associated with autoimmunity.

Keywords: autoimmune diseases, cancer, inflammation

Introduction

The unregulated inflammatory process leads to the development of two devastating conditions, cancer and autoimmune diseases. Cancer arises as a

---

* Corresponding Author's Email: eladelikgoz@gmail.com.

In: Autoimmunity and Cancer
Editors: Soner Şahin and Kenan Demir
ISBN: 978-1-68507-937-6

result of uncontrolled growth due to many mutations and changes in the metabolic balance of the tumor cell and its surroundings. Inflammation is indispensable in this process. The tumor microenvironment, which is formed by the reciprocal interactions between tumor cells, the surrounding stromal, and inflammatory cells, promotes tumorigenesis by influencing each step, including tumor angiogenesis, proliferation, and progression (Grivennikov et al., 2010). Autoimmune diseases are chronic inflammatory disorders characterized by immune-mediated self-tissue destruction due to loss of self-tolerance (Qiu et al., 2020). In autoimmune diseases, damage occurs in one or more organs as a result of inappropriate activation of T cells, B cells, or both (Davidson and Diamond, 2001). In addition, autoantibody production is a characteristic feature of autoimmune diseases.

Although the exact mechanism is not yet clearly understood, it is known that autoimmune diseases are associated with a high risk of malignancy. Similar inflammatory conditions are involved in the development of cancer and autoimmune diseases. In the emergence of these two diseases, the immune system is triggered through some biological pathways, and they gain the ability to proliferation, increased cell survival, and migration with growth factors and cytokine interactions.

The relationship between cancer and autoimmune diseases is bidirectional. While an increased risk of malignancy has been observed in various autoimmune diseases to date, autoimmune conditions have been described in patients with neoplastic diseases. In this article, it is aimed to discuss the relationship between the most common autoimmune diseases and malignancies and to mention the increasing cancer types associated with autoimmunity.

Systemic Lupus Erythematosus

Systemic lupus erythematosus (SLE) is an autoimmune disease that can cause mild to life-threatening damage to many organs such as joints, skin, brain, lungs, kidneys, and blood vessels. The etiology of SLE is not clearly known, but environmental, genetic, and hormonal changes are among the known causes. With the new treatment approaches in the management of SLE, the life expectancy of patients has increased, so late complications associated with the disease are observed and diagnosed more frequently. Known factors in the etiopathogenesis of the disease and chronic inflammation are common factors that also predispose to the emergence of malignancy in this patient population

(Bernatsky et al., 2002). It was observed that the frequency of hematologic malignancies, lung, thyroid, and skin cancers increased in SLE. On the other hand, it has been determined that the risk of cervical and prostate cancer is reduced.

Multicenter observational studies to estimate the cancer risk in SLE compared to the general population have shown an increased risk of malignancy in SLE patients. According to the Swedish National Cancer Registry, in a population-based cohort study that included 5715 SLE patients between 1964 and 1995, 443 malignancies were followed over a 15-year observation period. When the results were evaluated, the overall risk increased by 25% (standardized incidence ratio (SIR) 1.25, confidence interval (CI) 95% 1.14-1.37). An increased risk of non-Hodgkin lymphoma (NHL), lung cancer, and squamous cell skin cancer was observed. While the highest risk was observed in NHL (SIR: 2.86, CI 95% 1.96-4.04) with an approximately 3-fold increase, lung (SIR: 1.73, CI 95% 1.25-2.32) and squamous cell skin cancers (SIR:1.53, CI 95% 0.98 -2.28) were also frequently detected (Bjornadal et al., 2002).

In order to estimate the cancer risk in SLE according to the general population, 644 cancers were detected in a cohort study of 16409 patients from 30 centers. The increased risk of malignancy in patients with SLE has been confirmed with the estimated SIR was 1.15 (CI 95% 1.05-1.27). Similarly to Swedish data, the risk of hematologic malignancy was found to be higher, especially the incidence of NHL (SIR 4.39, 95% CI 3.46, 5.49) and leukemia. In addition, it was determined that the risk of solid cancers such as vulva (SIR: 3.78, 95% CI 1.52-7.78), lung (SIR: 1.30, 95% CI 1.04-1.60), thyroid (SIR: 1.76, 95% CI 1.13-2.61) and possibly liver (SIR: 1.87, 95% CI 0.97-3.27) was high. On the other hand, a reduced risk of breast (SIR: 0.73, 95% CI 0.61-0.88), endometrial (SIR: 0.44, 95% CI 0.23-0.77), and possibly ovarian cancer (SIR: 0.64, 95% CI 0.34-1.10) has been reported (Bernatsky et al., 2013).

The Danish cohort study, with the same endpoint, has recently published results assessing cancer risk in cutaneous lupus erythematosus (CLE) or SLE. When the follow-up results of 5310 patients were examined, it was reported that the frequency of hematologic, pancreatic, lung and skin cancers increased, especially the risk of NHL was reported to be 3-4 times higher (Westermann et al., 2021).

In SLE, cytokines such as interleukin-6 (IL-6), 10 (IL-10) and B cell activating factor (BAFF) are associated with the B cell life cycle. As a result of chronic stimulation, BAFF levels increase, so the immune system continues to trigger. A similar mechanism is involved in the pathogenesis of B-cell-associated malignancy (Schivakumar and Ansell, 2006).

Patients with new-onset SLE and new-onset NHL diagnosed between 1998 and 2012 were included in a nationwide population-based study to evaluate whether there is a bidirectional association between SLE and NHL in Taiwan. Of the 16417 patients with SLE, 512 cancer occurred, including 34 with NHL. The data confirmed the highest SIR for NHL (SIR: 4.2, 95% CI 2.9-5.9). Of the 25069 patients with NHL, 14 SLE occurred with a high SIR (SIR: 2.0, 95% CI 1.1-3.4). In both cases the highest rates were reported in the first year after diagnosis of the disease (Wang et al., 2019).

The results of previous studies showed that the use of immunosuppressive drugs and anti-malarial drugs increased the risk of malignancy in SLE, but today it cannot be said that this effect is clearly related to the use of these agents (Bernatsky et al., 2005; Tincani et al., 2009). Comprehensive studies with higher number of patients and longer follow-up are needed to evaluate this effect clearly.

Despite the aforementioned increased risk of malignancy with SLE, a reduced risk of prostate cancer has also been observed in men with SLE. In the data of 6068 male patients diagnosed with SLE, the risk of developing prostate cancer was 0.72 (CI 95% 0.57-0.89) compared to the normal population. Decreased adrenal hormones are thought to be effective in this regard, as well as genetic alterations (Bernatsky et al., 2011).

Systemic Sclerosis (Scleroderma)

Systemic sclerosis (SSc) is an autoimmune connective tissue disease in which skin involvement is predominant, vessels, and multiple organs can also be affected. Fibroblast activation triggered by inflammation, the development of vascular damage, and fibrosis constitute the basic mechanism. Several combined factors such as genetics, viral exposures and environmental factors appear to influence the risk of developing scleroderma. The incidence of lymphoma, skin cancer, and lung cancer has increased significantly in scleroderma. Barrett's esophagus and pulmonary fibrosis, which can be seen in scleroderma, are predisposing factors to the development of malignancy.

The nationwide Danish National Register reported an incidence of cancer in 2040 SSc patients, with 222 cases of cancer identified. The incidence of cancer increased 1.5 times compared to the general population (SIR: 1.5, CI

95% 1.3-1.7). Lung (SIR: 1.6, CI 95% 1.2-2.0) and hematologic (SIR: 2.5, CI 95% 1.5-4.0) cancers were the most common types (Olesen et al., 2010).

In 2013, three meta-analyzes were published that analyzed the findings of several studies that evaluated the risk of developing SSc and malignancy. In the first meta-analysis, which included 6 studies, it was reported that the cancer risk increased 1.4 times (SIR: 1.41, 95% CI 1.18–1.68), and the risk was higher in men 1.85 (95% CI 1.49–2.31) than in women 1.33 (95% CI 1.18–1.49). When organ-specific results were evaluated, lung (SIR: 3.18, 95% CI 2.09–4.85), liver (SIR: 4.36, 95% CI 2.00–9.51), hematologic system (SIR: 2.57, 95% CI 1.79–3.68), and bladder (SIR: 2.00, 95% CI 1.06–3.77), as well as of NHL (SIR: 2.26, 95% CI 1.21–4.23) risks were found to be significantly more common. The risk has been reported to be higher in the first 12 months after the diagnosis of SSc (SIR: 2.79, 95% CI 1.81–4.31) (Onishi et al., 2013). The second meta-analysis pooled 16 studies, including more than 7000 patients, reported an increase in cancer risk with a relative risk of 1.75 (RR 95% CI 1.41–2.18). Lung (RR: 4.4, 95% CI 2.1–9.1) and hematologic (RR: 2.2, 95% CI 1.5–3.3) cancers had the highest incidence (Bonifazi et al., 2013). Finally, in a meta-analysis that included 7 studies involving 7183 patients, they reported SIRs for cancers of the lung, NHL, and hematopoetic cancer of 3.14 (95% CI 2.02–4.89), 2.68 (95% CI 1.58–4.56), and 2.57 (95% CI 1.79–3.68), respectively (Zhang et al., 2013).

In previous studies, it was stated that the presence of anti-RNA polymerase III increases the risk of malignancy in patients with scleroderma and shortens the development of cancer (Mecoli et al., 2021; Pontifex et al., 2007).

Factors such as male gender, smoking history, and being diagnosed with scleroderma at an older age, diffuse cutaneous involvement, are associated with an elevated risk of cancer in SSc. According to the results of previous studies, it may be possible to say that the severity of scleroderma is important in the development of malignancy and that the affected organ and the organ undergoing malignant transformation are the same. The frequency of Barrett's esophagus is increased in scleroderma, it is found in the etiology of esophageal cancer. Interstitial lung disease and pulmonary fibrosis are seen due to lung involvement in SSc, although it is a controversial issue, the presence of interstitial lung disease is considered a risk factor for lung cancer (Weeding et al., 2020).

Rheumatoid Arthritis

Rheumatoid arthritis (RA) is a chronic inflammatory disorder characterized by predominantly joint involvement, from inflammation to deformity. In addition, extra-articular findings such as skin, eyes, lungs, heart, and blood vessels are also frequently observed. As in other rheumatologic autoimmune diseases, the risk of lymphoma increases in patients with rheumatoid arthritis. It is known that the risk of lung cancer and malignant melanoma increases, on the other hand, colorectal and urogenital cancers are seen at a lower rate compared to the normal population.

According to cumulative evidence, the probability of developing cancer is known to be higher in the early years of the disease and in cases with more severe disease (Baecklung et al., 2006).

In an Asian cohort study, 935 of 23644 patients with RA developed malignancy. The risk of hematologic cancer was found to be high and young age was reported as a negative risk factor (Chen et al., 2011).

In a meta-analysis published by Smitten et al. in 2008, it was reported that the cancer risk increased in RA cases compared to the general population and increased the risk of lymphoma (SIR: 2.08, 95% CI 1.80-2.39), especially HL (SIR: 3.29, 95% CI 2.56-4.22). Lung cancer with an SIR of 1.63 (95% CI 1.43-1.87) was also found to increase. On the contrary, it was observed that the frequency of colorectal (SIR: 0.77, 95% CI 0.65-0.90) and breast cancer (SIR: 0.84, 95% CI 0.79-0.90) decreased (Smitten et al., 2008).

Data from a recently published prospective study were associated with an increased risk of lung cancer (HR: 1.71, 95% CI 1.28-2.28) and lymphoma (HR: 2.01, 95% CI 1.34-3.01) in patients with rheumatoid arthritis, however, the risk of prostate (HR: 0.62, 95% CI 0.41-0.94) and breast (HR: 0.64, 95% CI 0.46-0.89) cancers has been shown to be reduced, confirming the results of previous studies (He et al., 2022).

Sjögren Syndrome

Sjögren's syndrome (SS) is one of the most common autoimmune diseases characterized by lymphocyte infiltration into the lacrimal and salivary glands and impairing the function of their secretory units. The risk of lymphoproliferative cancer in patients with primary Sjögren's syndrome, especially various types of lymphoma, is higher than other autoimmune diseases, with an increase of more than 6 times (Smedby et al., 2006).

Exposure to infectious agents such as Helicobacter pylori, p53 mutation and B cell-related disorders are among the possible risk factors for this transformation.

In a meta-analysis evaluating the results of 14523 pSS patients, including 14 studies, the risk of NHL (pooled RR: 13.76, 95% CI 8.53-18.99) and thyroid cancer (pooled RR: 2.58, 95% CI 1.14-4.03) risk were found to be significantly higher. The overall cancer rate also increased compared to the general population (pooled RR: 1.53 95% CI 1.17-1.88), although it is not yet clear whether this increase is a reflection of an increased risk of NHL, a point noted by the authors (Liang et al., 2014).

In the Korean study that evaluated the risk of malignancy in patients with pSS, 6369 patients over 50 years of age were included and 310 of these patients developed solid and 47 hematologic malignancies. Site-specific malignancy SIR values for NHL, multiple myeloma and oropharynx are 6.45 (95% CI 4.05-8.83), 4.88 (95% CI 2.00-7.76), 4.16 (95% CI 1.90-6.42), respectively. Also, lung cancer in men (SIR: 2.50, 95% CI 1.02-3.99) and thyroid cancer in women (SIR: 1.44, 95% CI 1.04-1.84) were increased. The authors emphasized the increased risk of NHL, especially in patients over 50 years of age, as well as the risk of oropharyngeal, lung, and thyroid cancer (Kang et al., 2020).

It also affects survival rates in patients with pSS who develop lymphoma. In the meta-analysis evaluating the risk of mortality in pSS patients. In addition to cardiovascular diseases, solid organ and lymphoid malignancies have been reported to be the leading causes of mortality (Singh et al., 2015).

The underlying causes of lymphoma development in pSS are still unclear. Many theories have been proposed to explain this relationship, exposure to environmental factors (EBV, cytomegalovirus, hepatitis C virus, or ultraviolet radiation), and genetic susceptibility through HLA-related immune system changes.

Mucosal-associated lymphoid tissue lymphoma (MALT) is the most common type of lymphoma in SS, H pylori is the infectious agent involved in the pathogenesis of MALT (Routsias et al., 2013). Systemic extraepithelial manifestations, low complement component C4 serum levels, and mixed type II cryoglobulinemia are among other high-risk factors for lymphoma development (Stergiou et al., 2020).

Idiopathic Inflammatory Myopathy

Idiopathic inflammatory myopathies (IIM) are a group of rare disorders that include polymyositis (PM), dermatomyositis (DM), and autoimmune necrotizing myopathies, characterized by inflammation of the skeletal muscles. The risk of cancer in patients with IIM is greatly increased compared to the general population. Adenocarcinomas of the lung, ovaries, breast, pancreas, bladder, cervix, and gastrointestinal tract, as well as hematologic malignancies, including Hodgkin lymphoma, are cancers associated with myositis. While malignancy can be detected simultaneously with the diagnosis of IIM, it can usually be detected within the first 3 years after diagnosis. There is a strong link between dermatomyositis and malignancy. In some cases, myositis, which regresses with cancer treatment, may reappear with tumor recurrence.

According to cohort studies and meta-analyses conducted to date, the risk of cancer in DM is at least 2 times higher than in PM. In a meta-analysis that included case-control and cohort studies with 1078 IIM patients, the overall odds ratio (OR) for cancers related to DM and PM was 4.4 (95% CI 3.0-6.6) and 2.1 (95% CI 1.4-3.3), respectively (Zantos et al., 1994). A nationwide cohort study of 1655 IIM patients from Taiwan found that cancer risk was significantly higher in DM (SIR: 5.11, 95% CI 5.01-5.22) than PM (SIR: 2.15, 95% CI 2.08-2.22) (Chen et al., 2010). In a meta-analysis of 4538 patients with IIM from 5 studies, it was reported that overall relative risk increased with IIM, especially in DM (4.66 and 1.75). When examined by gender, the SIR was found to be 5.29 in men with DM and 4.56 in women, while the SIR was found to be 1.62 in men with PM and 2.02 in women. The risk of malignancy is highest in the first 3 years after diagnosis, and the risk continues thereafter (Qiang et al., 2017).

In another meta-analysis of 20 studies, the pooled RR for DM, PM and DM/PM were 5.50 (95% CI 4.31-6.70), 1.62 (95% CI 1.19-2.04) and 4.07 (95% CI 3.02-5.12), respectively, compared to the normal population. The risk of cancer was higher in the first year after diagnosis of myositis and in men (Yang et al., 2015).

The clinical factors that increase the risk of IIM-associated cancer and the requirements for cancer screening are outlined in a comprehensive newly published meta-analysis that included 69 studies. The DM subtype (RR 2.21), older age (weighted mean differences (WMD) 11.19), male sex (RR 1.53), cutaneous ulceration (RR 2.73), dysphagia (RR 2.09) and anti-TIF-1 gamma positivity (RR 4.66) have been found to be associated with cancer development. PM (RR 0.49) and clinically amyopathic DM (RR 0.44) subtypes, interstitial lung disease (RR 0.49), Raynaud's phenomenon (RR 0.61), high lactate dehydrogenase (WMD 336.52) or creatine kinase (WMD 1189.96) levels, and anti-EJ (RR 0.17) or anti-Jo1 (RR 0.45) positivity reduced the risk of cancer. The authors commented that the risk of cancer with PM was low, but the risk was still increased with PM compared to the general population. In addition, when the results of cancer screening studies were evaluated, it was seen that screening of IIM patients without symptoms with CT was beneficial in detecting occult malignancies (Oldroyd et al., 2021).

In another study, it was proven that the clinical risk factors such as older age at disease onset, male gender, cutaneous necrosis, dysphagia, ulceration and vasculitis, refractory myositis, rapid onset of myositis, and autoantibodies such as anti-TIF1-gamma and antinuclear matrix protein-2 increased cancer risk in IIM (Moghadam-Kia et al., 2020).

In the studies included in the meta-analysis of Yang et al., many types of cancer were reported to be associated with myositis rather than an increased risk in one or a few types. There is an increased risk in most malignancies, except stomach, prostate, endometrial cancers, lymphoma, Hodgkin's disease, and melanoma (Yang et al., 2015).

Although PM and DM have similar diseases within the IIM, the types of organ-specific cancers that can occur may be different, despite the increased risk of cancer. Lung, breast, kidney, endometrial, cervical, bladder, and thyroid cancers, lymphoma, myeloma, and brain tumor are among the PM related malignancies. Lung, breast, ovarian, colorectal, cervical, bladder, esophageal, pancreatic, nasopharyngeal, and kidney cancers are the cancer types whose frequency increases in patients with DM (Yang et al., 2015).

Inflammatory Bowel Disease

Inflammatory bowel disease (IBD) is divided into two subgroups called Ulcerative Colitis (UC) and Crohn's disease (CD) that are characterized by chronic inflammation of the gastrointestinal tract. Both CD and UC have been associated with an elevated risk of developing colorectal cancer (CRC) due to long-standing chronic inflammation. As far as we know, factors such as the duration of the disease and the widespread involvement constitute important factors that may predispose to the development of cancer in this process. The associated CRC in IBD appear at a younger age and at a more advanced stage than those that develop sporadically. CRC development is a major concern in the management of IBD.

Ulcerative Colitis

UC is a disease of the rectum and colon, which is the last part of the gastrointestinal tract. Inflammation is seen in the mucosal layer and damage that starts from the rectum continues toward the colon. It is known that the risk of developing CRC is high in patients with UC, but this issue has been controversial for a long time. The first study to clarify this issue in a comprehensive meta-analysis of 116 studies by Eaden et al. was published in 2001 (Eaden et al., 2001). The overall prevalence of CRC in UC was estimated to be 3.7% (95% CI 3.2-4.2). The outcomes were classified according to 10-year intervals of duration of the disease. The cumulative risk of CRC was 2% at 10 years, 8% at 20 years, and 18% at 30 years.

However, subsequent studies show that the incidence of CRC in UC patients is reduced compared to the general population. Nevertheless, it is noted that the risk is still high in those with long-standing widespread colitis. In a meta-analysis of 81 studies including 181923 patients, the overall incidence rate of CRC in patients with UC was 1.58 per 1000 py (95% CI 1.39-1.76). Similarly, when the CCR risk was analyzed according to the duration of the disease, it was found to be the highest in the third 10-year interval (4.55/1000 py 95% CI 2.64–6.46) (Castaño-Milla et al., 2014).

In the meta-analysis published in 2017, data from 44 studies that examined the relationship between ulcerative colitis and CRC in the Asian population were presented. Of the 31287 UC patients, 293 developed CRC. The overall prevalence was 0.85% (95% CI 0.65-1.04). The risk of CRC at the time-specific assessment was 0.02% (95% CI 0.00-0.04), 4 81% (3.26-6.36) and 13.91% (7.09-20.72) at 10, 20, and 30 years, respectively (Bopanna et al., 2017).

Colorectal cancer is a substantial complication that contributes significantly to morbidity and mortality. Because of this awareness, patients diagnosed with UC should have regular follow-up and endoscopic examinations according to the guidelines. A systematic review and meta-analysis results of 164 studies conducted to determine the risk factors that may be associated with the development of colorectal neoplasia in IBD patients have been published recently. In univariate analysis, extensive disease was the only risk factor that was found to be strongly significant. Low-grade dysplasia, concomitant primary sclerosing cholangitis, strictures, postinflammatory polyps, family history of CRC and UC were defined moderate risk factors. Any dysplasia, aneuploidy, resection of the colon segment, male gender and age were determined as a low-risk group. Colonoscopic surveillance, 5-Aminosalicylic Acid, thiopurines, statin use and smoking are stated as protective factors (Wijnands et al., 2021).

A recent study published in JAMA Oncology, used data from 478753 participants to explore the relationship between cancers and "immune-mediated diseases", including many autoimmune diseases. In addition, the association of organ-specific immune-mediated disease with local and extralocal cancer risk was also tested. It has been shown that there is a stronger relationship between organ-specific immune-mediated diseases and local cancer risk, while in some immune-mediated diseases, there is an increased risk of cancer in nearby or distant organs or in different systems. According to study findings, some autoimmune diseases and local cancer risk are as follows: celiac disease for small intestine cancer (HR: 6.89, 95% CI 2.18-21.75), primary biliary cholangitis for hepatobiliary cancer (HR: 42.12, 95% CI 20.76-85.44), and autoimmune hepatitis for hepatobiliary cancer (HR: 21.26, 95% CI 6.79-66.61). In ulcerative colitis, the risk of local cancer was higher, and the risk of extralocal cancer was also present (HR: 1.73, 95% CI 1.26-2.39; HR: 1.30, 95% CI 1.13-1.49) (He et al., 2022).

Crohn's Disease

Crohn's disease (CD) can involve any part of the gastrointestinal tract. It is characterized by healthy areas with a patchy appearance and damage to all layers of the intestinal wall. The risk of malignancy is not limited to a single segment, as in UC, due to the possibility that the disease is ubiquitous in the gastrointestinal tract. The risk of CRC appears to be slightly lower in CD than in UC. Patchy distribution of CD may explain the lower risk of CRC. In a 2006 meta-analysis, an increase was observed in gastrointestinal tract cancers, and the risk of colorectal, colon and ileal cancers was reported as 2.5 (95% CI 1.3-4.7), 4.5 (95% CI 1.3-14.9) and 1.1 (95% CI 0.8-1.5), respectively. The duration of the disease is a prognostic feature, as is UC. The cumulative incidence of CRC in patients diagnosed with CD was 2.9% (95% CI 1.5–5.3%) at 10 years, 5.6% (95% CI 3.1–10.4) at 20 years, and 8.3% (95% CI 4.5–15.1) at 30 years (Canavan et al., 2006).

It is known that there is a strong relationship between CD and small bowel cancer. Small bowel cancer is rarely seen among all cancers of the gastrointestinal system, so the absolute risk remains low. A 2007 meta-analysis of 60122 patients with CD found an increased risk of small bowel, colon, extraintestinal cancers, and lymphoma with relative risk ratios of 28.4, 2.4, 1.27 and 1.42 (von Roon et al., 2007). In the last published meta-analysis of 7344 patients, in which the relationship between intestinal cancer and CD was analyzed, the incidence rates of CRC and small bowel cancer were 2.08 (95% CI 1.43-3.02) and 22.01 (95% CI 9.10-53.25), the prevalence was 57/7344 (0.77%) and 17/7344 (0.23%), respectively (Uchino et al., 2021). Since there is no screening method for small bowel cancer, it is recommended to be careful in this regard.

On the other hand, anorectal cancers associated with CD are extremely rare (Slesser et al., 2013). Anorectal cancer is often diagnosed in an advanced stage, unfortunately it has a poor prognosis. In this respect, surveillance colonoscopy is extremely important for early diagnosis (Ueda et al., 2020).

Primary Sclerosing Cholangitis

Primary sclerosing cholangitis (PSC) is a rare, chronic, and progressive biliary tract disease as a result of inflammation and sclerosis that causes structural disorders such as stenosis of the bile ducts. This rare autoimmune disease is often seen together with IBD. Compared to the general population, patients with PSC have a markedly increased risk of hepatobiliary cancer, particularly cholangiocarcinoma. Colorectal cancer has also increased with PSC, especially if there is a concurrent diagnosis of IBD, this risk increases at least 4 times. Many studies have also shown an increased risk of pancreatic and small bowel cancers.

The most common malignancy in patients with PSC is cholangiocarcinoma, which can develop within the first year after the diagnosis of PSC at a rate of 30-50%. It has been reported in many studies that it may occur in patients with PSC, with an increased frequency compared to the normal population. The cumulative incidence according to the duration of the disease increases with each passing year, there are studies showing that it is 7% for 5 years, 8-11% for 10 years, and 9-20% for lifetime (Song et al., 2020).

A matched cohort study of 1432 PSC patients was recently published assessing the risk of both gastrointestinal and other cancers. 88% of PSC patients had concomitant IBD. Cancer in PSC patients increased significantly with HR 120.9 for hepatobiliary cancer, 7.5 for colorectal cancer, 8.0 for pancreatic cancer, 4.2 for gastric cancer, 21.1 for small bowel cancer, and 3.0 for lymphoma (Lundberg Båve et al., 2021).

Autoimmune Hepatitis

Autoimmune hepatitis (AIH) is a disease that results in progressive destruction of the hepatic parenchyma caused by loss of immunological tolerance to hepatocyte-specific autoantigens. There is a risk of hepatocellular carcinoma at any time in the course of AIH, especially after the development of cirrhosis. In an analysis of 11 studies involving 8460 AIH patients, 0-12.3% of patients developed HCC. Although the risk of HCC was reported to be 0.2%-12.3% in AIH-associated cirrhosis, this rate was reported to be 1.03% in cases without cirrhosis (Valean et al., 2019).

Risk of Malignancy Associated with Treatment of Autoimmune Diseases

To date, in many studies, drugs used in the treatment of autoimmune diseases have been identified as a potentially carcinogenic factor. In this respect, studies on certain drugs that have a risk in the development of cancer will be mentioned.

Disease-modifying antirheumatic drugs (DMARD) such as methotrexate (MTX) and azathioprine are used in the treatment of RA, but it is not yet clear whether treatment of RA with DMARD will affect the risk of cancer in RA. In 1997, Bologna et al. compared two groups that used and did not use MTX for the treatment of RA and stated that there was no difference between the arms in the development of malignancy triggered by MTX (Bologna et al., 1997). However, in the following years, studies were published reporting that it especially increased the risk of lymphoma (Franklin et al., 2006). Recently, in a study comparing patients with RA using and not using MTX in 2020, the risk of cancer was found to be higher in those who did not use MTX, contrary to expectations. Furthermore, the risk has been reported to be lower in those using medium and high doses than in those using low doses (Perng et al., 2020). In previous studies, the use of azathioprine in the treatment of RA has been shown to increase the risk of lymphoma (Matteson et al., 1991). It has also been reported that the daily dose of the drug is higher at doses greater than 300 mg.

Cyclophosphamide is an alkylating agent used in the treatment of RA, SLE, and vasculitis. During the 20-year follow-up period, the cancer risk was reported to increase in patients using Cyclophosphamide for the treatment of RA compared to the control group. It was observed that the frequency of bladder cancer and skin cancer increased, and the use of high doses significantly increased the risk of bladder cancer (Radis et al., 1995).

Biological agents are mainly used in RA and IBD therapy. Etanercept, Infliximab, Adalimumab, Certolizumab, and Golimumab are anti-TNF-α agents. In a study evaluating the cancer risk associated with the use of Anti-TNFα in 29555 patients, the majority of whom were patients with RA and IBD, it was shown that the cancer risk did not increase compared to other drugs (Haynes et al., 2013). Many meta-analyses have also supported that the use of these agents does not increase the risk of cancer in general (Ramiro et al., 2014; Bongartz et al., 2009). No significant increase in the risk of malignancy was observed in 3316 patients with RA using etanercept as an anti-TNF agent (Bongartz et al., 2009).

However, a meta-analysis published in 2006 showed an association between infliximab and adalimumab with an increased risk of cancer, particularly lymphoma, colorectal, breast, and lung types. The pooled odds ratio for malignancy was 3.3 (95% CI 1.2-9.1). Higher doses of anti-TNF antibodies associated with an increased cancer risk (Bongartz et al., 2006).

Conclusion

Although the cause cannot be fully explained, there is a strong relationship between autoimmune diseases and malignancy. In patients diagnosed with autoimmune disease, increasing types of cancer specific to that disease have been clearly explained in many studies. In addition, due to many drugs used in the treatment of autoimmune diseases, the development of malignancy may be triggered. In the individual management of these patients, it is extremely important to be aware of the risk of developing cancer, to detect possible cancer development early, and to pay attention to screening programs.

References

Baecklung, E., Iliadou, A. Askling, J. Ekbom, A. Backlin, C. Granath, F. Catrina, AI. Rosenguist, R. Feltelius, N. Sundström, C. and Klareskog, L. (2006). Association of chronic inflammation, not its treatment, with increased lymphoma risk in rheumatoid arthritis. *Arthritis & Rheumatology,* 54(3):692-701. doi: 10.1002/art.21675.

Bernatsky, S., Clarke, A. and Ramsey-Goldman, R. (2002). Malignancy and systemic lupus erythematosus. *Current Rheumatology Reports,* 4(4):351-358. doi: 10.1007/ s11926-002-0045-6.

Bernatsky, S., Ramsey-Goldman, R. and Clarke, A. (2005). Malignancy risk in autoimmune rheumatic diseases. *Discovery Medicine,* 5(30):534-537.

Bernatsky, S., Ramsey-Goldman, R. Gordon, C. and Clarke, AE. (2011). Prostate cancer in systemic lupus erythematosus. *The International Journal of Cancer,* 129(12): 2966-2969. doi: 10.1002/ijc.25956.

Bernatsky, S., Ramsey-Goldman, R. Labrecque, J. Joseph, L. Boivin, JF., et al. (2013). Cancer risk in systemic lupus: an updated international multi-centre cohort study. *The Journal of Autoimmunity,* 42:130-135. doi: 10.1016/j.jaut.2012.12.009.

Bjornadal, L., Lofstrom, B. Yin, L. Lundberg, IE. and Ekbom, A. (2002). Increased cancer incidence in a Swedish cohort of patients with systemic lupus erythematosus. *Scandinavian Journal of Rheumatology,* 31(2):66-71. doi: 10.1080/03009740252937 568.

Bologna, C., Picot, MC. Jorgensen, C. Viu, P. Verdier, R. and Sany, J. (1997). Study of eight cases of cancer in 426 rheumatoid arthritis patients treated with methotrexate. *Annals of the Rheumatic Diseases,* 56(2):97-102. doi: 10.1136/ard.56.2.97.

Bongartz, T., Sutton, AJ. Sweeting, MJ. Buchan, I. Matteson, EL. and Montori, V. (2006). Anti-TNF antibody therapy in rheumatoid arthritis and the risk of serious infections and malignancies: Systematic review and meta-analysis of rare harmful effects in randomized controlled trials. *JAMA,* 295(19):2275-2285. doi: 10.1001/jama.295. 19.2275.

Bongartz, T., Warren, FC. Mines, D. Matteson,L. Abrams, KR. and Sutton, AJ. (2009). Etanercept therapy in rheumatoid arthritis and the risk of malignancies: a systematic review and individual patient data meta-analysis of randomised controlled trials. *Annals of the Rheumatic Diseases*, 68(7):1177-1183. doi: 10.1136/ard.2008. 094904.

Bonifazi, M., Tramacere, I. Pomponio, G. Gabrielli, B. Avvedimento, EV. La Vecchia, C. Negri, E. and Gabrielli, A. (2013). Systemic sclerosis (scleroderma) and cancer risk: systematic review and meta-analysis of observational studies. *Rheumatology (Oxford),* 52(1):143–154. doi: 10.1093/rheumatology/kes303.

Bopanna, S., Ananthakrishnan, AN. Kedia, S. Yajnik, V. and Ahuja, V. (2017). Risk of colorectal cancer in Asian patients with ulcerative colitis: a systematic review and meta-analysis. *The Lancet Gastroenterology & Hepatology,* 2(4):269-276. doi: 10.1016/S2468-1253(17)30004-3. Epub 2017 Feb 21.

Canavan, C., Abrams, KR. and Mayberry, J. (2006). Meta-analysis: colorectal and small bowel cancer risk in patients with Crohn's disease. *Alimentary Pharmacology & Therapeutics, 15*;23(8):1097-1104. doi: 10.1111/j.1365-2036.2006.02854.x.

Castaño-Milla, C., Chaparro, M. and Gisbert, JP. (2014). Systematic review with meta-analysis: the declining risk of colorectal cancer in ulcerative colitis. *Alimentary Pharmacology & Therapeutics,* 39(7):645-659. doi: 10.1111/apt.12651.

Chen, YJ., Chang, YT. Wang, CB. and Wu, CY. (2011). The risk of cancer in patients with rheumatoid arthritis: A nationwide cohort study in Taiwan. *Arthritis & Rheumatology,* 63(2):352-358. doi: 10.1002/art.30134.

Chen, YJ., Wu, CY. Huang, YL. Wang, CB. Shen, JL. and Chang, YT. (2010). Cancer risks of dermatomyositis and polymyositis: a nationwide cohort study in Taiwan. *Arthritis Research and Therapy,* 12(2):R70. doi: 10.1186/ar2987.

Davidson, A., Diamond, B. Autoimmune diseases. (2001). *The New England Journal of Medicine,* 345(5):340-350. doi: 10.1056/NEJM200108023450506.

Eaden, JA., Abrams, KR. and Mayberry, JF. (2001). The risk of colorectal cancer inulcerative colitis: a meta-analysis. *Gut,* 48(4):526-535. doi: 10.1136/gut.48.4.526.

Franklin, J., Lunt, M. Bunn, D. Symmons, D. and Silman, A. (2006). Incidence of lymphoma in a large primary care derived cohort of cases of inflammatory poly-arthritis. *Annals of the Rheumatic Diseases,* 65(5):617-622. doi: 10.1136/ard.2005.04 4784.

Grivennikov, SI., Greten, R. and Karin, M. (2010). Immunity, inflammation, and cancer. *Cell,* 140 (6) 883–899. DOI: 10.1016/j.cell.2010.01.025.

Haynes, K., Beukelman, T. Curtis, JR. Newcomb, C. Herrinton, LJ. Graham, DJ. Solomon, DH. Griffin, MR. Chen, L. Liu, L. Saag, KG. Lewis, JD. and SABER Collaboration. (2013). Tumor necrosis factor alpha inhibitor therapy and cancer risk in chronic immune-mediated diseases. *Arthritis & Rheumatology*, 65(1):48-58. doi: 10.1002/ art.37740.

He, MM., Lo, CH. Wang, K. Polychronidis, G. Wang, L. Zhong, R. Knudsen, MD. Fang, Z. Song, M. (2022). Immune-mediated diseases associated with cancer risks. *JAMA Oncology,* 8(2):209-219. doi: 10.1001/jamaoncol.2021.5680.

Kang, J., Kim, H. Kim, J. Choi, S. Jung, SY. Jang, EJ. Cho, SK. and Sung, YK. (2020). Risk of malignancy in Korean patients with primary Sjögren's syndrome. *International Journal of Rheumatic Diseases,* 23(9):1240-1247. doi: 10.1111/1756-185X.13927.

Liang, Y., Yang, Z. Qin, B. and Zhong, R. (2014). Primary Sjögren's syndrome and malignancy risk: a systematic review and meta-analysis. *Annals of the Rheumatic Diseases,* 73(6):1151-6. doi: 10.1136/annrheumdis-2013-203305.

Lundberg Båve, A., Bergquist, A. Bottai, M. Warnqvist, A. von Seth, E. and Nordenvall, C. (2021). Increased risk of cancer in patients with primary sclerosing cholangitis. *Hepatology International,* 15(5):1174-1182. doi: 10.1007/s12072-021-10214-6.

Matteson, EL., Hickey, AR. Maguire, L. Tilson, HH. and Urowitz, MB. (1991). Occurrence of neoplasia in patients with rheumatoid arthritis enrolled in a DMARD registry. Rheumatoid arthritis azathioprine registry Steering Committee. *Journal of Rheumatology,* 18(6):809-814.

Mecoli, CA., Rosen, A. Casciola-Rosen, L. and Shah, A. (2021). Advances at the interface of cancer and systemic sclerosis. *Journal of Scleroderma and Related Disorders,* 6(1): 50–57. DOI: 10.1177/2397198320905983.

Moghadam-Kia, S., Oddis, CV. Ascherman, DP. and Aggarwal, R. (2020). Risk factors and cancer screening in myositis. *Rheumatic Disease Clinics of North America,* 46(3):565-576. doi: 10.1016/j.rdc.2020.05.006.

Oldroyd, AGS., Allard, AB. Callen, JP. Chinoy, H. Chung, L. Fiorentino, D. George, MD. Gordon, P. Kolstad, K. Kurtzman, DJB. Machado, PM. McHugh, NJ. Postolova, A. Selva-O'Callaghan, A. Schmidt, J. Tansley, S. Vleugels, RA. Werth, VP. and Aggarwal, R. Systematic review and meta-analysis to inform cancer screening guidelines in idiopathic inflammatory myopathies. *Rheumatology (Oxford).,* 60(6): 2615-2628. doi:10.1093/rheumatology/keab166.

Perng, WT., Hung, YM. Chang, R. Lin, CL. Chiou, JY. Chen, HH. Kao, CH. and Wei, JC. (2020). Methotrexate at middle and high accumulative doses might be associated with lower risk of new-onset cancers in patients with rheumatoid arthritis: a nationwide population-based cohort study. *Therapeutic Advances in Musculoskeletal Disease,* 29;12:1759720X20981221. doi: 10.1177/1759720X20981221.

Pontifex, EK., Hill, CL. and Roberts-Thomson, P. (2007). Risk factors for lung cancer in patients with scleroderma: a nested case-control study. *Annals of the Rheumatic Diseases,* 66(4):551-553. doi: 10.1136/ard.2006.056424.

Qiang, JK., Kim, WB. Baibergenova, A. and Alhusayen, R. (2017). Risk of malignancy in dermatomyositis and polymyositis. *Journal of Cutaneous Medicine and Surgery,* 21(2):131–136. doi: 10.1177/1203475416665601. Epub 2016 Aug 20.

Qiu, R., Zhou, L. Ma, Y. Zhou, L. Liang, T. Shi, L. Long, J. and Yuan, D. (2018). Regulatory t cell plasticity and stability and autoimmune diseases. *Clinical Reviews in Allergy & Immunology*, 2020 Feb,58(1).52-70. https://doi.org/10.1007/s12016-018-8721-0.

Olesen, AB., Svaerke, C. Farkas, DK. and Sorensen, HT. (2010). Systemic sclerosis and the risk of cancer: A nationwide populationbased cohort study. *British Journal of Dermatology,* 163:800-6. doi: 10.1111/j.1365-2133.2010.09861.x.

Onishi, A., Sugiyama, D. Kumagai, S. and Morinobu, A. (2013). Cancer incidence in systemic sclerosis: meta-analysis of population-based cohort studies. *Arthritis & Rheumatology,* 65(7):1913-1921. doi: 10.1002/art.37969.

Radis, CD., Kahl, LE. Baker, GL. Wasko, MC. Cash, JM. Gallatin, A. Stolzer, BL. Agarwal, AK. Medsger, TA. and Kwoh, CK. (1995). Effects of cyclophosphamide on the development of malignancy and on long-term survival in patients with rheumatoid arthritis: a 20-year follow-up study. *Arthritis & Rheumatology,* 38(8):1120-1127. doi: 10.1002/art.1780380815.

Ramiro, S., Gaujoux-Viala, C. Nam, JL. Smolen, JS. Buch, M. Gossec, L. van der Heijde, D. Winthrop, K. and Landewe, R. (2014). Safety of synthetic and biological DMARDs: a systematic literature review informing the 2013 update of the EULAR recommendations for management of rheumatoid arthritis, *Annals Of The Rheumatic Diseases,* 73(3):529-535. doi: 10.1136/annrheumdis-2013-204575.

Routsias, JG., Goules, JD. Charalampakis, G. Tzima, S. Papageorgiou, A. and Voulgarelis, M. (2013). Malignant lymphoma in primary Sjögren's syndrome: an update on the pathogenesis and treatment. *Seminars in Arthritis and Rheumatism,* 43(2):178-186. doi: 0.1016/j.semarthrit.2013.04.004.

Schivakumar, L. and Ansell, S. (2006). Targeting B-lymphocyte stimulator/B-cell activating factor and a proliferation-inducing ligand in hematologic malignancies. *Clinical Lymphoma Myeloma,* 7(2):106-108. doi: 10.3816/CLM.2006.n.046.

Singh, AG., Singh, S. and Matteson, EL. (2016). Rate, risk factors and causes of mortality in patients with Sjögren's syndrome: a systematic review and meta-analysis of cohort studies. *Rheumatology (Oxford).*, 55(3):450-460. doi: 10.1093/rheumatology/kev354.

Slesser, AA., Bhangu, A. Bower, M. Goldin, R. and Tekkis, PP. (2013). A systematic review of anal squamous cell carcinoma in inflammatory bowel disease. *Surgical Oncology,* 22(4): 230–237.

Smedby, KE., Hjalgrim, H. Askling, J. Chang, ET. Gregersen, H. Porwit-MacDonald, A. Sundström, C. Akerman, M. Melbye, M. Glimelius, B. Adami, HO. (2006). Autoimmune and chronic inflammatory disorders and risk of non hodgkin lymphoma by subtype. *Journal of the National Cancer Institute*, 98(1):51-60. doi: 10.1093/jnci/djj004.

Smitten, A., Simon, TA. Hochberg, MC. and Suissa, S. (2008). A meta-analysis of the incidence of malignancy in adult patients with rheumatoid arthritis. *Arthritis Research and Therapy,* 10(2):R45. doi: 10.1186/ar2404.

Song, J., Li, Y. Bowlus, CL. Yang, G. Leung, PSC. and Gershwin, ME. (2020). Cholangiocarcinoma in Patients with Primary Sclerosing Cholangitis (PSC): a Comprehensive Review. *Clinical Reviews in Allergy & Immunology,* 58(1):134-149. doi: 10.1007/s12016-019-08764-7.

Stergiou, IE., Poulaki, A. and Voulgarelis, M. (2020). Pathogenetic mechanisms implicated in Sjögren's Syndrome Lymphomagenesis: a review of the literature. *Journal of Clinical Medicine,* 24;9(12):3794. doi: 10.3390/jcm9123794.

Tincani, A., Taraborelli, M. and Cattaneo, R. (2009). Antiphospholipid antibodies and malignancies. *Autoimmunity Reviews,* 9(4):200-202. doi: 10.1016/j.autrev.2009.04.001.

Uchino, M., Ikeuchi, H. Hata, K. Minagawa, T. Horio, Y. Kuwahara, R. Nakamura, S. Watanabe, K. Saruta, M. Fujii, T. Kobayashi, T. Sugimoto, K. Hirai, F. Esaki, M. Hiraoka, S. Matsuoka, K. Shinzaki, S. Matsuura, M. Inoue, N. Nakase, H. and Watanabe, M. (2021). Intestinal cancer in patients with Crohn's disease: A systematic review and meta-analysis *Journal of Gastroenterology and Hepatology,* 36(2):329-336. doi: 10.1111/jgh.15229.

Ueda, T., Inoue, T. Nakamoto, T. Nishigori, N. Kuge, H. Sasaki, Y. Fujii, H. and Koyama, F. (2020). Anorectal cancer in crohn's disease has a poor prognosis due to its advanced stage and aggressive histological features: a systematic literature review of Japanese patients. *Gastrointestinal Cancer,* 51(1):1-9. doi: 10.1007/s12 029-018-0180-6.

Valean, S., Acalovschi, M. Dumitrascu, DL. Ciobanu, L. Nagy, G. and Chira, R. (2019). Hepatocellular carcinoma in patients with autoimmune hepatitis - a systematic review of the literature published between 1989-2016. *Medicine and Pharmacy Reports,* 92(2):99-105. doi: 10.15386/mpr-1228.

von Roon, AC., Reese, G. Teare, J. Constantinides, V. Darzi, AW. and Tekkis, PP. (2007). The risk of cancer in patients with Crohn's disease. *Diseases of the Colon and Rectum,* 50(6):839–855. doi: 10.1007/s10350-006-0848-z.

Wang, LH., Wang, WM. Lin, SH. and Shieh, CC. (2019). Bidirectional relationship between systemic lupus erythematosus and non-Hodgkin's lymphoma: a nationwide population-based study. *Rheumatology (Oxford),* 58(7):1245-1249. doi: 10.1093/rheumatology/kez011.PMID: 30726952.

Weeding, E., Casciola-Rosen, L. and Shah, AA. (2020). Cancer and scleroderma. *Rheumatic Disease Clinics of North America,* 46(3): 551–564. doi: 10.1016/j.rdc.2020.03.002.

Westermann, R., Zobbe, K. Cordtz, R. Haugaard, JH. and Dreyer, L. (2021). Increased cancer risk in patients with cutaneous lupus erythematosus and systemic lupus erythematosus compared with the general population: A Danish nationwide cohort study. *Lupus,* 30(5):752-761. doi: 10.1177/0961203321990106. Epub 2021 Jan 26.

Wijnands, AM., Jong, ME. Lutgens, M. WMD. Hoentjen, F. Elias, SG. Oldenburg, B. and Dutch Initiative on Crohn and Colitis (ICC). (2021). Prognostic factors for advanced colorectal neoplasia in inflammatory bowel disease: systematic review and meta-analysis. *Gastroenterology*, 160(5):1584-1598. doi: 10.1053/j.gastro.2020.12.036.

Yang, Z., Lin, F. Qin, B. Liang, Y. and Zhong, R. (2015). Polymyositis/dermatomyositis and malignancy risk: a metaanalysis study. *The Journal of Rheumatology,* 42(2):282-291. doi:10.3899/jrheum.140566.

Zantos, D., Zhang, Y. and Felson, D. (1994). The overall and temporal association of cancer with polymyositis and dermatomyositis. *The Journal of Rheumatology,* 21(10):1855–1859.

Zhang, JQ., Wan, YN. Peng, WJ. Yan, JW. Li, BZ. Mei, B. Chen, B. Yao, H. Yang, GJ. Tao, JH. and Wang, J. (2013). The risk of cancer development in systemic sclerosis: a meta-analysis. *Cancer Epidemiology,* 37(5), 523–527. doi: 10.1016/j.canep.2013.04.014.

Chapter 10

Paraneoplastic Syndromes

Tuğçehan Sezer Akman*
Alaca State Hospital,
Department of Anesthesiology and Reanimation,
Çorum, Turkey

Abstract

Paraneoplastic syndromes (PNSs) are conditions arising from cytokines, hormones, and peptides released from tumor tissue or from the cross-immune interaction between normal tissue and malignant tissue and progress with dysfunction in various organs and systems far from the tumor. They may appear with different clinical pictures, particularly involvement of the endocrine, neurological, hematological, dermatological, and rheumatological system.

Recognition of PNSs enables the detection of the underlying malignancy at a treatable stage and increases survival time. Moreover, the diagnosis and treatment of PNSs, an important cause of morbidity, improve the patient's quality of life. The main principle in treatment is to treat the underlying malignancy. Furthermore, immunosuppression and correction of electrolyte-hormonal disorders are also among treatment options.

Keywords: paraneoplastic syndromes, paraneoplastic antibodics, tumors, autoimmune

* Corresponding Author's Email: tgchnszr@gmail.com.

In: Autoimmunity and Cancer
Editors: Soner Şahin and Kenan Demir
ISBN: 978-1-68507-937-6

Introduction

Paraneoplastic syndromes (PNSs) are rare systemic signs or symptoms that manifest themselves far from tumor tissue, independently of tumor size, metastasis status, and invasion (Henry, 2019; El Rassy et al., 2019). These syndromes can lead to dysfunction of various organs. They can induce changes in many systems, such as neurological, rheumatological, hematological, dermatological, and endocrine system disorders (El Rassy et al., 2019). Immunological or non-immunological reasons can be the cause of this situation (Thapa & Ramphul, 2021).

With advancing medicine, the effective diagnosis and treatment of PNSs improve clinical outcomes. The presence of PNSs is sometimes noticed before the diagnosis of primary cancer. Recognition of these syndromes may help identify an occult tumor at an early and treatable stage, and this case is generally encountered in neurological PNSs (Thapa & Ramphul, 2021; Pelosof & Gerber, 2010). PNSs can be diagnosed simultaneously with the diagnosis of the tumor or after its removal (Henry, 2019).

Developments in the early diagnosis and treatment of tumors will allow improving the prognosis of PNSs and associated tumors, detecting recurrence early and following up the response to treatment (Henry, 2019).

History

More than 100 years ago, it was observed that there were various completely independent symptoms that did not result from invasion or compression of primary cancer (Pelosof & Gerber, 2010). In 1865, Strauss revealed the existence of migratory venous thrombi associated with gastric carcinoma, which is today called the 'Strauss Migratory Thrombophlebitis Syndrome.' In 1888, Oppenheim reported symptoms not associated with tumor spread and invasion. However, the term 'polyradiculoneuritis' was used until Guichard and Vignon used the term 'Paraneoplastic Syndrome' in 1949 (Henry, 2019). Paraneoplastic syndrome is defined as 'a tissue/organ disorder induced by cancer but not directly induced by cancer invasion' in the book of Darnell and Posner (Henry, 2019).

Definition

PNSs are conditions not associated with tumor size, invasion, direct spread, and metastases but caused by their systemic effects. Believed to be rare in the past, PNSs have now come into prominence as the cause of symptoms in undiagnosed cancer patients. The definition of PNSs does not include infections, treatment effects, and nutritional deficiencies (Henry, 2019).

Etiology

Nowadays, the most well-defined PNSs are based mainly on two reasons. They either occur due to functional hormones, active peptides, cytokines, or enzymes secreted from the tumor or as a result of the autoimmune and immunological mechanisms that occur with a cross-immune reaction between tumor tissue and normal host tissue (Henry, 2019; Pelosof & Gerber, 2010).

Among PNS-associated malignancies, there are often small cell lung cancer, medullary thyroid cancer, prostate cancer, gynecological tumors, hematologic malignancies, and breast cancer (Thapa & Ramphul, 2021; Pelosof & Gerber, 2018). PNS-associated tumors are mostly lung tumors and thymoma (Henry, 2019).

Epidemiology

The exact incidence of PNSs is unknown. However, there are sources indicating that about 8% to 15% of cancer patients have PNSs, but this rate will increase as the life expectancy of cancer patients increases with the development of diagnostic methods (Thapa & Ramphul, 2021; Pelosof & Gerber, 2010; Pelosof & Gerber, 2018). Both genders are affected equally (Thapa & Ramphul, 2021). Recently, a better understanding of the pathophysiology of PNSs has been helpful in the recognition of new PNSs and PNS-associated tumors (Henry, 2019). However, PNSs may clinically show similarity to diseases other than neoplasia (Henry, 2019). This similarity can be distinguished due to the latest developments in serological tests and radiographic techniques (Pelosof & Gerber, 2018).

Pathophysiology

PNSs can appear due to immunological and nonimmunological reasons. Immunogenic tumor cells activate humoral and cell-mediated immune systems. Cytotoxic T cells recognize and attack antigens in tumor cells. They can also produce antibodies against tumor cells (Thapa & Ramphul, 2021). Autoimmune mechanisms, including the formation of onconeural tumor-specific antibodies, may damage normal tissue components because of shared tissue antigens (Henry, 2019).

In nonimmunological PNSs, tumor cells may produce hormones or cytokines and cause metabolic disorders. For example, conditions such as ADH-induced hyponatremia and hypercalcemia induced by parathyroid hormone-associated peptides may arise. Moreover, hematologic malignancies may affect the peripheral nervous system by producing immunoglobulin and result in neuropathy (Thapa & Ramphul, 2021).

PNSs affect multiple organ systems in the body, and clinicians may encounter them in different clinical manifestations. The clinical manifestation is not related to the stage and prognosis of malignancy (Thapa & Ramphul, 2021).

Classification

PNSs affect different organ systems. They can be examined under the main headings of endocrine, neurological, hematologic, dermatological, and rheumatological PNSs (Pelosof & Gerber, 2010). In addition to these systems, clinical PNSs have also been identified (Brown & Skarin, 2006).

Endocrine PNSs

The endocrine PNSs depend on the production of bioactive substances by neoplastic cells of endocrine or neuroendocrine origin. The distinctive characteristic of these syndromes is that symptoms cannot be ascribed to the presence of a secretory neoplastic lesion associated with the anatomical region from which symptoms originate, and secreted amines, peptides, and other bioactive substances are considered ectopic (Dimitriadis et al., 2017). Most endocrine PNSs are the result of nonendocrine neoplasms (Daskalakis et al., 2019). Since tumors without endocrine differentiation may also produce bioactive substances, they may present a clinically similar appearance (Dimitriadis et al., 2017).

Histopathological classification of endocrine tumors originating from different endocrine tissues (gastrointestinal neuroendocrine tumors, adreno-medullary-adrenocortical tumors, lung neuroendocrine tumors, thyroid, and skin tumors) came into existence when trying to obtain information on the malignant potential of these tumors. Severe lung, prostate, ovarian, breast, colon, skin, and hematologic malignancies are the cause of a great majority of endocrine PNSs originating from nonendocrine tumors (Dimitriadis et al., 2017). However, it should be remembered that tumors that lead to endocrine PNSs can range from benign to highly malignant tumors (Daskalakis et al., 2019).

Endocrine PNSs may influence the prognosis by complicating the patient's clinical course and treatment response (Daskalakis et al., 2019).

The presence of an endocrine or metabolic disorder in a tumor patient, remission after successful treatment of the patient, recurrence of the endocrine syndrome, abnormally high hormone levels, detection of hormone in tumor extracts, recognition of the relevant hormone mRNA in tumor tissue, synthesis and secretion of the relevant hormone in vitro by tumor cells help diagnose endocrine PNSs (Dimitriadis et al., 2017).

The most common endocrine PNSs are humoral hypercalcemia of malignancy (HHM), Cushing's syndrome, and syndrome of inappropriate ADH. Less common endocrine PNSs are non-islet cell tumor hypoglycemia, and gynecomastia/virilization. Rare endocrine PNSs are acromegaly, hypertension, ovarian hyperstimulation syndrome, hyperprolactinemia, hyper-thyroidism, secretory diarrhea, osteomalacia, ileus and acute inflammatory reaction/pyrexia (Dimitriadis et al., 2017).

Hypercalcemia

Cancer-associated hypercalcemia occurs in up to 10% of cancer patients in advanced stages and is associated with a poor prognosis. In cancer patients with hypercalcemia, the 1-month mortality rate is approximately 50% (Pelosof & Gerber, 2010). The cause of 80% of hypercalcemia in cancer patients is the release of PTH-related protein by the tumor. It is mostly seen in squamous cell carcinomas. Twenty percent of the cause is the osteolytic activity directly associated with bone metastasis. It may rarely develop due to the secretion of vitamin D secretion of the tumor. Patients may present with nausea, vomiting, lethargy, coma, and renal failure. The severity of symptoms depends on the calcium level (> 14 mg/dl), onset rate, and the patient's initial neurological and renal status. Treatment should be planned considering all these factors (Pelosof & Gerber, 2010).

The optimal treatment is the treatment of the underlying malignancy. If possible, medications that can elevate calcium levels (such as calcium, thiazide diuretics, vitamin D, lithium) should be discontinued. If the patient has persistent hypercalcemia, saline should be administered to the patient to increase the glomerular filtration rate (GFR) and prevent renal calcium absorption. After an adequate volume is replaced, loop diuretics can be given to the patient to prevent renal calcium absorption. Other treatment options are IV bisphosphonates (zoledronate, pamidronate), calcitonin, mithramycin, gallium nitrate, and hemodialysis (Pelosof & Gerber, 2010).

Cushing's Syndrome

Cushing's syndrome, which presents with high cortisol levels, may have endogenous or exogenous causes. The exogenous cause is the administration of high-dose glucocorticoid therapy, while endogenous causes can be examined in two groups as ACTH-dependent and independent causes. ACTH-dependent causes constitute 80% of all, and there are two main reasons. The first is Cushing's disease, and the second is ectopic corticotropin syndrome, which arises from nonpituitary tumors that secrete ACTH or CRH. These tumors are small cell lung cancer, bronchial carcinoid tumor, thymic neuroendocrine tumors, and thymoma (Guilmette & Nosé, 2019).

They increase glucocorticoid secretion from the adrenal glands as excessive ACTH secretion in pituitary adenoma. Uncontrolled glucocorticoid production may also occur in adrenal tumors. They may clinically present with hypercortisolism, central fat deposition, hypertension, striae, hirsutism, facial plateau, menstrual irregularity, and lower extremity edema. Research tests consist of urinary free cortisol, nocturnal salivary cortisol, overnight dexamethasone suppression test, or low-dose dexamethasone suppression test for 48 hours. If an endogenous tumor is the cause, first-line treatment is curative surgery. Secondary treatments are medical treatment, radical surgery, radiation therapy, and bilateral adrenalectomy (Guilmette & Nosé, 2019).

Syndrome of Inappropriate ADH (SIADH)

This syndrome, resulting from water retention due to ADH secretion, is characterized by euvolemic hyponatremia, low serum and high urine osmolality, and continued urinary sodium excretion. The relationship of this syndrome with malignancy was first identified in patients with bronchogenic carcinoma in 1957 (Iyer et al., 2017).

It is seen in 1-2% of patients with malignant tumors, while 70% of malignancy-associated SIADH has been reported to originate from small cell lung cancer (Dimitriadis et al., 2017; Iyer et al., 2017). Furthermore, it has been associated with lymphoma, mesothelioma, thymoma, Ewing's sarcoma, and head and neck squamous cell tumors (Iyer et al., 2017). The presence of SIADH in small cell lung cancer has been associated with an elevated possibility of CNS metastasis, advanced cancer, and poor response to treatment (Dimitriadis et al., 2017)

In the treatment of paraneoplastic SIADH, the optimal approach is to treat the underlying tumor, but it will take weeks for the sodium level to return to normal. ADH receptor antagonists can be used to eliminate the symptoms of hyponatremia. Tolvaptan, which is a V-2 receptor antagonist, is used particularly in patients with lung malignancies. However, more studies are needed on the safety of its chronic use (Dimitriadis et al., 2017).

Hypoglycemia

Paraneoplastic hypoglycemia emerges rather secondary to hepatocellular carcinoma, leiomyoma, and leiomyosarcoma. The exact cause of this syndrome is unknown, but it is believed that cancer cells accelerate glucose consumption or induce hypoglycemia by secreting insulin / insulin-like peptides. In the presence of hepatic neoplasia, it may also develop with a disorder of glycogenolysis or gluconeogenesis. In addition to symptomatic treatment, the underlying cancer must be treated to achieve long-term control (Morgan et al., 2018).

Neurological PNSs

It is believed that a significant part of PNSs that can affect the central, peripheral, and autonomic nervous systems develops due to immune-mediated mechanisms (Höftberger et al., 2015; Leypoldt & Wandinger, 2014). The immune response is determined with antineuronal antibodies measured in CSF and serum most of the time, and these antibodies are used to diagnose the paraneoplastic origin of these syndromes and sometimes certain tumor types (Höftberger et al., 2015). Paraneoplastic neurologic syndromes were classified as 'classical' and 'nonclassical' syndromes. Classical syndromes were specified as conditions with a high probability of paraneoplastic etiology (Leypoldt & Wandinger, 2014). Onconeural antibodies are generated as a result of the immune system's response to the neuronal antigen expressed ectopically by tumor tissue. The subtype ‘classical antibodies’ is aimed at intracellular antigens and is strongly linked to malignancy. Antibodies generated against cell surface antigens have a weaker relationship with the tumor (Gozzard & Maddison, 2010). However, only 60% of PNSs associated with the central nervous system and less than 20% of PNSs associated with the peripheral nervous system were found to be associated with antineuronal antibodies. These antibodies can be observed at low titers in people without PNSs, and false positives and negatives can be encountered, depending on the testing method or the preference of serum / CSF. In addition, the antibody titer can be high in the CSF, while serum can be negative in some cases of PNSs that affects the CNS and dorsal root ganglia. Therefore, the clinical and antibody test results should be evaluated together (Höftberger et al., 2015).

However, the PNS-Care panel gathered in September 2019 and revised the PNSs criteria for 2004. The panel suggested the use of “high-risk phenotypes” instead of “classical syndromes” for cancer and introduced the concept of “intermediate-risk phenotypes.” The term “onconeural antibodies” was replaced by “high-risk (>70% cancer-associated)” and “intermediate-risk (30-70% cancer-associated)” antibodies (Graus et al., 2021).

In the differential diagnosis of neurological PNSs, there are conditions such as autoimmune diseases, infections, neurodegenerative diseases, and metabolic-toxic disorders. These conditions, which are epidemiologically more common than PNSs in general terms, should be differentiated according to the clinical picture and demographic characteristics. Three levels of evidence - definite, probable, and possible - were defined with the PNS-Care Score by the current panel. The PNS-Care score is obtained by a joint evaluation of the clinical phenotype, the presence of cancer, the type of antibody and the follow-up time. The definitive diagnosis of PNSs other than opsoclonus-myoclonus syndrome requires the presence of intermediate or high-risk antibodies (Graus et al., 2021).

There are no definitive pathognomonic neurological findings associated with PNSs, but it is acknowledged that clinical conditions formerly known as “classical syndromes” and now called “high-risk phenotypes” are frequently associated with the paraneoplastic condition. If these phenotypes are detected, the presence of an underlying malignancy should be investigated, paying attention to the patient’s age, sex, and type of antibody. High-risk phenotypes are encephalomyelitis, limbic encephalitis, rapidly progressive cerebellar syndrome, opsoclonus-myoclonus syndrome, sensory neuronopathy, gastro-intestinal pseudo-obstruction (enteric neuropathy), and Lambert-Eaton myasthenic syndrome (Graus et al., 2021). High-risk antibodies are Hu

(ANNA-1), CV2/CRMP5, Yo (PCA-1), PCA 2 (MAP1B), Ri (ANNA-2), Tr/DNER, Ma proteins, Amphiphysin, SOX1 and KLHL 11 (Graus et al., 2021).

Intermediate-risk phenotypes involve neurological disorders with or without underlying cancer. If they cannot be explained for any other reason, PNSs should be considered and specific neuronal antibodies should be investigated. If rapid progression is observed at onset (< 3 months), and if there are inflammatory findings in CSF or brain/spine MRI, the intermediate-risk phenotype should be regarded. These antibodies are NMDAR, AMPAR, GABA(B)R, CASPR2, mGluR5 and P/Q VGCC. If encephalitides other than well-defined limbic encephalitis meet the diagnostic criteria for possible autoimmune encephalitis and if high- or intermediate-risk antibodies are detected, the intermediate-risk phenotype can be considered (Graus et al., 2021).

Low-risk antibodies are mGluR1, GABA(A)R, CASPR2, GFAP, GAD65, LGI1, DPPX, GlyR, AQP4 and MOG. This group of antibodies has a very weak relationship with cancer (<30%) or has no relationship (Graus et al., 2021).

Treatment includes diagnosing and treating the causing tumor, immunosuppression, and symptomatic treatment. Immunosuppression therapy consists of two steps according to the response. The first step includes the use of steroids, IV immunoglobulin (0.4 mg/kg/day, 5 days) and/or plasmapheresis. If no response to treatment is achieved within 2-3 weeks, rituximab (375 mg/m^2 once a week for 4 weeks) and/or cyclophosphamide (750 mg/m^2) are used as a second step. The healing process is slow. 80% of patients with anti-NMDAR encephalitis have been reported to recover almost completely with treatment within 24 months. Characteristics such as the type of surface antibodies and the patient's age affect the rate of response to treatment (Grativvol et al., 2018).

Hematological PNSs

They are rarely symptomatic syndromes, generally detected after cancer diagnosis (El Rassy et al., 2019; Pelosof & Gerber, 2010). The second most common cause of death in cancer patients is hemorrhagic and thrombotic complications (Rodríguez et al., 2017). Symptoms such as fatigue, paleness, venous thromboembolism, and dyspnea may sometimes develop (Pelosof & Gerber, 2010). They are observed together with advanced disease. They disappear with the treatment of the underlying malignancy (Pelosof & Gerber, 2010).

Multiple hematological paraneoplastic syndromes have been reported in cases of cancer of unknown primary. These syndromes are thrombotic thrombocytopenic purpura, Trousseau syndrome, microangiopathic hemolytic anemia, and leukoerythroblastosis (El Rassy et al., 2019).

Hematologic PNSs are eosinophilia, granulocytosis, pure red cell aplasia, and thrombocytosis (Pelosof & Gerber, 2010). Disseminated intravascular coagulation and leukemoid reactions may also be observed (Thapa & Ramphul, 2021).

Eosinophilia

PNSs correspond to secondary eosinophilia resulting from eosinophil growth factors IL 3, IL 5 and GM-CSF produced by the tumor (Pelosof & Gerber, 2010). Primary eosinophilia is a condition induced by direct hematologic neoplasia. In cases associated with secondary eosinophilia, serum levels of GM-CSF, IL 2, IL 3 and IL 5 may be high. Collagen vascular diseases, allergic reactions, and parasitic infections are other causes of secondary eosinophilia. Paraneoplastic eosinophilia is most often observed in leukemia and lymphomas, while it can also be observed together with lung, GIS, and gynecological tumors (Pelosof & Gerber, 2010; Rodríguez et al., 2017). Although usually asymptomatic, it can sometimes cause respiratory problems (Pelosof & Gerber, 2010; Rodríguez et al., 2017). However, these respiratory problems respond to corticosteroid therapy (Pelosof & Gerber, 2010).

Remaining eosinophilia after successful completion of cancer treatment may be a sign of recurrence (Pelosof & Gerber, 2010).

Granulocytosis

It is seen in about 15% of patients with solid tumors. White blood cell count typically ranges between 12- 30 10^9/L, whereas it may sometimes exceed 50 $\times 10^9$/L. Various reasons can lead to the elevation of white cell count in cancer patients. In addition to paraneoplastic syndromes, hematopoietic growth factors, infection, glucocorticoids, and vasopressors may cause this elevation.

Paraneoplastic granulocytosis may also be associated with breast, brain, kidney, gynecological, and GIS malignancies, particularly large cell lung cancer. Its exact mechanism is not known, but the production of substances with colony-stimulating activity by tumors has been held responsible. Special treatment is not required (Pelosof & Gerber, 2010).

Pure Red Cell Aplasia

It is mostly observed with thymoma, but it may also be seen in leukemia and lymphomas (Pelosof & Gerber, 2010). It is a paraneoplastic autoimmune syndrome. Autoantibodies disrupt erythroid differentiation, and reduction or absence of erythroid precursors is observed (Geng et al., 2020). Its treatment is cancer therapy and immunosuppression. In addition to corticosteroids, azathioprine, cyclosporine A, antithymocyte globulin, cyclophosphamide, and monoclonal antibodies (alemtuzumab, rituximab), androgen therapy and plasma exchange have also been used in treatment. Attention should be paid to immunosuppression therapy in cases associated with premalignant disorders and myelodysplasia because it accelerates malignant transformation. In PNSs cases caused by thymoma, it is necessary to administer immunosuppression therapy after thymectomy (Pelosof & Gerber, 2010). Chronic lymphocytic leukemia (CLL) and thymoma are neoplasms that are observed the most together (Geng et al. 2020).

Thrombocytosis

Platelet count higher than 400×10^9 /L in 35% of patients is associated with malignancy. Paraneoplastic thrombocytosis is assumed to arise due to cytokines such as IL-6 produced by the tumor. Thrombohemorrhagic complications and vasomotor symptoms are rare in paraneoplastic thrombocytosis. Special treatment is not required (Pelosof & Gerber, 2010).

Migratory Thrombophlebitis (Trousseau Sign)

The tumor generates procoagulant factors and pro-inflammatory cytokines. Cancer becomes prone to hypercoagulability. Thus, the risk of venous thromboembolism increases. It mostly develops in the presence of pancreatic mucinous carcinoma, stomach, and lung tumors (Rodríguez et al., 2017).

Migratory thrombophlebitis is a rare disease with an influence on the rib cage and upper extremities. It can be considered a warning sign in advanced malignancies of the lung and pancreas. Some cases have also been reported in stomach, rectum, and colon cancers (Rodríguez et al., 2017).

Dermatological and Rheumatological PNSs

They are generally clinical prior to the diagnosis or recurrence of cancer. Their response to treatment is weaker than their non-PNS equivalents (Pelosof & Gerber, 2010).

Acanthosis Nigricans

Acanthosis nigricans, which is described as the prototype of papulosquamous skin disorders of the PNSs, can be observed together with gastric neoplasms (most often gastric adenocarcinomas) or lymphoproliferative diseases (Pelosof & Gerber, 2010; Zappasodi et al., 2006). This condition involves small hyperpigmented and hyperkeratotic lesions in flexural areas such as the back of the neck and axilla, in intertriginous areas such as the area under the breast and groin, and in the palmar region. Mucosal regions (such as the periocular area, lips, anus) are typically involved in the PNSs form (Zappasodi et al., 2006). Up to 90% of the cases of acanthosis nigricans seen in the palm have been suggested to be associated with malignancy (Pelosof & Gerber, 2010). These lesions do not respond well to symptomatic treatment, such as topical steroids. Appropriate treatment for malignancy may heal them (Pelosof & Gerber, 2010).

Dermatomyositis

Dermatomyositis progresses with proximal and symmetric muscle weakness following multiple skin changes. Typically, it is a clinical inflammatory myopathy that develops with heliotropic rash on the upper eyelids, erythema on the face, neck, back, chest, and shoulders, periungual telangiectasia, itchy scalp eruptions, and Gottron papules (erythematous papules over the phalangeal joints) (Pelosof & Gerber, 2010; Zappasodi et al., 2006). Of the cases, 10-25% are paraneoplastic (Pelosof & Gerber, 2010). It may be encountered in lung, breast, ovarian, prostate cancers, and non-Hodgkin's lymphoma (NHL). It is diagnosed with a high creatine phosphokinase level, electromyography, and muscle biopsy (Pelosof & Gerber, 2010; Zappasodi et al., 2006). It generally appears before the diagnosis of cancer (Zappasodi et al., 2006).

Arthropathies

Carcinomatous polyarthritis (CP) is a disease associated with lymphoproliferative diseases in addition to oropharynx, esophagus, stomach, colon, lung, larynx, breast, ovary, and pancreas malignancies. It is independent of the tumor mass and metastasis effect. It is usually observed in people over 50 years of age and progresses rapidly (Khan et al., 2020).

Diseases such as seronegative spondyloarthropathies (enteric and reactive arthritis, etc.) and crystal arthropathies should be excluded. It is necessary to establish the differential diagnosis of CP and rheumatoid arthritis (RA) since the incidence of both increases with age, possibly resulting in a similar clinical picture. Despite exceptions, CP generally involves the joints in the legs asymmetrically and differs from RA because rheumatoid factor (RF) and anti-cyclic citrullinated peptide (CCP) antibodies are seronegative in CP. The recurrence of arthritis may indicate the recurrence of cancer (Khan et al., 2020).

Hypertrophic osteoarthropathy (HOA) can be a primary disease, whereas it can also be secondary to GIS and pulmonary system malignancies (especially non-small cell lung cancer). In large joints, it causes proliferation of bone and skin associated with effusion. It induces leg pain with a bilateral and progressive periostosis of the tubular bones. On physical examination, it presents with digital clubbing represented by swelling in the distal of the fingers and convex deformity of the nails. Hypertrophy may be observed on the skin of the facial and nail bed. A reduction in white blood cell count and an increase in viscosity are observed in the analysis of synovial fluid on the effusion of large joints. HOA may also regress when the underlying cancer is treated (Khan et al., 2020). About 90% of cases are associated with neoplasms. Treatment involves opioids, NSAIDs, bisphosphonates, local radiation, and treatment of primary cancer (Pelosof & Gerber, 2010).

Remitting seronegative symmetric synovitis with pitting edema (RS3PE) may be observed secondary to malignancy. Moreover, the incidence of malignancy is high in patients with RS3PE. It may develop in the colon, prostate, stomach, ovary, endometrial malignancies, lymphoma, leukemia, and myelodysplasia. Fever, weight loss, and insufficient response to steroid therapy are observed. Bilateral edema occurs in the hands and feet at an advanced age. The hands may have a boxing glove appearance. There is an increase in CRP and Erythrocyte sedimentation rate (ESR). Anti-CCP and RF antibodies are negative (Khan et al., 2020).

Polymyalgia rheumatica is a disease seen in the elderly, involving pain, stiffness and fatigue in the proximal muscles, increased ESR, and chronic disease anemia. Characteristically, it gives a dramatic response to a moderate steroid dose of 20 mg. Its atypical characteristics may indicate underlying cancer. Its atypical characteristics are asymmetric involvement, onset less than 50 years of age, deep anemia, proteinuria, ESR > 100 mm/h or < 40 mm/hour, and inadequate response to steroid treatment. It can be observed in lung, colon, kidney, and multiple myeloma malignancies. It can be seen up to about 1 year before cancer diagnosis. It regresses when the underlying malignancy is treated (Khan et al., 2020).

Gout is inflammatory arthritis, which may be observed primarily, but may also develop due to hyperuricemia following nucleic acid degradation secondary to CT and RT. It can be seen in the presence of hematologic malignancies. The severity of gout may increase if the liver is involved (Khan et al., 2020).

Amyloidosis is a disease that is caused by the accumulation of amyloid proteins, can lead to organ failure, and affects the synovium and periarticular space. It mostly causes pain in the shoulders, wrists, and knees. Low-level but significant asymmetric arthritis can be observed in multiple myeloma and Waldenstrom macroglobulinemia (Zappasodi et al., 2006).

Vasculitis

It is a group of diseases that progress with necrosis of blood vessels, rather seen in hematologic malignancies such as hairy cell leukemia, lymphoma, myelodysplastic syndrome (MDS), and CML. Approximately 5% of cases are associated with neoplasms. Leukocytoclastic vasculitis and polyarteritis nodosa (PAN) have been reported to be the most associated with hematological malignancies (Zappasodi et al., 2006). Leukocytoclastic vasculitis is a disease that involves the small vessels of the skin and often progresses with palpable purpura in the lower extremities (Zappasodi et al., 2006). Tumor-associated antigens involved in the circulation have been demonstrated as the cause (Pelosof & Gerber, 2010). PAN, on the other hand, is a disease characterized by linear subcutaneous nodules with medium-small artery involvement, progresses with livedo reticularis, ulceration, erythematous papules and necrosis in the distal finger, and creates systemic findings (abdominal pain, peripheral neuropathy, asymmetric polyarteritis). Treatment includes systemic steroids and treatment of the underlying neoplasm (Zappasodi et al., 2006).

Paraneoplastic Pemphigus (PNP)

It is a rare and serious autoimmune bullous disease that may accompany benign and malignant tumors. It mostly accompanies hematologic and lymphomatoid malignancies (CLL, Castleman disease, B-cell lymphoma, Waldenstrom macroglobulinemia, thymoma). Although the pathogenesis is not known exactly, autoantibodies developed against desmosomal and hemidesmosomal antigens are held responsible. The removal of benign tumors results in recovery, but the disease progresses more severely in malignant tumors and may not respond to treatment (Wieczorek & Czernik, 2016).

It is often observed between the ages of 45-70, while it accompanies Castleman disease, especially in children (Wieczorek & Czernik, 2016). Hemorrhagic painful polymorphic oral lesions appear and the first symptom is observed in the vermilion and tongue. It may develop as blisters, spots, papules, plaques, and erosions. Nikolsky's sign may be positive. Cutaneous lesions are generally seen after mucous lesions and involvement of the upper region is common. Furthermore, pemphigus vulgaris, erythema multiforme, mucous membrane pemphigoid, Stevens-Johnson syndrome, herpes simplex virus infection, lichen planus, and graft-versus-host disease are included in the differential diagnosis (Wieczorek & Czernik, 2016). If PNP is suspected in a patient without known malignancy, blood cell count, flow cytometry, LDH tests, and chest, abdomen, and pelvic CT should be requested. In one-third of patients, first PNP and then malignancy is diagnosed. If it is an operable malignancy, surgical treatment will also help with the remission of PNP. If it is not in an operable condition, there are treatment methods such as glucocorticosteroids, immunosuppressants (such as cyclosporine, azathioprine), rituximab, and IVIG. However, PNP is usually resistant to treatment and the mortality rate ranges between 75-90%. The main cause of mortality is respiratory failure. Quick diagnosis and early treatment are crucial (Wieczorek & Czernik, 2016).

Paraneoplastic Autoimmune Multiorgan Syndrome (PAMS)

PAMS is an autoimmune syndrome that targets the tegumental epithelium and internal organs. Both cellular and humoral immune mechanisms are responsible (Czernik et al., 2011). Autoantibodies target plakins, alpha-2-macroglobulin like 1 (A2ML1), cadherins, plaquephilin-3, BP180, and various neuromuscular antigens. PAMS is a multiorganopathy with many different characteristics from pemphigus vulgaris. It is associated with neoplasia and has a different predisposition to the HLA-II allele compared to classical pemphigus. The underlying cause is a malignancy or lympho-proliferative disorder. Hematological disorders (NHL, CLL, Castleman disease, respectively) have been observed in 84% of cases, and carcinomas, sarcomas, and malignant melanoma have been detected in 16% of nonhematologic malignancies, respectively (Amber et al., 2018).

Sweet's Syndrome

Sweet's syndrome, first described in 1964, is a dermatosis whose etiology has not been fully clarified and may be idiopathic or associated with certain clinical conditions. Autoimmune diseases, inflammatory bowel diseases, vaccination, infection, drug use, or malignancies may lead to this syndrome. It mostly accompanies hematological cancers (especially acute myeloid leukemia) and solid tumors of the genitourinary system (GUS).

Approximately 21% of the disease is associated with malignancy; hematologic neoplasms are seen in 85% of cases, and GUS neoplasms are observed in 15% (Cunha et al., 2018).

It is characterized by fever, cutaneous lesions, and neutrophilia. Lesions are generally located on the face, neck, and upper extremities. It appears as asymmetrically located papules, nodules, and painful and tense erythematous plaques. It usually responds well to corticosteroids, while complete remission can be achieved with the treatment of underlying neoplasia (Cunha et al., 2018).

Other PNS-Related Conditions

Kidney Involvement

In PNSs, renal involvements usually manifest themselves as nephrotic syndrome. It is suggested that about 10% of patients recently diagnosed with idiopathic nephrotic syndrome have malignancy and most patients with carcinoma have membranous glomerulonephritis (Brown & Skarin, 2006).

In Hodgkin's disease, 80% of glomerular lesions are lipoid nephrosis or minimal change disease, and 20% are typical membranous or membranoproliferative glomerulonephritis and focal sclerosis in patients with nephrotic syndrome. Nephrotic syndrome can also be encountered in other lymphomas, particularly in CLL. This situation has been associated with monoclonal immunoglobulins or cryoglobulins involved in the circulation. This condition also disappears with CLL treatment (Brown & Skarin, 2006).

Nephrotic syndrome is observed less frequently in NHL. However, it may be seen in diffuse large cell lymphoma or Burkitt lymphoma (Brown & Skarin, 2006).

GIS Involvement

Cancer patients often experience problems such as taste loss, anorexia, cachexia, and weight loss. This clinical picture generally emerges before tumor diagnosis and may regress with treatment. Experiments on mice have revealed that tumor cell production of TNF-α (cachectin) and IL-1β by tumor cells may be associated with this condition. TNF-α may facilitate the occurrence of anorexia and cachexia by inhibiting lipoprotein lipase (Brown & Skarin, 2006).

Intestinal obstruction may develop in patients with occult lymphoma with acquired angioedema. C1 inhibitor deficiency is observed in this disease. The resulting angioedema emerges in various parts of the body and may lead to pseudo-obstruction in the intestines. Acquired angioedema often arises from circulating paraproteins as a result of a C1 inhibitor deficiency in low-grade B-cell lymphoma. Danazol can treat angioedema by enhancing C1 inhibitor synthesis (Brown & Skarin, 2006).

Treatment

Treatment is specified on the basis of the severity, type, and location of the disease. The primary objective is to treat cancer, which is the cause of the disease, with surgery, chemotherapy, or radiotherapy. Corticosteroids, immunosuppressants, IVIG, plasma exchange, and plasmapheresis are other options (Thapa & Ramphul, 2021). Immunosuppression therapy can be administered in neurological, rheumatological, and dermatological syndromes. Elimination of hormonal-electrolyte disorders can be ensured in the endocrine PNSs (Pelosof & Gerber, 2010).

Conclusion

PNSs are clinical tumor-related conditions, but are independent of tumor tissue size, metastasis, and invasion. These syndromes are thought to be based on bioactive substances produced by tumor tissue and the autoimmune response. The incidence of PNSs will increase as the number of cancer patients increases and the lifetime of cancer patients is prolonged. PNSs can make the physician suspicious by revealing themselves before cancer diagnosis, enabling early treatment of the underlying tumor with early diagnosis, and improving the patient's quality of life. In addition, studies on these syndromes will help to better understand cancer development, proliferation, and care.

References

Amber, K. T., Valdebran, M., & Grando, S. A. (2018). Paraneoplastic autoimmune multiorgan syndrome (PAMS): Beyond the single phenotype of paraneoplastic pemphigus. *Autoimmunity reviews*, 17(10), 1002–1010. https://doi.org/10.1016/j.autrev.2018.04.008

Brown, J. R., Skarin, A. T. (2006). Paraneoplastic syndromes. George P. Canellos, T. Andrew Lister, Bryan D. Young (Eds.) *The Lymphomas* -Second Edition. (pp 139-145). https://doi.org/10.1016/B978-0-7216-0081-9.50011-X.

Cunha, D. G., Campos-do-Carmo, G., Marujo, J. M., & Verardino, G. C. (2018). Paraneoplastic Sweet's syndrome. *Anais Brasileiros de Dermatologia*, 93(4), 576–578. https://doi.org/10.1590/abd1806-4841.20187353.

Czernik, A., Camilleri, M., Pittelkow, M. R., & Grando, S. A. (2011). Paraneoplastic autoimmune multiorgan syndrome: 20 years after. *International Journal of Dermatology*, 50(8), 905–914. https://doi.org/10.1111/j.1365-4632.2011.04868.x.

Daskalakis, K., Chatzelis, E., Tsoli, M., Papadopoulou-Marketou, N., Dimitriadis, G. K., Tsolakis, A. V., & Kaltsas, G. (2019). Endocrine paraneoplastic syndromes in patients with neuroendocrine neoplasms. *Endocrine*, 64(2), 384–392. https://doi.org/10.1007/s12020-018-1773-3.

Dimitriadis, G. K., Angelousi, A., Weickert, M. O., Randeva, H. S., Kaltsas, G., Grossman, A. (2017). Paraneoplastic endocrine syndromes. *Endocr Relat Cancer*. Jun;24(6): R173-R190. https://doi.org/10.1530/ERC-17-0036.

El Rassy, E., Assi, T., Kattan, J., & Pavlidis, N. (2019). Paraneoplastic syndromes in cancers of unknown primary: An unknown field for oncologists. *Bulletin du Cancer*, 106(6), 590–603. https://doi.org/10.1016/j.bulcan.2019.03.011.

Geng, G., Yu, X., Jiang, J., & Yu, X. (2020). Aetiology and pathogenesis of paraneoplastic autoimmune disorders. *Autoimmunity Reviews*, 19(1), 102422. https://doi.org/10.1016/j.autrev.2019.102422.

Gozzard, P., & Maddison, P. (2010). Which antibody and which cancer in which paraneoplastic syndromes? *Practical Neurology*, 10(5), 260–270. https://doi.org/10.11 36/jnnp.2010.224105.

Grativvol, R. S., Cavalcante, W., Castro, L., Nitrini, R., & Simabukuro, M. M. (2018). Updates in the diagnosis and treatment of paraneoplastic neurologic syndromes. *Current Oncology Reports*, 20(11), 92. https://doi.org/10.1007/s11912-018-0721-y.

Graus, F., Vogrig, A., Muñiz-Castrillo, S., Antoine, J. G., Desestret, V., Dubey, D., Giometto, B., Irani, S. R., Joubert, B., Leypoldt, F., McKeon, A., Prüss, H., Psimaras, D., Thomas, L., Titulaer, M. J., Vedeler, C. A., Verschuuren, J. J., Dalmau, J., & Honnorat, J. (2021). Updated diagnostic criteria for paraneoplastic neurologic syndromes. *Neurology(R) Neuroimmunology & Neuroinflammation*, 8(4), e1014. https://doi.org/10.1212/NXI.0000000000001014.

Guilmette, J., Nosé, V. (2019). Paraneoplastic syndromes and other systemic disorders associated with neuroendocrine neoplasms. *Semin Diagn Pathol*. 36(4):229-239. https://doi.org/10.1053/j.semdp.2019.03.002.

Henry, K. (2019). Paraneoplastic syndromes: Definitions, classification, pathophysiology and principles of treatment. *Seminars in Diagnostic Pathology*, 36(4), 204–210. https://doi.org/10.1053/j.semdp.2019.01.002.

Höftberger, R., Rosenfeld, M. R., & Dalmau, J. (2015). Update on neurological paraneoplastic syndromes. *Current Opinion in Oncology*, 27(6), 489–495. https://doi.org/10.1097/CCO.0000000000000222.

Iyer, P., Ibrahim, M., Siddiqui, W., & Dirweesh, A. (2017). Syndrome of inappropriate secretion of anti-diuretic hormone (SIADH) as an initial presenting sign of non small cell lung cancer-case report and literature review. *Respiratory Medicine Case Reports*, 22, 164–167. https://doi.org/10.1016/j.rmcr.2017.08.004.

Khan, F., Kleppel, H., Meara, A. (2020). Paraneoplastic musculoskeletal syndromes. *Rheum Dis Clin North Am*, 46: 577-586 [PMID: 32631605 DOI: 10.1016/j.rdc.2020.04.002].

Leypoldt, F., & Wandinger, K. P. (2014). Paraneoplastic neurological syndromes. *Clinical and Experimental Immunology*, 175(3), 336–348. https://doi.org/10.1111/cei.12185.

Morgan, R. K., Cortes, Y., & Murphy, L. (2018). Pathophysiology and aetiology of hypoglycaemic crises. *The Journal of Small Animal Practice*, 59(11), 659–669. https://doi.org/10.1111/jsap.12911.

Pelosof, L. C., & Gerber, D. E. (2010). Paraneoplastic syndromes: an approach to diagnosis and treatment. *Mayo Clinic Proceedings*, 85(9), 838–854. https://doi.org/10.4065/mcp.2010.0099.

Pelosof, L. C., & Gerber, D. E. (2018). Paraneoplastic syndromes. The American Cancer Society's oncology in practice, 661–674. doi:10.1002/9781118592168.ch45.

Rodríguez, L., Yurgaky, J., Otero, W., Faizal, M. (2017). Review of Paraneoplastic Syndromes in Gastrointestinal tumors. *Rev. Colomb.* Gastroenterol. 32;226-40. https://doi.org/10.22516/25007440.155.

Thapa, B., Ramphul, K. (2021). *Paraneoplastic Syndromes*. In: StatPearls [Internet]. Treasure Island (FL): StatPearls Publishing; 2021 Jan-. Available from: https://www.ncbi.nlm.nih.gov/books/NBK507890/.

Wieczorek, M., & Czernik, A. (2016). Paraneoplastic pemphigus: a short review. *Clinical, Cosmetic and Investigational Dermatology*, 9, 291–295. https://doi.org/10.2147/CCID.S100802.

Zappasodi, P., Forno, C., Corso, A., & Lazzarino, M. (2006). Mucocutaneous paraneoplastic syndromes in hematologic malignancies. *International Journal of Dermatology*, 45(1), 14–22. https://doi.org/10.1111/j.1365-4632.2005.02668.x.

Chapter 11

Autoimmune Diseases in Cancer

Sidika Tapsin*
Department of Immunology,
School of Medicine, Marmara University,
Istanbul, Turkey

Abstract

The connection between autoimmunity and cancer is dynamic and bidirectional. The oncoming and encouragement of cancer may be contributed by the various autoimmune diseases. However, during cancer prognosis or cancer therapies, an autoimmune response can be triggered due to the immunogenic environment. Such nonspecific immunologic activations can further promote immune-related adverse events (irAEs) and autoimmune diseases. In this chapter, the origin of autoimmune responses during the cancer prognosis, as well as irAEs secondary to the cancer prognosis and treatments, is discussed. The factors that play a role in irAEs secondary to cancer, the incidence of irAEs in solid cancers, and treatment considerations are highlighted.

Keywords: autoimmunity, immune related adverse effects, autoimmune diseases, cancer immunotherapy, tumor antigens, cancer, autoantibodies

Introduction

The immune system has long been considered to be able to distinguish and attack only nonself-antigens because of its safeguard property against

* Corresponding Author's Email: sidika.tapsin@marmara.edu.tr.

In: Autoimmunity and Cancer
Editors: Soner Şahin and Kenan Demir
ISBN: 978-1-68507-937-6

autoimmunity. Since cancer cells are made up of the cells of the body, the destructive power of the immune system would be ineffective against cancer cells. However, the hypothesis fails when the immune system does not attack the microorganism that is found ubiquitously in the body. Then, the hypothesis has revisited the way that the immune system can only recognize and attack harmful molecules over harmless molecules such as self-antigens and microbes that started living in the body very early in life (Bareke et al., 2021). This change in hypothesis allowed researchers to think of the possibility of an immune response against harmful tumor progression by targeting antitumor antigens. Further research in immunosuppressed individuals and immune-compromised severe combined immunodeficiency (SCID) mice revealed that immune cells can, indeed, distinguish cancer cells under the right pro-immunogenic conditions. However, activation of the immune system against cancer cells can drive loss of self-tolerance and induce autoimmunity (Burkholder et al., 2014).

The Origin of the Autoimmune Response in Cancer

The autoimmune response in cancer can originate from cumulative reasons such as genetic factors, inflammatory conditions, and the intervention of cancer treatments.

Shared Genetic Factors may Lead the Autoimmune Response during the Cancer Prognosis

Cancer and autoimmune diseases share genetic components which could be a loss- or gain of function mutations and single nucleotide polymorphisms (SNPs). These components may be protein-coding genes and may play a role in tumor and autoimmunity progression, such as evading apoptosis. Apoptosis is one of the hallmarks of cancer, and mutations in anti- or pro-apoptotic genes can enable the evasion of cancer cells from apoptosis. On the other hand, the same apoptotic factors may play a role in the evasion of auto-reactive lymphocytes from cell death during negative selection.

TP53 is one of the pro-apoptotic genes and the protein encoded from this gene, called p53, plays a role in DNA repair, induction of apoptosis to secure genomic stability, and cell cycle arrest (Kandoth et al., 2013). Mutations in TP53 that inactivate p53 cause genomic instability and allow tumorigenic cells to escape from the cancer treatments as well as the reaction of the immune system. Interestingly, it is shown that the down-regulation of p53 expression increases autoimmune vulnerability in mice (Leech et al., 2008; Okuda et al., 2003). Briefly, CD4+ T cells have subpopulations named conventional helper T (Th) cells and regulatory T (Treg) cells. Th cells control adaptive immunity by activating other effector immune cells against cancer cells and pathogens (Corthay, 2009). Treg cells suppress the immune response by inhibiting cytokine production and T cell proliferation, thus maintaining self-tolerance and preventing autoimmune diseases. In rheumatoid arthritis patients, lower expression of p53 is associated with a higher number of Th17 cells, suggesting that p53 may shift the balance from Treg to Th17 cells and plays a role in disease prognosis (Park et al., 2013). SNPs that are down-regulating the expression of p53 are also associated with an elevated risk of autoimmune diseases such as inflammatory bowel disease (Volodko et al., 2015). Autoantibodies (aAbs) are immune proteins that react against self-antigens, therefore, individuals' own tissues and organs (Ludwig et al., 2017). aAbs that react against down-regulation of p53 called MDM2 are detected in both lung cancer patients as well as autoimmune disease individuals as systemic lupus erythematosus (SLE) and Sjogren's syndrome (Li et al., 2016; Liu et al. 2015; Liu et al., 2017). In addition, these aAbs are further used as biomarkers in both cancer and autoimmune diseases (Himoto et al., 2012; Li et al., 2005). Since down-regulation of p53 is a hallmark of cancer, as well as associated with autoimmune diseases, p53 can be called a shared genetic factor that may be playing a role in autoimmune disease development during the cancer prognosis.

Bcl-2 is an antiapoptotic protein located in mitochondria that plays a role in cell survival (Tischner et al., 2010). Bcl-2 overexpression is associated with a cancer prognosis in many types of cancer (Consortium, 2017; Wong, 2011). Interestingly, certain genotypes are linked to autoimmune diseases such as SLE (Mehrian et al., 1998). In a study, Bcl-2 down-regulation prevented CD8+ T cells from apoptosis that reacts to ovalbumin (OVA), a self-antigen, and thereby protected from the autoimmune response (Davey et al., 2002). In light of such examples, we can conclude that the overexpression of Bcl-2 that occurs during the cancer prognosis may promote an autoimmune response.

Akt is a protooncogene that belongs to the PI3K pathway and suppresses apoptosis while promoting migration and proliferation. It is the second most commonly mutated gene after TP53 and its overexpression is linked to many cancer types such as breast and pancreatic cancers (Kandoth et al., 2013; Revathidevi & Munirajan, 2019). Its protective effect against death can also help cells of the immune system evade immune tolerance. Researchers showed that Akt overexpression in mice is associated with B and T cell accumulation in the lymph nodes and spleen, increased T cell activation, and systemic autoimmunity (Parsons et al., 2001). Higher Akt activity is associated with lower Treg activity, leading to lymphoproliferative disorder, autoimmune encephalomyelitis, and kidney defect (Huynh et al., 2015). In a human study, pemphigus vulgaris patients exhibited overexpression of Akt, its phosphorylated form, members of the PI3K pathway, and a higher number of Th2 cells than control groups (Lai et al., 2021). In summary, overexpression of members of PI3K pathway decreases Treg differentiation while protecting cancer cells and helper T cells from apoptosis, which presents another pathway involved in cancer prognosis and promotes the autoimmune response.

Epigenetic changes are reversible, and sometimes heritable gene expression changes affect the reading of DNA without altering the DNA sequence. Epigenetic changes severely exist in cancer that affect gene transcription and histone stability (Portela & Esteller, 2010). Nucleosomes are the regions of DNA that are surrounded by proteins that further form highly organized DNA complexes and proteins called chromosomes. In autoimmune diseases, aAbs against nucleosomes are reported, as 88% of SLE patients carry anti-nucleosome antibodies (Pradhan et al., 2010). It has been discovered that severe anticancerogenic treatments that induce massive apoptosis may promote antinucleosome aAbs, and thus autoimmunogenity can be induced by the apoptotic epigenetic structure of nucleosomes (Portela & Esteller, 2010).

Microbiota Changes may Modulate the Autoimmune Response during Cancer Prognosis

The microbiota is the sum of commensal, symbiotic or pathogenic bacteria, viruses, protozoans, fungi, and archaea living in or on the multicellular organism (Peterson et al., 2009). They are mainly located on mucosal surfaces and skin, and the interaction between microbiota members and with the host shapes immune tolerance and response to diseases (Ruff et al., 2020). The microbiota shows its immunological effect by modulating immune system cells using immune components such as cytokines, microbial metabolites, and microbiota-trained immune cells (Ruff et al., 2020). An imbalance in the gut microbial community, called gut dysbiosis, is related to many diseases such as respiratory diseases, rheumatoid arthritis, and Crohn's disease (Dumas et al., 2018; Itzhaki et al., 2013). Gut dysbiosis also plays an important role in the immune-based cancer response, and microbiota content can be used as a predictor of the efficiency of cancer treatment (Routy et al., 2018). It is shown that the imbalance in gut dysbiosis caused by antibiotics administered before ICI therapy causes a reduction in survival in patients with renal cell carcinoma (Young et al., 2018). Similarly, it has been shown that a higher number of *A. muciniphila* which is the reason for increased interferon gamma (IFN-γ) secretion by Th1 is significantly related to a favorable outcome of ICI treatment in non-small cell lung carcinoma and renal cell carcinoma (Routy et al., 2018). In a recent study, a fecal microbiota transplant (FMT) was performed in patients with metastatic melanoma. FMT includes the transfer of normal flora from the stool of a donor to the colon of a recipient to transform their gut microbiota. Transformation in the gut microbiota of the patients decreased resistance to anti-PD-1 therapy and reversed resistance to ICI in 6 out of 15 patients (Davar et al., 2021). The gut microbiota can also modulate the induction of Immune-Related Adverse Events (irAEs) caused by ICI therapy. It has been shown that an increased number of *Bacteroidetes* phylums has been shown to protect against colitis in CTLA-4 treatment, whereas *Faecalibacterium* phylum induces colitis in ipilimumab treatment (Khan & Gerber, 2020). The gut microbiota may also support the autoimmune response during tumorigenesis. In a mouse model, the induction of T helper differentiation toward Th17 by microbiota shift worsened autoimmunity. In turn, the microbiota changes as a result of a deficiency in TH17A protected from experimental autoimmune encephalomyelitis (Brevi et al., 2020; Regen et al., 2021). According to this study, it can be speculated that autoimmune responses can be observed if the microbiota supports protumorigenic factors during tumorigenesis.

Self-Antigens and Autoantibodies can Potentially Trigger Autoimmune Responses

Immune system cells identify cancer cells using tumor-associated antigens or self-responsive lymphocytes such as CD8+ cytotoxic T lymphocytes (CTLs) and natural killer (NK) cells. However, the lysis of cancer cells by these lymphocytes releases a large number of self-antigens and pro-inflammatory components that can induce an autoimmune response. Autoimmune diseases and cancer share common aAbs that may have pathophysiological importance such that antitumor immune responses might decrease immune tolerance (Herkel et al., 2001). As an example, aAbs against p53 are observed in breast, lung, ovarian, and colorectal cancers (Fortner et al. 2017; Mu et al., 2020; Pagaza-Straffon et al., 2020; Wang, Li et al., 2019), while some other aAbs against cell cycle proteins such as c-myc and cyclin B1 are reported in ovarian and lung cancer (Benvenuto et al., 2017; Fortner et al., 2017). Interestingly, these aAbs are also detected in SLE patients, suggesting that shared aAbs in both autoimmune diseases and cancer may play a role in the prognosis of autoimmune diseases in cancer (Benvenuto et al., 2017; Herkel et al., 2001).

Autoimmune Diseases that are Observed as a Consequence of Oncoimmunotherapies

Immune system cells are trained to identify and remove cells that have undergone malignant status. In some instances, the immune system could not successfully eliminate tumorigenic cells, and thus malignancy grows and reaches the size that can be detected clinically (Schreiber et al., 2011). In addition to surgical, chemical, and radiological treatments, immunotherapeutic agents are also being used to boost the destructive power of the immune system. Current oncoimmunotherapies aim to elevate the quality and quantity of effector cells, direct the immune response by specific tumor antigens, or stop the immunological surveillance and destructive mechanisms that tumors develop to escape from the immune response (Schreiber et al., 2011).

Immune Checkpoint Inhibitor (ICI) Therapy in Cancer

Immune checkpoints are the regulators of the immune system that play critical roles in maintaining self-tolerance and preventing autoimmunity (Pardoll, 2012). T cell exhaustion contributes to loss of immune surveillance and thereby to tumor development (Tocut et al., 2018). ICIs block checkpoint inhibition on T cells and hence enhance the antitumor immunity (Friedman et al., 2016). However, removal of self-tolerance elevates the risk of an autoimmune response, which may result in immune-driven inflammatory toxicity called immune related adverse events (irAEs) (Day & Hansen, 2016).

To date, the United States Food and Drug Administration (FDA) has approved three ICI targets, but many other immunomodulatory agents are being developed, including drugs targeting programmed death ligand (PD-L1), T cell immunoglobulin and mucin domain 3 (TIM-3), and lymphocyte activation gene 3 (LAG-3) (Keir et al., 2008; Okazaki et al., 2013; Topalian et al., 2015). ICIs are named according to their checkpoint inhibition targets as cytotoxic T lymphocytes-associated antigen 4 (CTLA-4), anti-programmed death (PD)-1, and PD-ligand (L)-1. CTLA-4 and PD-1/PD-L1 show their effects on the distinctive points of T cell activation. CTLA-4 attaches to antigen-presenting cells using CD80-CD86, limits the binding of costimulatory CD28 and thus decreases T cell activation (Kostine et al., 2017). PD-1/PD-L1, on the other hand, induces apoptosis of already activated T cells and thus makes exhausted effector cells respond (Kostine et al., 2017).

There are six FDA-approved ICIs in recent years: atezolizumab, avelumab, durvalumab, ipilimumab, nivolumab, and pembrolizumab. Ipilimumab (Yervoy) is a CTLA-4 inhibitor that increases co-stimulation of T cells. Nivolumab (Opdivo) and pembrolizumab (Keytruda) are PD-1 inhibitors, while atezolizumab (Tecentriq), avelumab (Bavencio) and durvalumab (Imfinzi) are PD-L1 inhibitors that inhibit induced effector T cell death (Tocut et al., 2018).

ICI therapy has great success in a variety of cancer groups, such as renal cell carcinoma (RCC), non-small cell lung cancer (NSCLC), and melanoma (Cappelli et al., 2017). Ipilimumab, nivolumab, and pembrolizumab have a higher survival benefit of up to 25-31% in 5 years compared to chemotherapy (Buchbinder & McDermott, 2015; Ivashko & Kolesar, 2016). In patients with NSCLC, nivolumab therapy has a higher survival rate of 51% at 12 months compared to docetaxel with 39%. Similarly, in patients with RCC, nivolumab therapy increases the survival rate up to 6 months after chemotherapy (Brahmer et al., 2015; Motzer et al., 2020). In combinatory therapies, survival rates are even higher: treatment of ipilimumab and nivolumab for metastatic melanoma had a response of 60% compared to ipilimumab alone with 11% (Postow et al., 2015). Despite the success of ICI therapy in cancer, the development of irAEs as a consequence of ICI therapy is also higher compared to traditional cancer therapy approaches.

Incidence of Autoimmune irAEs Caused by ICIs Treatment

IrAEs are observed in 60% of patients receiving ICI administration (Sibaud, 2018). The development time course of irAEs is variable and can emerge either after one dose or after several months of therapy (Weber et al., 2012). The incidence rate of irAEs caused by ICIs treatment changes according to the type of ICIs treatment utilized, its dosage, and its administration type such as alone or in a combinatory form (Tocut et al., 2018). For example, patients treated with CTLA-4 inhibitors have a higher incidence of irAEs compared to patients treated with one of the PD-1/PD-L1 inhibitors (Larkin et al., 2015). Similarly, combinatory treatment with CTLA-4 and one of the PD-1/PD-L1 ICIs has a higher incidence of irAEs compared to the mono ICIs treatment (Dyck & Mills, 2017). Moreover, the occurrence of irAEs in the case of CTLA-4 ICIs therapy is dose dependent, but not in the case of PD-1/PD-L1 ICIs therapy (Tocut et al., 2018).

Arthritis and arthralgia are the most common musculoskeletal and rheumatic irAEs reported in clinical trials of ICIs, and their incidence depends on the ICIs used. In a study, the incidence of arthralgia as a consequence of monotherapy with ipilimumab or nivolumab is reported to be in the range of 5 to 16% (Brahmer et al., 2015). This ratio increases in combinatory ICI treatments, since the combinatory therapy group showed a 10.5% incidence, while mono-ICI therapies of ipilimumab and nivolumab were 6.1% and 7.7%, respectively (Larkin et al., 2015).

Sicca syndrome is another irAEs induced ICIs therapy. Recent studies observed that between 3% and 4% of patients developed dry eyes after ipilimumab therapy in combination (Hodi et al., 2014; Le et al., 2013). Similarly, dry mouth was observed in 4 to 7% of patients in a trial of pembrolizumab versus ipilimumab in advanced melanoma (Robert et al., 2015).

Muscle weakness and myalgia have also been reported as irAEs after ICI treatment in clinical trials. Muscle weakness is observed in 1% of patients who had ipilimumab treatment with or without sargramostim, while myalgia was reported in 2 to 18% of patients treated with nivolumab and ipilimumab, respectively (Borghaei et al., 2015; Gibney et al., 2015; Hodi et al., 2014).

Vasculitis is a rare irAE that has been reported in a single case among 74 patients in whom ipilimumab was used in mono- or combinatory treatment together with dacarbazine for melanoma (Hersh et al., 2011).

Lupus nephritis is another rare irAE that has been observed in a case in which melanoma patients are treated with CTLA-4 inhibitor and ipilimumab (Fadel et al., 2009).

Organ-specific irAEs, besides classical autoimmune irAEs as mentioned above, are also reported:

Dermatological irAEs are the most common irAEs in patients with melanoma treated with ICIs. Rash is the most common outcome in up to 30-35% of patients treated with PD-1 inhibitors in patients with melanoma. Vitiligo, erythema, psoriasis, bullous pemphigoid, DRESS syndrome, and

Stevens-Johnson syndrome have also been reported after ICI treatment (Beck et al., 2016; Carlos et al., 2015; Hwang et al., 2016; Jour et al., 2016).

Gastrointestinal irAEs such as diarrhea (frequently in anti-CTLA-4 therapy) and inflammatory colitis mimicking Crohn's disease are observed with a high incidence (Kostine et al., 2017). Pancreatitis, gastritis, and celiac disease have also been observed (Kostine et al., 2017).

Endocrine irAEs such as hypothyroidism (observed in anti-PD-1 therapy that affects mainly the thyroid gland), and less frequently hyperthyroidism are reported (Kostine et al., 2017). Hypophysitis, adrenal insufficiency, and type 1 diabetes are also observed (Corsello et al., 2013; Hansen et al., 2016).

Pulmonary irAEs, such as inflammatory lung diseases, contain sarcoidosis and BOOPs and less frequently pleural effusions are reported (Nishino et al., 2016).

Finally, more rare irAEs such as neurological (like peripheral neuropathy, aseptic meningitis, Guillain-Barre syndrome, myelitis, encephalitis, myasthenia gravies), hematological (hemolytic anemia, thrombocytopenia, neutropenia, aplastic anemia, acquired hemophilia), cardiac (pericarditis, myocarditis), and ophthalmological (episcleritis, uveitis, retinitis) are also associated with treatment of ICI (Kostine et al., 2017).

Autoimmune Response in Cancer Therapies Other than ICIs

Cytokine Therapy in Cancer

The first oncoimmunotherapy, named recombinant interleukin 2 (IL-2), was administered in the 1980s for metastatic melanoma (Coley, 1891). IL-2, which is a potent T cell activator, and interferon alpha (IFN-α) are used for adjuvant cancer therapy for solid cancers such as melanoma, renal cell carcinoma, and colorectal cancers. These cytokines work by triggering T cell activation and effector cell function; however, their induction is associated with severe irAEs such as RA and SLE (Ascierto et al., 2013; Gogas et al., 2010). IFN-α administration is associated with pernicious anemia in midgut carcinoid tumors. Vitiligo that occurs as a consequence of an autoimmune response against melanocytes was also observed after IL-2 treatment (Amos et al., 2011). Furthermore, it has been reported that cytokine administration causes colorectal damage, inducing inflammation and immune activation (Young et al., 2018).

Vaccine Therapy in Cancer

Cancer vaccines that aim to enhance antitumor immune response revolutionized the field of cancer therapy. One type of cancer vaccine, called multipeptide vaccine (gp100, MART-1, and NY-ESO-1 with Montanide ISA 51 VG) aims to enhance the activation of antitumor immunity (Donninger et al., 2021). In a study, it has been reported that combinatory therapies of cancer vaccines with immunotherapies have a higher incidence of developing arthralgia at a rate of 43% (Gibney et al., 2015). Sicca syndrome has also been observed in multipeptide vaccine treatment. Dry mount was reported in 24% of patients who have combinatory administration of nivolumab and multipeptide vaccine in metastatic melanoma (Gibney et al., 2015). Myalgia and muscle weakness have also been reported in 12% of patients who had nivolumab and multipeptide vaccine treatment (Gibney et al., 2015).

Adoptive T Cell Therapy in Cancer

Adoptive T cell therapy includes stimulation of patient-derived T cells and their transfer to patients to overcome the lack of T cell activation (Itzhaki et al., 2013). During therapy, lymphodepletion can be administered to patients to give them a competitive advantage over reinfused T cells, however, an autoimmune response can be induced after such interventions. As an example, in a study, adoptive T cell therapy has been shown to induce ocular attack and vitiligo in patients with melanoma (Amos et al., 2011).

One type of adoptive T cell therapy, named Chimeric Antigen Receptor (CAR) T cell therapy, contains custom production of T cell receptors (TCR) with the desired specificity using gene modification techniques. CAR T cell therapy aims to overcome the lack of naturally occurring antigen-specific T cells; however, the autoimmune response can be triggered due to this treatment. In a study, carbonic anhydrase IX – specific CAR T cell therapy has been reported to cause grade 3-4 liver toxicities that indicate irAEs occur with CAR T cell therapies for solid cancers (Lamers et al., 2006).

Autoimmune Response in Conventional Cancer Therapies

Chemotherapy is one of the conventional cancer therapies that targets cell cycle components and counteracts uncontrolled cell growth in cancer. Massive apoptosis, especially immunologic cell death, caused by chemotherapy creates an immunological environment and makes the peptides available to self-reactive lymphocytes (Gebremeskel & Johnston, 2015). For example, bleomycin, which is a chemotherapeutic agent that causes DNA damage, can induce sclerosis in cancer (Egiziano et al., 2016). Drug therapies and aromatase inhibitors used in estrogen receptor positive breast cancer (ER +) have also been reported to cause syndromes similar to lupus and RA (Cappelli & Shah, 2020; Egiziano et al., 2016; Valencia et al., 2019). In another study, it has also been observed that bleomycin and gemcitabine trigger skin sclerosis and also play a role in the development or exacerbation of Raynaud's phenomenon and ischemic digits (Alias et al., 2012).

Radiotherapy is another conventional cancer therapy that kills cells by ionizing radiation locally. It can induce an autoimmune response, as seen in the abscopal effect. The abscopal effect refers to a phenomenon that causes a decrease in tumor size not only in the tumor region targeted by radiotherapy or chemotherapy, but also in untreated tumors located elsewhere in the body (Ashrafizadeh et al., 2020). The precise mechanism of the abscopal effect is still unknown; however, the immunostimulatory environment produced by radiation therapy is considered to play an important role in its development. On the other hand, radiotherapy has been reported to promote localized scleroderma in patients (Egiziano et al., 2016).

Conclusion

The autoimmune responses observed in solid tumors are complex. They can be developed due to shared genetic factors, changes in the microbiota, and the toxicity of oncotherapies. Understanding the main factors of the autoimmune response would shed light on the general concept of immune tolerance, as well as the basic immunology in irAEs induced by oncotherapies. Novel cancer immunotherapy approaches have a better survival rate compared to conventional cancer therapies, with increasing immune toxicity. Further investigations in the immunology of the bidirectional relationship between cancer and autoimmune diseases would, we hope, help the development of optimal strategies for the treatment of cancer and the management of autoimmune diseases.

References

Alias, A., Rodriguez, E. J., Bateman, H. E., Sterrett, A. G., & Valeriano-Marcet, J. (2012). Rheumatology and oncology. *Bulletin of the NYU Hospital for Joint Diseases*, *70*(2), 109-114.

Amos, S. M., Duong, C. P., Westwood, J. A., Ritchie, D. S., Junghans, R. P., Darcy, P. K., & Kershaw, M. H. (2011). Autoimmunity associated with immunotherapy of cancer. *Blood*, *118*(3), 499-509. doi: 10.1182/blood-2011-01-325266.

Ascierto, P. A., Gogas, H. J., Grob, J. J., Algarra, S. M., Mohr, P., Hansson, J., & Hauschild, A. (2013). Adjuvant interferon alfa in malignant melanoma: an interdisciplinary and multinational expert review. *Critical Reviews in Oncology/Hematology*, *85*(2), 149-161.

Ashrafizadeh, M., Farhood, B., Eleojo Musa, A., Taeb, S., Rezaeyan, A., & Najafi, M. (2020). Abscopal effect in radioimmunotherapy. *Int Immunopharmacol*, *85*, 106663. doi: 10.1016/j.intimp.2020.106663.

Bareke, H., Juanes-Velasco, P., Landeira-Viñuela, A., Hernandez, A.-P., Cruz, J. J., Bellido, L., Góngora, R. (2021). Autoimmune responses in oncology: causes and significance. *International Journal of Molecular Sciences*, *22*(15), 8030.

Beck, K. M., Dong, J., Geskin, L. J., Beltrani, V. P., Phelps, R. G., Carvajal, R. D., Gartrell, R. D. (2016). Disease stabilization with pembrolizumab for metastatic acral melanoma in the setting of autoimmune bullous pemphigoid. *Journal for ImmunoTherapy of Cancer*, *4*(1), 1-5.

Benvenuto, M., Mattera, R., Masuelli, L., Tresoldi, I., Giganti, M. G., Frajese, G. V., Bei, R. (2017). The crossroads between cancer immunity and autoimmunity: antibodies to self antigens. *Front Biosci (Landmark Ed)*, *22*, 1289-1329.

Borghaei, H., Paz-Ares, L., Horn, L., Spigel, D. R., Steins, M., Ready, N. E., Holgado, E. (2015). Nivolumab versus docetaxel in advanced nonsquamous non–small-cell lung cancer. *New England Journal of Medicine*, *373*(17), 1627-1639.

Brahmer, J., Reckamp, K. L., Baas, P., Crino, L., Eberhardt, W. E., Poddubskaya, E., Spigel, D. R. (2015). Nivolumab versus docetaxel in advanced squamous-cell non-small-cell lung cancer. *N Engl J Med*, *373*(2), 123-135. doi: 10.1056/NEJMoa1504627.

Brevi, A., Cogrossi, L. L., Grazia, G., Masciovecchio, D., Impellizzieri, D., Lacanfora, L., Bellone, M. (2020). Much more than IL-17A: cytokines of the IL-17 family between microbiota and cancer. *Frontiers in Immunology*, *11*, 2914.

Buchbinder, E. I., & McDermott, D. F. (2015). Cytotoxic T-lymphocyte antigen-4 blockade in melanoma. *Clin Ther*, *37*(4), 755-763. doi: 10.1016/ j.clinthera.2015.02.003.

Burkholder, B., Huang, R.-Y., Burgess, R., Luo, S., Jones, V. S., Zhang, W., Zhang, Y.-M. (2014). Tumor-induced perturbations of cytokines and immune cell networks. *Biochimica et Biophysica Acta (BBA)-Reviews on Cancer*, *1845*(2), 182-201.

Cappelli, L. C., & Shah, A. A. (2020). The relationships between cancer and autoimmune rheumatic diseases. *Best Practice & Research Clinical Rheumatology*, *34*(1), 101472.

Cappelli, L. C., Shah, A. A., & Bingham, C. O., 3rd. (2017). Immune-related adverse effects of cancer immunotherapy- implications for rheumatology. *Rheum Dis Clin North Am*, *43*(1), 65-78. doi: 10.1016/j.rdc.2016.09.007.

Carlos, G., Anforth, R., Chou, S., Clements, A., & Fernandez-Peñas, P. (2015). A case of bullous pemphigoid in a patient with metastatic melanoma treated with pembrolizumab. *Melanoma Res*, *25*(3), 265-268.

Coley, W. B. (1891). II. Contribution to the knowledge of sarcoma. *Annals of Surgery*, *14*(3), 199.

Consortium, A. P. G. (2017). AACR Project GENIE: powering precision medicine through an international consortium. *Cancer Discovery*, *7*(8), 818-831.

Corsello, S. M., Barnabei, A., Marchetti, P., De Vecchis, L., Salvatori, R., & Torino, F. (2013). Endocrine side effects induced by immune checkpoint inhibitors. *J Clin Endocrinol Metab*, *98*(4), 1361-1375. doi: 10.1210/jc.2012-4075.

Corthay, A. (2009). How do regulatory T cells work? *Scandinavian Journal of Immunology*, *70*(4), 326-336.

Davar, D., Dzutsev, A. K., McCulloch, J. A., Rodrigues, R. R., Chauvin, J.-M., Morrison, R. M., Pagliano, O. (2021). Fecal microbiota transplant overcomes resistance to anti–PD-1 therapy in melanoma patients. *Science*, *371*(6529), 595-602.

Davey, G. M., Kurts, C., Miller, J. F., Bouillet, P., Strasser, A., Brooks, A. G., Heath, W. R. (2002). Peripheral deletion of autoreactive CD8 T cells by cross presentation of self-antigen occurs by a Bcl-2–inhibitable pathway mediated by Bim. *The Journal of Experimental Medicine*, *196*(7), 947-955.

Day, D., & Hansen, A. R. (2016). Immune-related adverse events associated with immune checkpoint inhibitors. *BioDrugs*, *30*(6), 571-584.

Donninger, H., Li, C., Eaton, J. W., & Yaddanapudi, K. (2021). Cancer vaccines: promising therapeutics or an unattainable dream. *Vaccines (Basel)*, *9*(6). doi: 10.3390/vaccines9060668.

Dumas, A., Bernard, L., Poquet, Y., Lugo-Villarino, G., & Neyrolles, O. (2018). The role of the lung microbiota and the gut–lung axis in respiratory infectious diseases. *Cellular Microbiology*, *20*(12), e12966.

Dyck, L., & Mills, K. H. (2017). Immune checkpoints and their inhibition in cancer and infectious diseases. *European Journal of Immunology*, *47*(5), 765-779.

Egiziano, G., Bernatsky, S., & Shah, A. A. (2016). Cancer and autoimmunity: Harnessing longitudinal cohorts to probe the link. *Best Pract Res Clin Rheumatol*, *30*(1), 53-62. doi: 10.1016/j.berh.2016.03.001.

Fadel, F., Karoui, K. E., & Knebelmann, B. (2009). Anti-CTLA4 antibody–induced lupus nephritis. *New England Journal of Medicine*, *361*(2), 211-212.

Fortner, R. T., Damms-Machado, A., & Kaaks, R. (2017). Systematic review: Tumor-associated antigen autoantibodies and ovarian cancer early detection. *Gynecol Oncol*, *147*(2), 465-480. doi: 10.1016/j.ygyno.2017.07.138.

Friedman, C. F., Proverbs-Singh, T. A., & Postow, M. A. (2016). Treatment of the immune-related adverse effects of immune checkpoint inhibitors: a review. *JAMA Oncology*, *2*(10), 1346-1353.

Gebremeskel, S., & Johnston, B. (2015). Concepts and mechanisms underlying chemotherapy induced immunogenic cell death: impact on clinical studies and considerations for combined therapies. *Oncotarget*, *6*(39), 41600-41619. doi: 10.18632/oncotarget.6113.

Gibney, G. T., Kudchadkar, R. R., DeConti, R. C., Thebeau, M. S., Czupryn, M. P., Tetteh, L., Fisher, K. J. (2015). Safety, correlative markers, and clinical results of adjuvant nivolumab in combination with vaccine in resected high-risk metastatic melanoma. *Clinical Cancer Research*, *21*(4), 712-720.

Gogas, H., Kirkwood, J. M., Falk, C. S., Dafni, U., Sondak, V. K., Tsoutsos, D., Spyropoulou-Vlachou, M. (2010). Correlation of molecular human leukocyte antigen typing and outcome in high-risk melanoma patients receiving adjuvant interferon. *Cancer, 116*(18), 4326-4333.

Hansen, E., Sahasrabudhe, D., & Sievert, L. (2016). A case report of insulin-dependent diabetes as immune-related toxicity of pembrolizumab: presentation, management and outcome. *Cancer Immunology, Immunotherapy*, *65*(6), 765-767.

Herkel, J., Mimran, A., Erez, N., Kam, N., Lohse, A. W., Märker-Hermann, E., Cohen, I. R. (2001). Autoimmunity to the p53 protein is a feature of systemic lupus erythematosus (SLE) related to anti-DNA antibodies. *Journal of Autoimmunity*, *17*(1), 63-69.

Hersh, E. M., O'Day, S. J., Powderly, J., Khan, K. D., Pavlick, A. C., Cranmer, L. D., Weber, J. S. (2011). A phase II multicenter study of ipilimumab with or without dacarbazine in chemotherapy-naive patients with advanced melanoma. *Investigational New Drugs*, *29*(3), 489-498.

Himoto, T., Yoneyama, H., Kurokohchi, K., Inukai, M., Masugata, H., Goda, F., Masaki, T. (2012). Clinical significance of autoantibodies to p53 protein in patients with autoimmune liver diseases. *Canadian Journal of Gastroenterology*, *26*(3), 125-129.

Hodi, F. S., Lee, S., McDermott, D. F., Rao, U. N., Butterfield, L. H., Tarhini, A. A., Kirkwood, J. M. (2014). Ipilimumab plus sargramostim vs ipilimumab alone for treatment of metastatic melanoma: a randomized clinical trial. *JAMA*, *312*(17), 1744-1753. doi: 10.1001/jama.2014.13943.

Huynh, A., DuPage, M., Priyadharshini, B., Sage, P. T., Quiros, J., Borges, C. M., Sharpe, A. H. (2015). Control of PI (3) kinase in Treg cells maintains homeostasis and lineage stability. *Nature Immunology*, *16*(2), 188-196.

Hwang, S. J., Carlos, G., Chou, S., Wakade, D., Carlino, M. S., & Fernandez-Penas, P. (2016). Bullous pemphigoid, an autoantibody-mediated disease, is a novel immune-related adverse event in patients treated with anti-programmed cell death 1 antibodies. *Melanoma Res*, *26*(4), 413-416.

Itzhaki, O., Levy, D., Zikich, D., Treves, A. J., Markel, G., Schachter, J., & Besser, M. J. (2013). Adoptive T-cell transfer in melanoma. *Immunotherapy*, *5*(1), 79-90.

Ivashko, I. N., & Kolesar, J. M. (2016). Pembrolizumab and nivolumab: PD-1 inhibitors for advanced melanoma. *Am J Health Syst Pharm*, *73*(4), 193-201. doi: 10.2146/ajhp1 40768.

Jour, G., Glitza, I. C., Ellis, R. M., Torres-Cabala, C. A., Tetzlaff, M. T., Li, J. Y., Ivan, D. (2016). Autoimmune dermatologic toxicities from immune checkpoint blockade with anti-PD-1 antibody therapy: a report on bullous skin eruptions. *Journal of Cutaneous Pathology*, *43*(8), 688-696.

Kandoth, C., McLellan, M. D., Vandin, F., Ye, K., Niu, B., Lu, C., Ding, L. (2013). Mutational landscape and significance across 12 major cancer types. *Nature*, *502* (7471), 333-339. doi: 10.1038/nature12634.

Keir, M. E., Butte, M. J., Freeman, G. J., & Sharpe, A. H. (2008). PD-1 and its ligands in tolerance and immunity. *Annu. Rev. Immunol., 26*, 677-704.

Khan, S., & Gerber, D. E. (2020). *Autoimmunity, Checkpoint Inhibitor Therapy and Immune-Related Adverse Events: A Review.* Paper presented at the Seminars in Cancer Biology.

Kostine, M., Chiche, L., Lazaro, E., Halfon, P., Charpin, C., Arniaud, D., Richez, C. (2017). Opportunistic autoimmunity secondary to cancer immunotherapy (OASI): an emerging challenge. *La Revue de Médecine Interne, 38*(8), 513-525.

Lai, K., Zhang, W., Li, S., Zhang, Z., Xie, S., Xu, M., Zeng, K. (2021). mTOR pathway regulates the differentiation of peripheral blood Th2/Treg cell subsets in patients with pemphigus vulgaris. *Acta Biochimica et Biophysica Sinica, 53*(4), 438-445.

Lamers, C., Sleijfer, S., Vulto, A. G., Kruit, W., Kliffen, M., Debets, R., Oosterwijk, E. (2006). Treatment of metastatic renal cell carcinoma with autologous T-lymphocytes genetically retargeted against carbonic anhydrase IX: first clinical experience. *Journal of Clinical Oncology: Official Journal of the American Society of Clinical Oncology, 24*(13), e20-22.

Larkin, J., Chiarion-Sileni, V., Gonzalez, R., Grob, J. J., Cowey, C. L., Lao, C. D., Rutkowski, P. (2015). Combined nivolumab and ipilimumab or monotherapy in untreated melanoma. *New England Journal of Medicine, 373*(1), 23-34.

Larkin, J., Chiarion-Sileni, V., Gonzalez, R., Grob, J. J., Cowey, C. L., Lao, C. D., Wolchok, J. D. (2015). Combined nivolumab and ipilimumab or monotherapy in untreated melanoma. *N Engl J Med, 373*(1), 23-34. doi: 10.1056/NEJMoa1504030.

Le, D. T., Lutz, E., Uram, J. N., Sugar, E. A., Onners, B., Solt, S., Laheru, D. A. (2013). Evaluation of ipilimumab in combination with allogeneic pancreatic tumor cells transfected with a GM-CSF gene in previously treated pancreatic cancer. *J Immunother, 36*(7), 382-389. doi: 10.1097/CJI.0b013e31829fb7a2.

Leech, M., Xue, J. R., Dacumos, A., Hall, P., Santos, L., Yang, Y., Morand, E. F. (2008). The tumour suppressor gene p53 modulates the severity of antigen-induced arthritis and the systemic immune response. *Clinical & Experimental Immunology, 152*(2), 345-353.

Li, P., Shi, J.-X., Dai, L.-P., Chai, Y.-R., Zhang, H.-F., Kankonde, M., Zhang, J.-Y. (2016). Serum anti-MDM2 and anti-c-Myc autoantibodies as biomarkers in the early detection of lung cancer. *Oncoimmunology, 5*(5), e1138200.

Li, Y., Karjalainen, A., Koskinen, H., Hemminki, K., Vainio, H., Shnaidman, M., Brandt-Rauf, P. W. (2005). p53 autoantibodies predict subsequent development of cancer. *International Journal of Cancer, 114*(1), 157-160.

Liu, Y., Dai, L., Liu, W., Shi, G., & Zhang, J. (2015). Autoantibody to MDM2: a potential serological marker of systemic lupus erythematosus. *Journal of Immunology Research, 2015*.

Liu, Y., Liao, X., Wang, Y., Chen, S., Sun, Y., Lin, Q., & Shi, G. (2017). Autoantibody to MDM2: a potential serological marker of primary Sjogren's syndrome. *Oncotarget, 8*(9), 14306.

Ludwig, R. J., Vanhoorelbeke, K., Leypoldt, F., Kaya, Z., Bieber, K., McLachlan, S. M., Hammers, C. M. (2017). Mechanisms of autoantibody-induced pathology. *Frontiers in Immunology*, 603.

Mehrian, R., Quismorio Jr, F. P., Strassmann, G., Stimmler, M. M., Horwitz, D. A., Kitridou, R. C., Jacob, C. O. (1998). Synergistic effect between IL-10 and bcl-2 genotypes in determining susceptibility to systemic lupus erythematosus. *Arthritis & Rheumatism: Official Journal of the American College of Rheumatology*, *41*(4), 596-602.

Motzer, R. J., Escudier, B., George, S., Hammers, H. J., Srinivas, S., Tykodi, S. S., Tannir, N. M. (2020). Nivolumab versus everolimus in patients with advanced renal cell carcinoma: Updated results with long-term follow-up of the randomized, open-label, phase 3 CheckMate 025 trial. *Cancer*, *126*(18), 4156-4167. doi: 10.1002/cncr.33033.

Mu, Y., Xie, F., & Sun, T. (2020). Clinical value of seven autoantibodies combined detection in the diagnosis of lung cancer. *J Clin Lab Anal*, *34*(8), e23349. doi: 10.1002/jcla.23349.

Nishino, M., Ramaiya, N. H., Awad, M. M., Sholl, L. M., Maattala, J. A., Taibi, M., Hodi, F. S. (2016). PD-1 inhibitor–related pneumonitis in advanced cancer patients: radiographic patterns and clinical course. *Clinical Cancer Research*, *22*(24), 6051-6060.

Okazaki, T., Chikuma, S., Iwai, Y., Fagarasan, S., & Honjo, T. (2013). A rheostat for immune responses: the unique properties of PD-1 and their advantages for clinical application. *Nature Immunology*, *14*(12), 1212-1218.

Okuda, Y., Okuda, M., & Bernard, C. C. (2003). Regulatory role of p53 in experimental autoimmune encephalomyelitis. *J Neuroimmunol*, *135*(1-2), 29-37. doi: 10.1016/s0165-5728(02)00428-9.

Pagaza-Straffon, C., Marchat, L. A., Herrera, L., Diaz-Chavez, J., Avante, M. G., Rodriguez, Y. P., Lopez-Camarillo, C. (2020). Evaluation of a panel of tumor-associated antigens in breast cancer. *Cancer Biomark*, *27*(2), 207-211. doi: 10.3233/CBM-190708.

Pardoll, D. M. (2012). The blockade of immune checkpoints in cancer immunotherapy. *Nature Reviews Cancer*, *12*(4), 252-264.

Park, J. S., Lim, M. A., Cho, M. L., Ryu, J. G., Moon, Y. M., Jhun, J. Y., Kim, H. Y. (2013). p53 controls autoimmune arthritis via STAT-mediated regulation of the Th17 cell/Treg cell balance in mice. *Arthritis Rheum*, *65*(4), 949-959. doi: 10.1002/art.37841.

Parsons, M. J., Jones, R. G., Tsao, M.-S., Odermatt, B., Ohashi, P. S., & Woodgett, J. R. (2001). Expression of active protein kinase B in T cells perturbs both T and B cell homeostasis and promotes inflammation. *The Journal of Immunology*, *167*(1), 42-48.

Peterson, J., Garges, S., Giovanni, M., McInnes, P., Wang, L., Schloss, J. A., Deal, C. (2009). The NIH human microbiome project. *Genome Research*, *19*(12), 2317-2323.

Portela, A., & Esteller, M. (2010). Epigenetic modifications and human disease. *Nature Biotechnology*, *28*(10), 1057-1068.

Postow, M. A., Chesney, J., Pavlick, A. C., Robert, C., Grossmann, K., McDermott, D., Hodi, F. S. (2015). Nivolumab and ipilimumab versus ipilimumab in untreated melanoma. *N Engl J Med*, *372*(21), 2006-2017. doi: 10.1056/ NEJMoa1414428.

Pradhan, V., Patwardhan, M., & Ghosh, K. (2010). Anti-nucleosome antibodies as a disease marker in systemic lupus erythematosus and its correlation with disease activity and other autoantibodies. *Indian Journal of Dermatology, Venereology and Leprology, 76*(2), 145.

Regen, T., Isaac, S., Amorim, A., Núñez, N. G., Hauptmann, J., Shanmugavadivu, A., Yogev, N. (2021). IL-17 controls central nervous system autoimmunity through the intestinal microbiome. *Science Immunology*, *6*(56), eaaz6563.

Revathidevi, S., & Munirajan, A. K. (2019). *Akt in Cancer: Mediator and More.* Paper presented at the Seminars in Cancer Biology.

Robert, C., Schachter, J., Long, G. V., Arance, A., Grob, J. J., Mortier, L., Investigators, K.-. (2015). Pembrolizumab versus ipilimumab in advanced melanoma. *N Engl J Med, 372*(26), 2521-2532. doi: 10.1056/NEJMoa1503093.

Routy, B., Le Chatelier, E., Derosa, L., Duong, C. P., Alou, M. T., Daillère, R., Roberti, M. P. (2018). Gut microbiome influences efficacy of PD-1–based immunotherapy against epithelial tumors. *Science*, *359*(6371), 91-97.

Ruff, W. E., Greiling, T. M., & Kriegel, M. A. (2020). Host–microbiota interactions in immune-mediated diseases. *Nature Reviews Microbiology*, *18*(9), 521-538.

Schreiber, R. D., Old, L. J., & Smyth, M. J. (2011). Cancer immunoediting: integrating immunity's roles in cancer suppression and promotion. *Science*, *331*(6024), 1565-1570.

Sibaud, V. (2018). Dermatologic reactions to immune checkpoint inhibitors: skin toxicities and immunotherapy. *Am J Clin Dermatol*, *19*(3), 345-361. doi: 10.1007/ s40257-017-0336-3.

Tischner, D., Woess, C., Ottina, E., & Villunger, A. (2010). Bcl-2-regulated cell death signalling in the prevention of autoimmunity. *Cell Death & Disease*, *1*(6), e48-e48.

Tocut, M., Brenner, R., & Zandman-Goddard, G. (2018). Autoimmune phenomena and disease in cancer patients treated with immune checkpoint inhibitors. *Autoimmunity Reviews*, *17*(6), 610-616.

Topalian, S. L., Drake, C. G., & Pardoll, D. M. (2015). Immune checkpoint blockade: a common denominator approach to cancer therapy. *Cancer Cell*, *27*(4), 450-461.

Valencia, J. C., Egbukichi, N., & Erwin-Cohen, R. A. (2019). Autoimmunity and cancer, the paradox comorbidities challenging therapy in the context of preexisting autoimmunity. *Journal of Interferon & Cytokine Research*, *39*(1), 72-84.

Volodko, N., Salla, M., Eksteen, B., Fedorak, R. N., Huynh, H. Q., & Baksh, S. (2015). TP53 codon 72 Arg/Arg polymorphism is associated with a higher risk for inflammatory bowel disease development. *World Journal of Gastroenterology: WJG*, *21*(36), 10358.

Wang, H., Li, X., Zhou, D., & Huang, J. (2019). Autoantibodies as biomarkers for colorectal cancer: A systematic review, meta-analysis, and bioinformatics analysis. *The International Journal of Biological Markers*, *34*(4), 334-347.

Weber, J. S., Kahler, K. C., & Hauschild, A. (2012). Management of immune-related adverse events and kinetics of response with ipilimumab. *J Clin Oncol*, *30*(21), 2691-2697. doi: 10.1200/JCO.2012.41.6750.

Wong, R. S. (2011). Apoptosis in cancer: from pathogenesis to treatment. *Journal of Experimental & Clinical Cancer Research*, *30*(1), 1-14.

Young, A., Quandt, Z., & Bluestone, J. A. (2018). The balancing act between cancer immunity and autoimmunity in response to immunotherapy. *Cancer Immunology Research*, *6*(12), 1445-1452.

Chapter 12

Autoantibodies in Cancer

Nese Cabuk Celik*, MD
Department of Rheumatology,
Cumhuriyet University, Sivas, Turkey

Abstract

Cancer is the most frightening and undesirable group of diseases among almost all diseases. However, autoimmunity is a principle operation in our body with a complex mechanism in our body, and we are not yet sure of its starting point. So what is the relationship between autoantibodies and cancer?

This section will discuss the increased potential association between autoantibodies and cancer. Autoantibodies against tumor antigens are a response of the humoral immune system. Autoantibodies may emerge before tumor development. Therefore, identifying antigens that affect an autoantibody response limited to any cancer has excellent potential for early detection. Numerous strategies are currently available to discover tumor antigens from circulating autoantibodies.

There are advantages and disadvantages of testing in all existing approaches during the extensive discovery of antigenic epitopes. Therefore, this section aims to review established or new strategies and methodologies and highlight their potential applications in cancer. In addition, of course, more detailed and cohort studies are needed to reveal the links between cancer and autoimmunity to lay the foundation for chance stratification and targeted cancer detection.

Keywords: autoimmune disease, autoimmunity, autoantibodies, cancer, rheumatic diseases

---

* Corresponding Author's Email: nesecabuk@gmail.com.

In: Autoimmunity and Cancer
Editors: Soner Şahin and Kenan Demir
ISBN: 978-1-68507-937-6

Introduction

Cancer is the second most common cause of death worldwide (Yach et al., 2004). In 2002, it was reported that there were 11 million new cancer patients and 7 million cancer-related deaths, and roughly 25 million people survived cancer (Parkin et al., 2005). Unfortunately, even today, despite the new strategies developed, many countries, including the USA and the UK, still cannot prevent high rates of cancer-related deaths (Jemal et al., 2008; Olsen et al., 2008). To meet this challenge, early cancer detection in advanced stages of cancer and often before it becomes incurable has been the focus of current medicine (Etzioni et al., 2003).

In addition, tumor-infiltrating B lymphocytes have been observed in most cancers in studies (Tsou et al., 2016). The B cell response occurs early during tumor development. This event is achieved by autoantibodies developed against cell surface and intracellular antigens (Hanash, 2003; le Naour, 2007; Pereira-Faca et al., 2007). In some cancers, this production of autoantibodies against neural cell proteins leads to paraneoplastic neurological symptoms that precede diagnosis (Leypoldt & Wandinger, 2014; Tschernatsch et al., 2009). In most patients, unfortunately, the presence of autoantythyrosis does not initiate symptoms, and, after all, it can not raise suspicion in the clinician. In early diagnosis, autoantythyra were seropositive formed during tumor development with humoral response to tumor antigens. Therefore, it can be used for cancer detection. In addition, antigenic epitopes can be used for immunotherapy and vaccine development.

The immune system determines the changes caused by cancer in cells and aims to destroy these damaged cells. During tumor formation, the protein patterns of normal cells change, and cancer begins to form. As a result, the tumor cell with a different code activates the immune system and humoral immunity is activated. Unfortunately, the immune system cannot detect antigens in the early period. On the other hand, it is possible to detect antibodies produced in response to the antigen early. Therefore, auto-antibodies play an important role in early cancer diagnosis.

Today, the autoantibodies formed can be detected thanks to several high-level featured methods. Currently, autoantibodies screening methods for cancer detection include serological proteome analysis (SERPA), serological analysis, expression cDNA libraries (SEREX), multiple affinity protein profiling (MAPPing) and phage display (H. T. Tan et al., 2009; Zaenker & Ziman, 2013). Moreover, recent advances in proteomic techniques to identify neo-epitopes of simultaneously discovered tumor-associated autoantigens have extended a new field of 'immuno-proteomics' that presents tumor-associated autoantibody signatures and informs to redefine the function of tumorigenesis (Heo et al., 2012).

Tumor-associated autoantibodies have different properties. These autoantibodies have very long half-lives. In addition, it can be easily controlled by a blood test. However, it is challenging to detect antigens formed in the early period of tumor formation in the blood. On the contrary, antibodies against a small antigen can be detected early as a robust immune system response. In addition, thanks to recently developed proteomic technology, simultaneous autoantibodies and autoantigens can be detected (Anderson & LaBaer, 2005; Kang et al., 2011). In this way, the TAA panel can be determined (Zhang et al., 2003).

Tumor-Associated Autoantibodies under the Control of the Immune System

The immune system, in which several interrelated mechanisms work simultaneously and in connection, fights external factors, such as viruses or bacteria, when our body encounters them. For example, cancer cells separate and multiply uncontrollably, composing malignant tumors and invading the body. Although tumor formation occurs cellularly, it is another important immune system target. Remodeling of the tumor cell in tumorigenesis and secretion of different proteins from normal cells causes changes in protein expression patterns and tumor microenvironments. In addition, microvesicles detached from tumor cells or proteins leftover from destroyed tumor cells affect the microenvironment of cells (Murphy et al., 2012; H. T. Tan et al., 2009). In recent studies, it has been observed that the immune system, whose main task is to recognize and destroy the cancer cell, sometimes interacts for transformation as a tumor cell (Chaput et al., 2008; Whiteside, 2008). In the early stage of cancer, this mutual interaction is one of the steps in cancer formation. The stages of the interaction of cancer and the immune system consist of 3 phases. These 3 phases of elimination, escape, and immune destruction is called 'immunosurveillance' (Dunn et al., 2002, 2004).

Considering the first phase, elimination, if the organism's immune system is healthy, it recognizes and eliminates cancer precursor cells (Zitvogel et al., 2006). To give an example of tumor elimination, activation of the immune system by natural killer cells and special receptors on T cells against natural killer ligand group 2D (NKG2D) on tumor cells is an example of elimination.

(McGilvray et al., 2009; Waldhauer & Steinle, 2008). Tumor cells that escape elimination prepare zenumin to balance the immune system. Thus, the tumor cell creates a suitable environment for survival (Dunn et al., 2002). Although difficult to directly analyze, there is evidence to support the immune surveillance hypothesis in cancer. It is observed that the incidence of cancer subtypes is high in immunocompromised individuals (Salavoura et al., 2008).

The immune subversion phase is now the phase in which tumor cells completely suppress the immune system of the cancer cell. Analyses have shown that vascular endothelial growth factor (VEGF) removed from tumor cells suppresses dendritic cells in many stages. In addition, VEGF is a potent stimulator of immature dendritic cells (iDCs). In this way, it allows iDCs to migrate from the bone marrow to the tumor site. iDCs arriving at the tumor site induce immune destruction by disrupting T cell function (Yigit et al., 2010).

Other tumor-derived factors such as IL-6, M-CSF and IL-1β prevent MSCs from transforming into dendritic cells by involving myeloid suppressor cells (MSCs) in the immune response. Increasing numbers of MSCs then act on tumor-specific T cells, inhibiting T cell responses via nitric oxide (NO) synthesis (Zitvogel et al., 2006), balancing the formation of a pro-tumor environment (Lechner et al., 2005). Tumor cells that use these mechanisms can exert an immunosuppressive effect on the self-microenvironment. The interaction mechanisms between the immune system and cancer cells are interested in tumor progression.

Immunoproteomics, which is used to identify these different components, aims to improve prevention, understanding, diagnosis, classification, and therapy. Immunoproteomics plays a critical role in the formation of tumor autoantigens and specific autoantibodies against them.

One of the critical roles of immunoproteomics is tumor-associated antigens and organizations related to autoantibodies formed in response to the antigen. Antigens formed at a low titer cannot trigger immunity, but autoantibodies can trigger an immune response at a lower titer. However, autoantibodies may not be sufficient to induce a necessary response. In this way, cancer cells can escape from immune control. Therefore, alternative ways are needed to understand the patho-physiology of tumorigenesis and for early diagnosis (Murphy et al., 2012).

Baldwin first described the emergence of hundreds of TAAs (Baldwin, 1966) as an immune response against visceral tumors. With the product of new proteomic technologies for detecting tumor-associated antigens, more studies have been conducted on profiling the serum of cancer patients (Ran et al.,

2008). Advanced technologies using proteomics platforms have allowed the simultaneous discovery of many TAAs (Figure 1) (Heo et al., 2012). In addition, these approaches have helped to detect many antigens using a small number of serums.

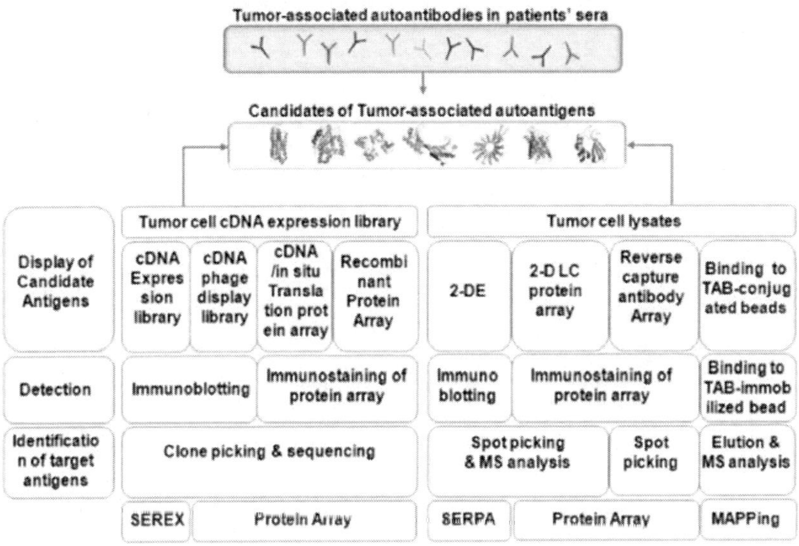

Figure 1. Systematic approaches for identifying tumor-associated autoantibodies (Heo et al., 2012).

Characteristics of Tumor-Associated Autoantigens (TAA) and Generation of Specific Humoral Immune Response

To date, many tumor-specific autoantibodies have been identified using various methods. The list of TAAs includes oncoproteins (e.g., HER-2/Neu, ras, and c-MYC), tumor suppressor proteins (e.g., p53), survival proteins (e.g., survivor), cell cycle regulatory proteins (e.g., cyclin B1), mitosis-associated proteins (e.g., centromere protein F), mRNA-binding proteins (e.g., p62, IMP1, and Koc) and differentiation and CTAs (e.g., tyrosinase and NY-ESO-1) (Table 1 and Table 2) (Desmetz et al., 2011; E. M. Tan & Zhang, 2008).

Table 1. Relationship between patient numbers and tumor-associated autoantigens in recent studies in 2011 (Heo et al., 2012)

Tumor-associated autoantigens	Patient number	Tumor type	Validation method	Specificity/ Sensitivity (%)
Phage display clones (N = 45)	235	Gastric cancer	Microarray	89.7/58.7
ABCC3	114	ESCC	ELISA	>95/13.2
HSP60, p53, Her2-Fc, NY-ESO-1, HSP70	29	Breast cancer	Microarray	82.7/–
NY-ESO-1, XAGE-1, ADAM29, MAGEC1	94	NSCLC	Microarray	89/36
GAL3, PAK2, PHB2, RACK1, RUVBL1	182	Breast cancer	ELISA	84/66
A1AT	25	Breast cancer	WB	–/96
NOLC1, MALAT1, HMMR, SMOX	65	NSCLC	ELISA	60/66.7
GRP78, AFP	76	HCC	ELISA	–/71.4
Ku86	58	HCC	ELISA	90/60.7
Lymphocyte antigen six complex locus K (LY6K)	62	ESCC	ELISA	78.7/80.6
p53, NY-ESO-1, CAGE, GBU4-5, SOX2, HuD, MAGE A4	235	Lung cancer	ELISA	91/41
BMI-1	67	Cervical cancer	ELISA	76/78
p53, p16, p62, survivin, Koc, IMP1	23	Pancreatic cancer	ELISA	87/60.9
Phage display clones (N = 5)	60	Colon cancer	ELISA	91.7-93.3/90-92.7
RPH3AL	84	Colon cancer	WB	84.1 /72.6
NY-ESO-1, SSX-2,4, XAGE-1b, AMACR, p90, LEDGF + PSA	131	Prostate cancer	seroMAP	84/79
MMP-7	50	ESCC	ELISA	81/78
SEC61β	86	Colon cancer	WB	75/79
STK4/MST1, SULF1, NHSL1, SREBF2, GRN, GTF2	50	Colon cancer	ELISA	73.9/72
p53, NY-ESO-1, CAGE, Hu-D, SOX2, Annexin I, GBU4-5	243	SCLC	ELISA	99/42
Programmable protein clones (N = 28)	51	Breast cancer	Microarray	61.6/80.8

*An updated list of the most recent studies (2011-present).

Table 2. Characteristics of tumor-associated autoantigens in 2010 (Heo et al., 2012)

Autoantigens	Number of patients	Tumor type	Prognosis
ENOA 1, 2	120	Pancreatic cancer	Increased survival
MUC1	28	Ovarian	Decreased survival
MUC1	395	Breast	Increased survival
EpCAM	84	Ovarian	None
ALK	95	Anaplastic large cell lymphoma	Decreased recurrence
CDC25B phosphatase	134	Esophageal cancer	Decreased survival
p53	120	Ovarian cancer	Increased survival
The panel of 29 antigens	60/59	Ovarian cancer/Pancreatic cancer	Increased survival
MIA	34	Pancreatic cancer	Increased survival

*An updated list of the most recent studies (2010-present).

Clinical Use of Tumor-Associated Autoantibodies

Antibodies, one of the adaptive immune responses, have many functions in preventing pathogenic infections. Although autoantibodies formed from the adaptive immune system have many protective functions, the functions of those developing secondary to the tumor are not fully understood. Autoantibodies can cause complement-dependent cytotoxicity (CDC) and antibody-dependent cell-mediated cytotoxicity (ADCC). In addition, autoantibodies amplify T lymphocyte activation and antigen cross-presentation. Autoantibodies against growth factors or cell surface receptors can inhibit receptor/ligand interactions. Autoantibodies, in general, organize to mount a severe immune response against non-self proteins (Casal & Barderas, 2010).

Tumor-Associated Autoantibodies as Diagnostic Markers

The definitive test to be chosen for early diagnosis of cancer; should give an idea about the prognosis and be inexpensive and straightforward. For this reason, much work has been done in recent years to detect increased or newly formed biomarkers due to tumor cells. However, research has shown that the clinical trial phase cannot be exceeded despite all efforts. The most important reasons are proteome heterogeneity, short half-life, and low blood antigen level. Tumor-associated autoantibodies have many advantages over standard protein biomarkers (Murphy et al., 2012). Although antigens are long-lived, this is not the case for autoantibodies. The antibody response is stable and persistent. In addition, due to the nature of the immune system, even a tiny amount of autoantibody response to the antigen will be in more significant concentrations to trigger the immune response better (Hanash, 2003). Because of these advantages, autoantibodies are functional as biomarkers. Another positive feature is that ELISA is cheap. Diagnostic and clinical, they can be applied to related analyzes. It is easy to create a multiplex panel of autoantibodies that develop secondary to the tumor. In this way, it can be used in a quickly combined form. Thus, the heterogeneity of tumor cell proteomes is overcome. In one study, combined analysis of autoantibodies against p53, HER-2, IGFBP-2, and TOPO2α increased diagnostic specificity and sensitivity by up to 75% for breast cancer patients (Lu et al., 2008). A diagnostic panel using five autoantigens (p53, NY-ESO-1, CAGE, GBU4-5, Annexin 1) was conducted to study 600 patients with lung cancer. The panel thus identified showed remarkable specificity (90%), while the sensitivity remained relatively low at 40% (Murray et al., 2010). Autoantibody detection methods are often performed proteomically by forming a panel, that is, by combining them, and it is beneficial in early diagnosis (Table 1).

Tumor-Associated Autoantibodies as Prognostic Markers

Biomarkers are essential for identifying individuals at high risk for cancer or following the survival or prognosis of diagnosed cases (Järås & Anderson, 2011). Oncologically followed patients can be predicted prognostic according to various classification and staging criteria. Thanks to prognostic biomarkers that measure gene expression, it has broad applications for multiple types of cancer and discrimination of cancer types with similar histology (Sotiriou & Pusztai, 2009). Although autoantibodies were targeted and recommended as precursors to cancer progression, today autoantibodies are often used for prognosis (Järås & Anderson, 2011; Kobold et al., 2010).

Tumor-Associated Autoantibodies in Personalized Cancer Therapy

The primary purpose of the immune system is to find the protein that does not belong to it and destroy it. Based on this strategy, the immune system aims to destroy the protein antigens formed by the tumor cell. These proteins are also used as therapeutic targets (Casal & Barderas, 2010; E. M. Tan & Zhang, 2008). Thus, vaccines against tumor cells have been developed with humoral and cellular immune system mechanisms. However, the mechanism did not act perfectly on normal cells, or healthy cells were not affected by the vaccine side effect, and only tumor cells were targeted (Fuessel et al., 2006; Slovin et al., 2007). On the other hand, patient heterogeneity can cause conflicting treatment results (Heller et al., 2010; Neller et al., 2008). Therefore, personalized autoantibody profiles should be used in therapy when targeting tumor-associated antigens.

Cancer Overview in Autoantibody Positive Autoimmune Diseases

Numerous autoimmune rheumatic diseases have an improved risk of cancer than the widespread population (Shah et al., 2015). However, the severe relationship between cancer and autoimmune rheumatologic diseases is becoming more complex. Learning epidemiology, pathogenesis, and long-term studies of rheumatic diseases have shown more links between the two pathological conditions, with new therapies being developed to treat cancer and autoimmune diseases (Cappelli & Shah, 2020). In addition, there is a close relationship with malignancy in many autoimmune diseases that are autoantibody-positive. For example, numerous epidemiological studies have supported the association between inflammatory myopathy and malignancy, with the strongest association observed in patients with dermatomyositis (DM) (Fallah et al., 2014).

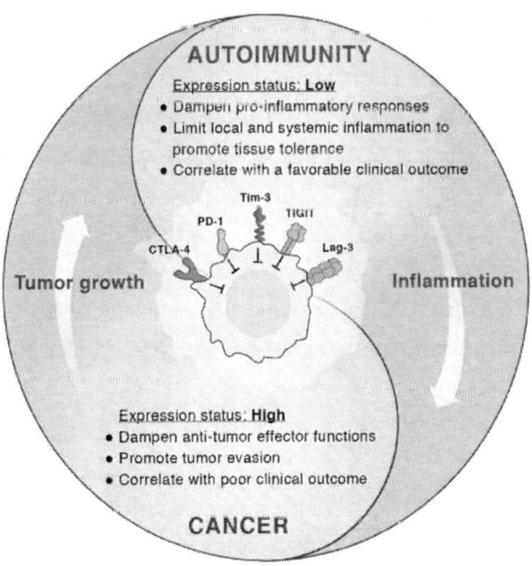

Figure 2. The dynamic and bidirectional link between autoimmunity and cancer (Masetti et al., 2021).

In addition to rheumatic diseases, such as inflammatory myopathies, which are much more well known to be associated with cancer, it has become evident that a wide range of rheumatic diseases is associated with certain types of cancer, increasing malignancy rates (Cappelli & Shah, 2020). Although the type of cancer and the type of rheumatic disease and the relationship between them are specific, research has shown that some types of cancer are sometimes associated with more than one autoimmune disease (Fallah et al., 2014). Furthermore, contrary to what has been known for years, as a result of studies conducted by centers with careful records and vital databases, it has been understood that there is almost no connection between anti-tumor necrosis factor (anti-TNF) therapy and certain malignancies. Moreover, these treatments have been shown to not cause an increase in cancer rates while treating autoimmune diseases (Liu et al., 2014; Wu et al., 2014). However, data indicate that chronic inflammation from rheumatic diseases or treatments can contribute to the initiation and progression of cancer. On the other hand, anti-tumor immune responses can initiate cross-reactions with their tissues, resulting in the development of autoimmunity (Figure 2) (Masetti et al., 2021).

Cancer Potential Mechanisms Secondary to Autoimmune Rheumatic Diseases

Various mechanisms can cause cancer to develop secondary to rheumatic diseases. These include chronic inflammation and tissue damage caused by autoimmunity, self-intolerance that develops while eliminating oncogenic viral infections, and long-term immunosuppressive treatments for rheumatic diseases (Roberts et al., 2020; Szekanecz et al., 2020; Xie et al., 2020).

Table 3. Mechanisms of cancer secondary to autoimmune rheumatic diseases (Masetti et al., 2021)

Type of autoimmune rheumatic disease	Mechanism	Effect
Systemic lupus erythematosus, Sjogren's syndrome, rheumatoid arthritis	Chronic inflammation and tissue damage	Failure of immune tolerance, production of cytokines and chemokines
Diseases requiring immunosuppressive therapies	Inability to clear oncogenic viral infection	Immune dysregulation
Diseases requiring immunosuppressive therapies	Prolonged immunosuppression	Immune dysregulation

Chronic Inflammation and Tissue Damage Caused by Autoimmunity

The immune system must maintain the integrity of the organism against all external threats (not from itself). In other words, the main task of the immune system here is to identify infective agents or tumors that the organism may encounter during its life cycle and to protect the organism against them. In this process, a healthy immune system can identify its antigens and does not create any reaction against them, which is called self-tolerance (Ruiz de Morales et al., 2020). CD4 (+) CD25 (+) Foxp3 (+) regulatory T cells (Tregs) are the mechanisms that provide immunological homeostasis. Both Tregs emanate directly from the thymus (natural Tregs) or from the periphery (peripheral Tregs). T lymphocytes stimulated by regulatory cytokines (i.e., TGF-β, IL-10) are responsible for terminating the immunological response, warning that the immune system is no longer required to function in an activated state against pathogens. Tregs are also responsible for eliminating self-responding lymphocytes that incorrectly evade central tolerance mechanisms through various suppressive mechanisms (Attridge & Walker, 2014; Campbell, 2015). These cells prevent tolerance and autoimmunity by inducing inhibitory cytokines, cytolysis, metabolic degradation, and activation or development of dendritic cells (DCs) (Karin et al., 2002). When immune tolerance mechanisms fail, autoimmunity and overall inflammation are activated. In other words, the failure of immune tolerance causes autoinflammation to be triggered, that is, the onset of chronic inflammation.

Chronic inflammation and tissue damage caused by autoimmunity; can produce cytokines and chemokines that trigger the development of malignancies through many mechanisms, including inactivation of tumor suppressor genes, DNA damage, stimulation of cellular growth and maintenance, enhancement of angiogenesis, and invasion. Often, this picture begins long before the development of the tumor structure. For example, various inflammatory cytokines, namely tumor necrosis factor (TNF)-α, interleukin (IL)-6, tumor growth factor (TGF)-β, and IL-10, have been shown to play a role in both the initiation and progression of cancer by initiating inflammation (Balkwill & Mantovani, 2001).

Inadequate Treatment of Oncogenic Viral Infections

Autoimmune diseases or immunosuppressive agents used to treat these diseases prevent the body from effectively dealing with oncogenic viral infections. As a result, it has been observed that many types of cancer develop secondary to specific viral agents. For example, in a study conducted on 576 patients with SLE in Denmark, an increased risk of virus-related cancer was observed. In particular, malignancies associated with human papillomavirus have been identified, including anal cancer, vaginal/vulvar cancer, cervical dysplasia, and non-melanoma skin. In addition, the risk of other potential viruses-associated cancers is also increased, including hepatocellular cancer (hepatitis B and C virus), bladder cancer (poliomavirus), and lymphoma (Epstein Barr virus) (Dreyer et al., 2011).

Rheumatological Treatments

The general principle of rheumatologic treatments is to suppress increased autoinflammation. For this reason, because of the immunosuppressive effect of almost all drugs used in the treatment of rheumatologic diseases, in addition to the above-mentioned mechanisms, drugs can cause cancer with specific effects. For example, cyclophosphamide, which has been used for many years to treat many rheumatological diseases and is still indispensable for rheumatologists, is well known as a side effect of bladder cancer, as evidenced by many studies (Monach et al., 2010). Mycophenolate use has been related to a possible increased risk of non-melanoma skin cancer and central nervous system lymphoma (Crane et al., 2015). The long-term use of azathioprine (>11 years or cumulative dose greater than 500 g) has been shown to generate the risk of skin squamous cell carcinoma and cervical atypia (van den Reek et al., 2014). A small, although significant, increase in the development of cutaneous malignant melanoma was observed in methotrexate-treated cases (Polesie et al., 2017). If we talk about anti-TNF therapy, which is one of the current treatment options and indispensable for rheumatology, we often encounter melanoma or non-melanoma skin cancer rather than visceral malignancies after these treatments. In addition, when patients with Rheumatoid Arthritis (RA) and those receiving anti-TNF therapy were examined, an increased incidence of lymphoma was observed (Solomon et al., 2012). On the other hand, it has been shown that there is no increase in the risk of malignancy after anti-TNF therapy in long-term studies with extensive follow-up (Emery et al., 2020).

Rarely, T cell lymphoma and hepatosplenic T cell lymphoma are increased in cases of inflammatory bowel disease using anti-TNF agents combined with thiopurines (azathioprine or 6-mercaptopurine) (Baecklund et al., 2014). In addition, some research has demonstrated that the use of thiopurine alone is linked to an improved risk of lymphoma (Wolfe & Michaud, 2004). Finally, a combination of methotrexate and anti-TNF agents has been observed to trigger a greater risk of non-melanoma skin cancer in RA (Eisenlohr & Rothstein, 2006).

Mechanisms of Autoimmune Rheumatic Diseases Secondary to Cancer

Table 4. Cancer risk of autoimmune rheumatic diseases (Masetti et al., 2021)

Type of autoimmune rheumatic disease	Cancer risk
Systemic lupus erythematosus	Non-Hodgkin's lymphoma
	Hodgkin's lymphoma
	Leukemia
	Laryngeal cancer
	Lung cancer
	Liver cancer
	Vaginal/vulvar cancer
	Thyroid malignancy
Scleroderma	Lung cancer
	Bladder cancer
	Hematological cancers
	Nonmelanoma skin cancers
Juvenile idiopathic arthritis	Lymphoproliferative malignancies
	Melanoma
	Solid-organ cancer
Sjogren's syndrome	Non-Hodgkin's lymphoma
Dermatomyositis	Nasopharyngeal carcinoma
	Ovarian carcinoma
	Lung cancer
	Colon cancer
	Pancreatic cancer
	Gastric cancer
Hashimoto's thyroiditis	Thyroid cancer

Although many patients have cancer due to autoimmunity, the opposite is possible (Table 4) (Masetti et al., 2021). In other words, some patients may have to struggle with a disease caused by autoimmune inflammation shortly after or before being diagnosed with cancer (Szekanecz et al., 2020). This pathology also develops through various mechanisms, like cancer that develops secondary to autoimmunity. These mechanisms arise from oncogenic inflammation, chemotherapy, radiation therapy, or immune-therapy.

Oncogenic Inflammation

Oncogene expression in target organ cells that develop after carcinogenesis can induce the release of innate chemokines, including NK (Natural Killer), NK T cells, macrophages, dendritic cells and neutrophils (Roberts et al., 2020; Xie et al., 2020). Factors secreted by the innate immune system cells can induce survival or apoptosis of neoplastic cells depending on the genes or pathways active in them. Self- or neoantigen-activated lymphocytes cause the let off of many cytokines, including interferon-γ, which lead to organ toxicity or dysfunction (Alias et al., 2012).

One of the most striking examples of oncogenic inflammation was scleroderma (Sc) when studies were examined. Examining Sc patients, increased expression of disease-associated antigens was found in specific subsets of cancer-associated autoantibodies comprehended as anti-RNA polymerase III in tumor tissues (Ioannou & Isenberg, 2000; Yang et al., 2015).

Chemotherapy, Radiation Therapy, and Immunotherapy

Chemotherapeutic agents can cause direct vascular toxicity and neurotoxicity. Therefore, endothelial dysfunction and abnormal sympathetic arterial vasoconstriction may develop due to these treatments. As a result of all these mechanisms, tumor tissue can cause new antigen formation. For example, a picture of skin sclerosis developed after using Bleomycin and Gemstabin, which are frequently used, chemotherapeutic agents. In addition, fingertip ischemia and associated exacerbations due to Raynaud's syndrome have been detected in some patients (Ioannou & Isenberg, 2000). Considering radiation therapy can induce severe skin thickening in patients with pre-existing Sc or newly developing localized Sc. Finally, as a result of IL-2 therapy, antitumor T cell infusions, cancer vaccines, immune checkpoint inhibitors, and all treatments aimed at strengthening the immunity of cancer patients or targeting the destruction of tumor cells through immunity, inflammatory rheumatological diseases can develop or inactive rheumatological diseases. May cause disease activation (Yang et al., 2015).

Immune checkpoint inhibitors (ICI) are among the most effective oncological treatments in recent years. Due to its precise and targeted working mechanism, global effects are not observed compared to classical treatments, and thus cancer cells are combated in a more localized area without affecting all organs. For many patients, these are treatment modalities that are more easily adapted than chemotherapy drugs. That is, they are more easily tolerated in terms of side effects. On the other hand, in addition to all these conveniences, immunotherapy also causes patients to encounter different problems due to autoimmune diseases that develop secondary to treatment. Anti-cytotoxic T lymphocyte-associated antigen (CTLA-4) agents (ipilimumab, tremelimumab), anti-PD-1 (nivolumab, pembrolizumab, cemiplimab) and anti-PD-L1 (atezolizumab, durvalumab, avelumab) are ICI class drugs. Considering the clinical benefits of ICI therapy, it causes serious autoinflammatory problems in patients. Studies have shown that ICIs cause new autoinflammatory diseases as side effects and activate existing but inactive autoinflammatory diseases (Xie et al., 2020).

Many autoantibodies are detected, especially when diagnosing patients with dermatomyositis (DM) and polymyositis (PM). Some of these autoantibodies indicate cancer for the clinician, while the presence of some indicates that suspicion of cancer should be avoided (Chinoy et al., 2007; Kaji et al., 2007; Targoff et al., 2006). Studies have shown that autoantibodies such as Transcription intermediary factor (TIF)-1 gamma, anti-p155, anti-p155/140, and nuclear matrix protein (NXP)-2 (anti-MJ or anti-p140) are closely associated with cancer. On the other hand, myositis-specific antisynthetase antibodies, antibodies such as anti-Mi-2, anti-SRP, anti-MDA5, and myositis-associated antibodies such as anti-RNP and anti-PM-Scl anti-Ku reduce the risk of cancer in DM but reduce the risk of interstitial cancer. On the other contrary, they were observed to cause an increase in lung diseases (Chinoy et al., 2007). Antinuclear antibodies (ANAs) are autoantibodies that react with various cytoplasmic and nuclear components of cells. They are serological markers of various autoimmune diseases such as systemic lupus erythematosus (SLE), Sjögren's syndrome (SS), scleroderma, polymyositis, or mixed connective tissue disease. In recent years, studies revealing the intricate relationship between autoimmunity and tumor development have focused on the role of autoantibodies in this mechanism. ANAs have been found in autoimmune diseases and in the serum of cases diagnosed with other cancers (Vlagea et al., 2018). These data mean that ANAs can recreate a role in the pathogenesis of cancer and premalignant diseases. In other words, studies have predicted that ANA becomes positive long before cancer or tumor formation and vice versa (Zou et al., 2015). Some cancer patients have been clinically misdiagnosed due to various serum autoantibodies and manifestations of rheumatism. Regardless of autoimmunity, ANA positivity can sometimes be detected in patients (Table 5) (Attar & Koshak, 2010).

This situation was related to prognosis in cancer cases, but also with autoantibody positivity, and it was observed that survival was higher in positive patients. Therefore, ANA positivity has been associated with progression-free and extended survival in patients with lung and colon cancer studies (Syrigos et al., 2000). Furthermore, in some studies, it has been observed that ANA values can be used to follow up on prognosis after immunotherapy treatment (Mitchell et al., 2015). Accordingly, some studies have shown that an autoimmune reaction is typical in patients with lung cancer and, as a precautionary measure, some asymptomatic patients may offer high levels of autoantibodies long before visceral tumors or related symptoms are noticed (Dellen & Seemayer, 1983). Furthermore, in another study, the spontaneous emergence of autoantibodies in some tumors, such as metastatic melanoma, was an excellent prognostic element in a prospective cohort (Maire et al., 2013). Therefore, types of cancer associated with ANAs classified according to their staining patterns are being investigated.

Table 5. Correlation between autoimmune disease, ANAs, and tumors with positive titer

Colagenosis	ANAs	Tumors related to a positive titer
SLE	Anti-DNA native y monocatenary Antihistones Anti-Sm Anti-Ro/SSA Anti-La/SSB Antiproteíns P ribosomals, Antifosfolípides Anti-PCNA.	Tymoma, lymphoma, lung cancer, MALT and NHL Lung, pancreatic, colon, and cervical cancer Lymphoma, myeloma, teratocarcinoma NHL, squamous cell carcinoma NHL Lymphoma
Scleroderma	Anticentromere, anti-DNA Topoisomerase I (Scl-70), Antinucleolar (PM/Scl, RNA polimerase, etc.)	Breast and lung cancer Lung cancer, ovarian and breast cancer Breast, lung, and haematologic cancer
Sjögren Syndrome	Anti-Ro/SSA Anti-La/SSB	NHL, squamous cell carcinoma NHL
Polimiositis	Antiaminoacil-sintetases t-RNA (Jo-1, etc.) Anti-Mi Anti-PM/Scl	Lung cancer, NHL, and renal cell cancer

Autoantibodies in Nuclear Staining Pattern

Staining Pattern AC-1 (Anti-ds DNA Antibodies)

Anti-ds DNA, double-stranded (ds) DNA, is essential for diagnosing SLE. In addition to SLE, anti-dsDNA antibodies may be positive secondary to some drugs such as minocycline, etanercept, infliximab, and penicillamine. These have been characterized as drug-induced lupus syndrome (arthritis, arthralgias, cutaneous vasculitis, and serositis) (Swaak et al., 1986). In 1978, Riska et al. found that these antibodies were also positive when working in malignant pleural effusions. In another study of 212 patients, it was observed that the principal risk of malignancy was thymoma and lymphoma in people without SLE (Attar & Koshak, 2010). Similar findings have been observed in recent studies, where the coexistence of lymphoproliferative diseases and rheumatological diseases is frequent, especially among lymphoma (MALT and diffuse B-cell large cell lymphoma) and anti-ds DNA positive individuals (titers >1/160) (Chloraki-Bobota et al., 2006).

Although anti-dsDNA antibodies are more specific for SLE, they can sometimes be noticed in malignant diseases unrelated to autoimmune diseases. However, these proteins' prognostic significance or therapeutic predictive value has not yet been clarified. For example, a recent article found that a high anti-ds DNA titer may increase the risk of thymoma recurrence (Cavagna et al., 2011). Similarly, a close relationship has been defined between the high-titer anti-ds DNA value and prognosis in cases diagnosed with colorectal cancer. Anti-histone protein antibodies are a subtype of ANAs and can be positive in approximately 50-70% of all cases with SLE. In addition, they often become positive in drug-induced SLE, which can occur due to procainamide, hydralazine, chlorpromazine, quinidine, and anticonvulsants (Katz & Zandman-Goddard, 2010). In colon cancer, anti-histone detection can be associated with colon cancer-associated p16 hypermethylation and serum screening results and can be used as a prognostic biomarker in these types of tumor, especially in stage II patients (Sakamoto et al., 2010). Accordingly, if these proteins are interpreted according to the results of the mentioned study, it was thought that they could be helpful for serum screening in colon cancer.

Staining Pattern AC-2 (Anti-DFS70 Antibodies)

Anti-DFS70, unlike other autoantibodies, is often negative in auto-inflammatory rheumatologic diseases (SARD). On the contrary, it was observed that it was more positive in the healthy population. They have also been related to different non-SARD conditions such as infections, atopic disease, asthma, inflammatory bowel disease, thyroid diseases, neurological disorders. DFS70-1 is an antiapoptotic protein associated with cellular stress. This protein is also involved in human immunodeficiency virus (HIV) infection (Syrigos et al., 2000).

When the relationship between malignancy and anti-DFS70 is examined, it has been observed that it is more frequently positive in prostate cancer. Furthermore, its changed expression has also been observed to be associated with cancer aggressiveness (Das et al., 2012).

Staining Pattern AC-3 (Anti-Centromere Antibodies)

Anticentromere antibodies with CREST and connective tissue diseases and cancer secondary to scleroderma. (SSc), has also been observed. An analysis based on the Asian population found that anticentromere antibody (ACA) positivity was a statistically influential cancer risk factor ($p < 0.05$) (Higuchi et al., 2000; Mccarty et al., 1983).

Staining Pattern AC-4 (Anti-Ro/SSA and Anti-La/SSB Antibodies)

After anti-Ds DNA, the most important antibodies to be analyzed in SLE screening are Anti-Ro/SSA antibodies. Although this antibody positivity is often associated with Sjögren's syndrome, it has also been closely associated with secondary non-Hodgkin lymphoma (Fragkioudaki et al., 2016). Again, this antibody negativity means that the risk of lymphoma is low (Quartuccio et al., 2015). Although several articles indicate a potential association between cutaneous lupus and cancer in anti-Ro/SSA-positive patients, further analysis is needed to provide this possible link. Laubli et al. reported the positivity of antinuclear anti-SSA/Ro and anti-SSB/La antibodies at high titers associated with autoimmune toxicity resulting in statistically significant results in cerebral vasculitis cases after AntiPDL1 treatment (Läubli et al., 2017).

Staining Pattern AC-5

Anti-Sm Antibodies

They can be found in approximately 25-30% of patients with high specificity in SLE. These antibodies have been caught in malignancies, primarily lymphoma and myeloma. In addition, some studies determined that this antibody was positive in mice with teratocarcinoma from visceral tumors (Kida et al., 1987).

Anti-RNP Antibodies

Many studies have determined a close relationship between anti-RNP and some visceral tumors. For example, Foster et al. described a metastatic undifferentiated carcinoma of unknown primary in a young patient who presented with musculoskeletal symptoms and high titers of anti-RNP antibodies. However, anti-RNP antibody positivity was not detected in patients with musculoskeletal symptoms until this study (Foster et al., 1997).

Anti-RNA Polymerase III

This antibody positivity in patients with scleroderma has been defined as a high risk of cancer. Shah et al. conducted a study on the increased cancer risk in scleroderma with high levels of anti-RNA polymerase III autoantibodies. A significant association has been found between probable cancer and autoimmunity in SSC patients (Bernal-Bello et al., 2017). As a result of the study conducted by the European League Against Rheumatism Scleroderma Research Group (EUSTAR), it was found that anti-RNAP3 positive patients with SSc have a high risk of malignancy. EUSTAR recommended that anti-RNAP3-positive SSc patients be screened regularly for cancer (Lazzaroni et al., 2017). In another study, in a cohort of patients with SSc, it was concluded that patients with SSc and positive anti-RNA P III were also predisposed to malignancy (Airo' et al., 2011).

Staining Pattern AC-13 (Anti-PCNA, Proliferating Cell Nuclear Antigen Antibodies)

This protein is a cofactor of the DNA-polymerase delta and is required for cell proliferation. The role of PCNA in cancer has been observed in many studies. Several studies have shown its expression to be positive in primary tumors and metastatic nodes. Conversely, no research has explained the association between anti-PCNA and PCNA in tumor tissue. Therefore, this antibody has not been accepted among ANA subtypes for its cancer relevance (Sidari et al., 2003). However, studies show that it is positive in skin cancers. In particular, it has been determined that it enables the determination of whether skin cancer is resistant to treatment and provides an early diagnosis of skin malignancies by determining the distribution of PCNA-positive cells in the skin (Kawahira, 1999).

Staining Pattern AC-14 (Anti-Centromere F)

CENP-F antibody positivity was highly correlated with neoplasia in malignant diseases when the studies were examined. Ratner et al. examined cancer incidence in patients with anti-CENP-F, a subtype of anticentromere antibodies. It was seen that 22 of 36 patients with CENP-F antibodies had neoplasms, of which 9 had breast cancer, and 5 had lung cancer. It has been concluded that individuals with CENP-F antibodies have a high incidence of neoplasia (Rattner et al., 1997). In another study, positive serum levels of anti-CENP-F were found to have a significantly high incidence in some histological subgroups of NHL patients. They also highlighted the utility of anti-CENP-F as a marker for NHL subgroups (Bencimon et al., 2005).

Staining Pattern AC -29 (Anti-SCL-70 or Anti-Topoisomerase I DNA Antibodies)

These antibodies are generally positive for visceral involvement and extensive systemic sclerosis. They are associated with pulmonary fibrosis and other connective tissue diseases (Bernal-Bello et al., 2017; Jablonska et al., 1992). High levels of these antibodies have been observed in some patients with cancer and paraneoplastic sclerosis. Although studies have shown a higher risk of cancer in patients with scleroderma positive, the possible risk factors for these cancers are unknown. In one study, 123 cases with systemic sclerosis with a median follow-up of 4 years were retrospectively analyzed and 14 cancer cases (11.3%) were found. Their distribution is lung 3, breast 2, ovary 2, skin 1, thyroid 1, rectum 1, cervix 1, larynx 1, pancreas 1, myelodysplasia 1 case (Gangopadhyay et al., 2013). In addition, Collaci et al. studied the relationship of tumors with Scleroderma (SSC) in patients with lung cancer. In patients with SSC positive for anti-Scl70 antibodies, the prevalence of lung cancer was 11.4% in the subgroup of patients with SSc, lung involvement compared to the general population. However, in the literature, the prevalence of lung cancer in an SSc series was 2.4%. At the end of the study, it was confirmed that there was a higher incidence of lung cancer. In another study, mean levels of anti-Scl-70 ($p = 0.023$), anti-Jo-1 ($p = 0.017$), and RF ($p = 0.046$) in newly diagnosed patients with NHL (Non-Hodgkin Lymphoma) were compared to other groups of patients without NHL significantly higher. This suggested that NHL has a potential role in the development of autoimmune disease. However, no significant relationship was found between autoantibodies and other clinical-pathological factors (Bilici et al., 2012). The association between ANAs and gastric cancer was investigated in 93 gastric cancer patients (stages I-IV) studied in a different study conducted in Africa. At the end of the study, anti-scl 70 autoantibody positivity was statistically significantly higher in cancer cases than in healthy controls (29% vs 5%, $p < 0.001$) (Lazzaroni et al., 2017).

Autoantibodies in Mitotic Staining Pattern

Staning Model AC-26: NuMA (MSA-1)

Nuclear mitotic apparatus proteins (NuMA) are proteins located in the cell nucleus in the interphase phase in response to external signals (such as hormones) that cause cell division, that is, apoptosis, thus inducing heat shock. Nuclear matrix protein (subtype 1), even learned as NuMA1, has been detected in the nuclear organization during the cell cycle in estrogen-sensitive MCF-7 breast cancer cells and androgen-sensitive LNCaP prostate cancer cells immunoelectron microscopy (Attar & Koshak, 2010). Additional studies are also underway on the possible use of nuclear matrix proteins as prostate cancer markers (Gobert et al., 2001).

Cytoplasmic Staining

Staining Model AC-15, 16 y 17 (Cytoskeletal Fibrils)

Anti-Actin Antibodies

Cytoskeleton: It is made of different proteins such as actin, actin-related proteins, cytokeratin, tropomyosin, and vimentin. Other studies have revealed connections between these proteins and various types of cancer. For example, Maroun MC et al. showed that cases of breast cancer have high anticentrosome antibodies in their serum. This study's targeted antigens, actin-induced protein, and HS actin gamma-1 were positive (Fernández-Madrid & Maroun, 2014). However, studies have shown that transgelin, an actin-induced protein, has tumor-suppressive activity. Transgelin has been shown to be repressed in pending prostate cancer progression and may play an essential function in the dysregulation of the actin cytoskeleton (Prasad et al., 2010). Some studies have been planned according to the mechanism of action of these proteins, which are potential targets for different drugs that can block tumor cell activity (Giganti & Friederich, 2003). When urothelial cancers are examined, different patterns in tumor cytoskeletal proteins (in tissue, not serum) such as Gelsolin and E-cadherin, have provided separate prognostic data for high-grade urothelial carcinomas (Rao et al., 2002).

Anti-Ribosomal P Protein Antibodies

This antibody targets ribonucleoproteins P0, P1, and P2. Specific for SLE, such as anti-dsDNA or anti-Sm, are available. However, they are found positive in only 10-30% of patients. Lupus patients are associated with psychosis, acute nephropathy, mononeuritis, or serositis. Autoantibodies against ribosomal proteins are usually positive in patients with systemic lupus erythematosus with active disease (Field et al., 1988).

Staining Model AC-20 (Anti-Jo1)

Antibodies are located in the nucleus and cytoplasm and target t-RNA. The most common subtype is anti-Jo 1 antibodies that bind to histidylsynthetase. They induce an enzymatic complex with a cytoplasmic pattern. It is associated with Anti-synthetase syndrome and polymyositis. Nakanishi et al. first described their relationship with cancer in prostate cancer. Anti-Jo1 positivity was observed in a patient with prostate cancer diagnosed with polymyositis (Nakanishi & Hatayama, 2006). Research has explained that cancer risk in polymyositis cases is associated with high antibodies (anti-Jo1, anti-PM-Scl, anti-U1-RNP, anti-U3-RNP, anti-Ku antibodies). It has also been susceptible to predicting cancer risk in these cases (Hochberg et al., 1984).

Staining Model AC-21 (AMA Anti-Mitochondrial Antibodies)

Immunohistochemical expression of these antibodies has been observed in various tumors with oncocytic differentiation (Ohtake et al., 2010). For instance, in one study, Anti-AMA113-1 was used to diagnose different salivary tumors (Vera-Sempere & Vera-Sirera, 2011). However, there are not many studies investigating the role of the AMA titer in cancerous tissue.

Conclusion

Mechanisms of the formation of tumor-associated autoantibodies and how their production is regulated have not been enterily determined. However, the known proof of TAAs and their characterization will lead us to a more precise understanding of the process of tumorigenesis and the interaction between tumor cells and the immune system. Autoantibodies are also very successful in identifying organizations that remodel or become disorganized at the cellular level. (Liu et al., 2011). When autoantibodies against these TAAs become early cancer markers, it is unclear whether anti-TAA antibody expression changes in advanced stages or with treatment. More detailed and further studies are also needed to find them. TAA autoantibodies have been investigated for their usefulness as a biomarker used in the early diagnosis of tumors, demonstrating therapeutic results, and monitoring the prognosis of the disease. (Hanash, 2003). Autoantibody profiles have already confirmed clinically complex cohorts of prostate cancer patients (Taylora et al., 2008). This classification may be helpful for personalized medicine.

Additionally, as mentioned above, autoantibodies such as ANAs are on the way to becoming a marker that can be used to specify patients with cancer risk and should be examined explicitly for early diagnosis. It is also very promising as a biomarker that can predict cancer prognosis. New diagnostic tools based on antibodies can decrypt these difficulties experienced in cancer and rheumatic diseases can be decrypted. Cancer development in cases with rheumatic diseases is a significant issue that requires long-term prospective follow-up studies in patients with rheumatic diseases. Several of the new biological immunotherapies can cause autoimmune diseases and ANAs can be possible identifications of effectiveness and toxicity.

References

Airo, P., Ceribelli, A., Cavazzana, I., Taraborelli, M., Zingarelli, S., & Franceschini, F. (2011). Malignancies in Italian patients with systemic sclerosis positive for anti-RNA polymerase III antibodies. *Journal of Rheumatology*, *38*(7), 1329–1334. https://doi.org/10.3899/jrheum.101144.

Alias, A., Rodriguez, E. J., Bateman, H. E., Sterrett, A. G., & Valeriano-Marcet, J. (2012). Rheumatology and oncology: An updated review of rheumatic manifestations of malignancy and anti-neoplastic therapy. *Bulletin of the NYU Hospital for Joint Diseases*, *70*(2), 109–114.

Anderson, K. S., & LaBaer, J. (2005). The sentinel within: Exploiting the immune system for cancer biomarkers. *Journal of Proteome Research*, *4*(4), 1123–1133. https://doi.org/10.1021/pr0500814.

Attar, S. M., & Koshak, E. A. (2010). Medical conditions associated with a positive anti-doublestranded deoxyribonucleic acid. *Saudi Medical Journal*, *31*(7), 781–787.

Attridge, K., & Walker, L. S. K. (2014). Homeostasis and function of regulatory T cells (Tregs) in vivo: Lessons from TCR-transgenic Tregs. *Immunological Reviews*, *259*(1), 23–39. https://doi.org/10.1111/imr.12165.

Baecklund, E., Smedby, K. E., Sutton, L. A., Askling, J., & Rosenquist, R. (2014). Lymphoma development in patients with autoimmune and inflammatory disorders - What are the driving forcesα. *Seminars in Cancer Biology*, *24*, 61–70. https://doi.org/10.1016/j.semcancer.2013.12.001.

Baldwin, R. W. (1966). Tumour-specific immunity against spontaneous rat tumours. In *Int. J. Cancer* (Vol. 1).

Balkwill, F., & Mantovani, A. (2001). Inflammation and cancer: Back to Virchow? *Lancet*, *357*(9255), 539–545. https://doi.org/10.1016/S0140-6736(00)04046-0.

Bencimon, C., Salles, G., Moreira, A., Guyomard, S., Coiffier, B., Bienvenu, J., & Fabien, N. (2005). Prevalence of anticentromere F protein autoantibodies in 347 patients with non-Hodgkin's lymphoma. *Annals of the New York Academy of Sciences*, *1050*, 319–326. https://doi.org/10.1196/annals.1313.034.

Bernal-Bello, D., Guillén-del Castillo, A., Selva-O'Callaghan, A., Fonollosa-Pla, V., de Tena, J. G., & Simeón-Aznar, C. P. (2017). Understanding the role of antibodies as markers of cancer-associated systemic sclerosis: comment on the article by Shah et al. *Arthritis and Rheumatology*, *69*(9), 1914–1914. https://doi.org/10.1002/art.40129.

Bilici, A., Yapici, H. S., Ercan, S., Seker, M., Oven Ustaalioglu, B. B., Salman, T., Orcun, A., & Gumus, M. (2012). The prevalence and significance of autoantibodies in patients with non-Hodgkin's lymphoma: Are they correlated with clinicopathological features? *Journal of B.U.ON.*, *17*(3), 502–507.

Campbell, D. J. (2015). Control of Regulatory T cell migration, function, and homeostasis. *The Journal of Immunology*, *195*(6), 2507–2513. https://doi.org/10.4049/jimmunol.1500801.

Cappelli, L. C., & Shah, A. A. (2020). The relationships between cancer and autoimmune rheumatic diseases. *Best Practice and Research: Clinical Rheumatology*, *34*(1), 1–14. https://doi.org/10.1016/j.berh.2019.101472.

Casal, J. I., & Barderas, R. (2010). Identification of cancer autoantigens in serum: Toward diagnosticprognostic testing? *Molecular Diagnosis and Therapy*, *14*(3), 149–154. https://doi.org/10.2165/11534760-000000000-00000.

Cavagna, L., Prisco, E., Montecucco, C., & Caporali, R. (2011). Association between anti-dsDNA titre increase and thymoma relapse. *Clinical and Experimental Rheumatology*, *29*(3), 599–600.

Chaput, N., Conforti, R., Viaud, S., Spatz, A., & Zitvogel, L. (2008). The Janus face of dendritic cells in cancer. *Oncogene*, *27*(45), 5920–5931. https://doi.org/10.1038/onc.2008.270.

Chinoy, H., Fertig, N., Oddis, C. v., Ollier, W. E. R., & Cooper, R. G. (2007). The diagnostic utility of myositis autoantibody testing for predicting the risk of cancer-associated myositis. *Annals of the Rheumatic Diseases*, *66*(10), 1345–1350. https://doi.org/10.1136/ard.2006.068502.

Chloraki-Bobota, A., Megalakaki, C., Repousis, P., Chalkiopoulou, I., Lalaki, I., Trafalis, D. T., Athanassiou, A. E., & Mitsouli-Mentzikof, C. (2006). Prevalence of auto-antibodies (ANA, anti ds-DNA, ENA, IMF) and rheumatic syndromes in patients with lymphoproliferative diseases. *Journal of B.U.ON.*, *11*(4), 485–489.

Crane, G. M., Powell, H., Kostadinov, R., Rocafort, P. T., Rifkin, D. E., Burger, P. C., Ambinder, R. F., Swinnen, L. J., Borowitz, M. J., & Duffield, A. S. (2015). Primary CNS lymphoproliferative disease, mycophenolate and calcineurin inhibitor usage. *Oncotarget*, *6*(32), 33849–33866. https://doi.org/10.18632/oncotarget.5292.

Das, N., Paul, S., Chatterjee, D., Banerjee, N., Majumder, N. S., Sarma, N., Sau, T. J., Basu, S., Banerjee, S., Majumder, P., Bandyopadhyay, A. K., States, J. C., & Giri, A. K. (2012). Arsenic exposure through drinking water increases the risk of liver and cardiovascular diseases in the population of West Bengal, India. *BMC Public Health*, *12*(1), 1–9. https://doi.org/10.1186/1471-2458-12-639.

Dellen, H., & Seemayer, N. H. (1983). Autoimmunity in patients with bronchogenic carcinomas: Occurrence of antibodies against nuclear antigens, chromosomes and dsdesoxy-ribonucleic acid. *Zentralblatt Fur Bakteriologie, Mikrobiologie Und Hygiene. 1. Abt. Originale B, Hygiene*, *177*(6), 451–468.

Desmetz, C., Mange, A., Maudelonde, T., & Solassol, J. (2011). Autoantibody signatures: Progress and perspectives for early cancer detection. *Journal of Cellular and Molecular Medicine*, *15*(10), 2013–2024. https://doi.org/10.1111/j.1582-4934.2011.01355.x.

Dreyer, L., Faurschou, M., Mogensen, M., & Jacobsen, S. (2011). High incidence of potentially virus-induced malignancies in systemic lupus erythematosus: A long-term follow-up study in a Danish cohort. *Arthritis and Rheumatism*, *63*(10), 3032–3037. https://doi.org/10.1002/art.30483.

Dunn, G. P., Bruce, A. T., Ikeda, H., Old, L. J., & Schreiber, R. D. (2002). Cancer immunoediting: from immunosurveillance to tumor escape. *Nature Immunology*, *3*(11), 991–998. https://doi.org/10.1038/ni1102-991.

Dunn, G. P., Old, L. J., & Schreiber, R. D. (2004). The three Es of cancer immunoediting. *Annual Review of Immunology*, *22*, 329–360. https://doi.org/10.1146/annurev.immunol.22.012703.104803.

Eisenlohr, L. C., & Rothstein, J. L. (2006). Oncogenic inflammation and autoimmune disease. *Autoimmunity Reviews*, *6*(2), 107–114. https://doi.org/10.1016/j.autrev.2006.04.002.

Emery, P., Furst, D. E., Kirchner, P., Melega, S., Lacey, S., & Lehane, P. B. (2020). Risk of malignancies in patients with rheumatoid arthritis treated with rituximab: analyses of global postmarketing safety data and long-term clinical trial data. *Rheumatology and Therapy*, *7*(1), 121–131. https://doi.org/10.1007/s40744-019-00183-6.

Etzioni, R., Urban, N., Ramsey, S., McIntosh, M., Schwartz, S., Reid, B., Radich, J., Anderson, G., & Hartwell, L. (2003). The case for early detection. *Nature Reviews Cancer*, *3*(4), 243–252. https://doi.org/10.1038/nrc1041.

Fallah, M., Liu, X., Ji, J., Försti, A., Sundquist, K., & Hemminki, K. (2014). Autoimmune diseases associated with non-Hodgkin lymphoma: a nationwide cohort study. *Annals of Oncology*, *25*(10), 2025–2030. https://doi.org/10.1093/annonc/mdu365.

Fernández-Madrid, F., & Maroun, M. C. (2014). Autoantibodies in breast cancer. *Advances in Clinical Chemistry*, *64*, 1–15. https://doi.org/10.1016/B978-0-12-800263-6.00005-7.

Field, M., Williams, D. G., Charles, P., & Maini, R. N. (1988). Specificity of anti-Sm antibodies by ELISA for systemic lupus erythematosus: Increased sensitivity of detection using purified peptide antigens. *Annals of the Rheumatic Diseases*, *47*(10), 820–825. https://doi.org/10.1136/ard.47.10.820.

Foster, H. E., Malleson, P. N., Petty, R. E., & Cabral, D. A. (1997). Anti-RNP antibody in a child with undifferentiated carcinoma and no evidence of mixed connective tissue disease. *British Journal of Rheumatology*, *36*(2), 289–291. https://doi.org/10.1093/rheumatology/36.2.289.

Fragkioudaki, S., Mavragani, C. P., & Moutsopoulos, H. M. (2016). Predicting the risk for lymphoma development in Sjogren syndrome. *Medicine (United States)*, *95*(25), 1–8. https://doi.org/10.1097/MD.0000000000003766.

Fuessel, S., Meye, A., Schmitz, M., Zastrow, S., Linné, C., Richter, K., Löbel, B., Hakenberg, O. W., Hoelig, K., Rieber, E. P., & Wirth, M. P. (2006). Vaccination of hormone-refractory prostate cancer patients with peptide cocktail-loaded dendritic cells: Results of a phase I clinical trial. *Prostate*, *66*(8), 811–821. https://doi.org/10.1002/pros.20404.

Gangopadhyay, A., Sen, S., Naskar, B., & Chatterjee, G. (2013). Anti-SCL-70 antibody positive systemic sclerosis in a patient with lung cancer: A paraneoplastic or a purely coincidental phenomenon? *Indian Journal of Dermatology*, *58*(5), 400–401. https://doi.org/10.4103/0019-5154.117326.

Giganti, A., & Friederich, E. (2003). The actin cytoskeleton as a therapeutic target: state of the art and future directions. *Progress in Cell Cycle Research*, *5*, 511–525.

Gobert, G. N., Hueser, C. N., Curran, E. M., Sun, Q. Y., Glinsky, V. v., Welshons, W. v., Eisenstark, A., & Schatten, H. (2001). Immunolocalization of NuMA and phosphorylated proteins during the cell cycle in human breast and prostate cancer cells as analyzed by immunofluorescence and post embedding immunoelectron micro-scopy. *Histochemistry and Cell Biology*, *115*(5), 381–395. https://doi.org/10.1007/s004180100260.

Hanash, S. (2003). Harnessing immunity for cancer marker discovery. *Nature Biotechnology*, *21*(1), 37–38. https://doi.org/10.1038/nbt0103-37.

Heller, A., Zörnig, I., Müller, T., Giorgadze, K., Frei, C., Giese, T., Bergmann, F., Schmidt, J., Werner, J., Buchler, M. W., Jaeger, D., & Giese, N. A. (2010). Immunogenicity of SEREX-identified antigens and disease outcome in pancreatic cancer. *Cancer Immunology, Immunotherapy*, *59*(9), 1389–1400. https://doi.org/10.1007/s00262010-0870-9.

Heo, C. K., Bahk, Y. Y., & Cho, E. W. (2012). Tumor-associated autoantibodies as diagnostic and prognostic biomarkers. *BMB Reports*, *45*(12), 677–685. https://doi.org/10.5483/BMBRep.2012.45.12.236.

Higuchi, M., Horiuchi, T., Ishibashi, N., Yoshizawa, S., Niho, Y., & Nagasawa, K. (2000). Anti centromere antibody as a risk factor for cancer in patients with systemic sclerosis. *Clinical Rheumatology*, *19*(2), 1–7. https://doi.org/10.1007/s100670050029.

Hochberg, M. C., Feldman, D., Stevens, M. B., Arnett, F. C., & Reichlin, M. (1984). Antibody to Jo-1 in polymyositis/dermatomyositis: Association with interstitial pulmonary disease. *Journal of Rheumatology*, *11*(5), 663–665.

Ioannou, Y., & Isenberg, D. A. (2000). Current evidence for the induction of autoimmune rheumatic manifestations by cytokine therapy. *Arthritis and Rheumatism*, *43*(7), 1431–1442. https://doi.org/10.1002/1529-0131(200007)43:7<1431::AID-ANR3>3.0.CO;2-E.

Jablonska, S., Blaszczyk, M., Chorzelski, T. P., Jarzabek-Chorzelska, M., Kumar, V., & Beutner, E. H. (1992). Clinical relevance of immunologic findings in scleroderma. *Clinics in Dermatology*, *10*(4), 407–421. https://doi.org/10.1016/0738-081X(92)90087-F.

Järås, K., & Anderson, K. (2011). Autoantibodies in cancer: Prognostic biomarkers and immune activation. *Expert Review of Proteomics*, *8*(5), 577–589. https://doi.org/10.1586/epr.11.48.

Jemal, A., Siegel, R., Ward, E., Hao, Y., Xu, J., Murray, T., & Thun, M. J. (2008). Cancer Statistics, 2008. *CA: A Cancer Journal for Clinicians*, *58*(2), 71–96. https://doi.org/10.3322/ca.2007.0010.

Kaji, K., Fujimoto, M., Hasegawa, M., Kondo, M., Saito, Y., Komura, K., Matsushita, T., Orito, H., Hamaguchi, Y., Yanaba, K., Itoh, M., Asano, Y., Seishima, M., Ogawa, F., Sato, S., & Takehara, K. (2007). Identifying a novel autoantibody reactive with 155 and 140 kDa nuclear proteins in patients with dermatomyositis: An association with malignancy. *Rheumatology*, *46*(1), 25–28. https://doi.org/10.1093/rheumatology/kel161.

Kang, J. G., Ko, J. H., & Kim, Y. S. (2011). Pros and cons of using aberrant glycosylation as companion biomarkers for therapeutics in cancer. *BMB Reports*, *44*(12), 765–771. https://doi.org/10.5483/BMBRep.2011.44.12.765.

Karin, M., Cao, Y., Greten, F. R., & Li, Z. W. (2002). NF-κB in cancer: From innocent bystander to major culprit. *Nature Reviews Cancer*, *2*(4), 301–310. https://doi.org/10.1038/nrc780.

Katz, U., & Zandman-Goddard, G. (2010). Drug-induced lupus: An update. *Autoimmunity Reviews*, *10*(1), 46–50. https://doi.org/10.1016/j.autrev.2010.07.005.

Kawahira, K. (1999). Immunohistochemical staining of proliferating cell nuclear antigen (PCNA) in malignant and nonmalignant skin diseases. *Archives of Dermatological Research*, *291*(7–8), 413–418. https://doi.org/10.1007/s004030050431.

Kida, K., Hayashi, M., Yamada, I., Matsuda, H., Yoshinaga, J., Takami, S., Yashiki, S., & Sonoda, S. (1987). Heterogeneity in myasthenia gravis: HLA phenotypes and autoantibody responses in ocular and generalized types. *Annals of Neurology*, *21*(3), 274–278. https://doi.org/10.1002/ana.410210309.

Kobold, S., Luetkens, T., Cao, Y., Bokemeyer, C., & Atanackovic, D. (2010). Prognostic and diagnostic value of spontaneous tumor-related antibodies. *Clinical and Developmental Immunology*, *2010*, 1–8. https://doi.org/10.1155/2010/721531.

Läubli, H., Hench, J., Stanczak, M., Heijnen, I., Papachristofilou, A., Frank, S., Zippelius, A., & Stenner-Liewen, F. (2017). Cerebral vasculitis mimicking intracranial metastatic progression of lung cancer during PD-1 blockade. *Journal for Immuno Therapy of Cancer*, *5*(1), 1–6. https://doi.org/10.1186/s40425-017-0249-y.

Lazzaroni, M. G., Cavazzana, I., Colombo, E., Dobrota, R., Hernandez, J., Hesselstrand, R., Varju, C., Nagy, G., Smith, V., Caramaschi, P., Riccieri, V., Hachulla, E., Balbir-Gurman, A., Chatelus, E., Romanowska-Próchnicka, K., Carolina Araújo, A., Distler, O., Allanore, Y., & Airo, P. (2017). Malignancies in patients with anti-RNA polymerase III antibodies and systemic sclerosis: Analysis of the EULAR scleroderma trials and research cohort and possible recommendations for screening. *Journal of Rheumatology*, *44*(5), 639–647. https://doi.org/10.3899/jrheum.160817.

Lechner, M., Lirk, P., & Rieder, J. (2005). Inducible nitric oxide synthase (iNOS) in tumor biology: The two sides of the same coin. *Seminars in Cancer Biology*, *15*(4), 277–289. https://doi.org/10.1016/j.semcancer.2005.04.004.

le Naour, F. (2007). Identification of tumor antigens by using proteomics. *Methods in Molecular Biology (Clifton, N.J.)*, *360*, 327–334. https://doi.org/10.1385/1-59745-165-7:327.

Leypoldt, F., & Wandinger, K. P. (2014). Paraneoplastic neurological syndromes. *Clinical and Experimental Immunology*, *175*(3), 336–348. https://doi.org/10.1111/cei.12185.

Liu, W., Peng, B., Lu, Y., Xu, W., Qian, W., & Zhang, J. Y. (2011). Autoantibodies to tumor-associated antigens as biomarkers in cancer immunodiagnosis. *Autoimmunity Reviews*, *10*(6), 331–335. https://doi.org/10.1016/j.autrev.2010.12.002.

Liu, Y., Fan, W., Chen, H., & Yu, M. X. (2014). Risk of breast cancer and total malignancies in rheumatoid arthritis patients undergoing TNF-α antagonist therapy: A meta-analysis of randomized control trials. *Asian Pacific Journal of Cancer Prevention*, *15*(8), 3403–3410. https://doi.org/10.7314/APJCP.2014.15.8.3403.

Lu, H., Goodell, V., & Disis, M. L. (2008). Humoral immunity directed against tumor-associated antigens as potential biomarkers for the early diagnosis of cancer. *Journal of Proteome Research*, *7*(4), 1388–1394. https://doi.org/10.1021/pr700818f.

Maire, C., Vercambre-Darras, S., Devos, P., D'Herbomez, M., Dubucquoi, S., & Mortier, L. (2013). Metastatic melanoma: Spontaneous occurrence of auto antibodies is a good prognosis factor in a prospective cohort. *Journal of the European Academy of Dermatology and Venereology*, *27*(1), 92–96. https://doi.org/10.1111/j.1468-3083.2011.04364.x.

Masetti, R., Tiri, A., Tignanelli, A., Turrini, E., Argentiero, A., Pession, A., & Esposito, S. (2021). Autoimmunity and cancer. *Autoimmunity Reviews*, *20*(9), 1–8. https://doi.org/10.1016/j.autrev.2021.102882.

McCarty, G. A., Rice, J. R., Bembe, M. L., & Barada Jr, F. A. (1983). Anticentromere antibody: clinical correlations and association with favorable prognosis in patients with scleroderma variants. *Arthritis and Rheumatism*, *26*(1), 1–7.

McGilvray, R. W., Eagle, R. A., Watson, N. F. S., Al-Attar, A., Ball, G., Jafferji, I., Trowsdale, J., & Durrant, L. G. (2009). NKG2D ligand expression in human colorectal cancer reveals associations with prognosis and evidence for immunoediting. *Clinical Cancer Research*, *15*(22), 6993–7002. https://doi.org/10.1158/1078-0432.CCR-09-0991.

Mitchell, D. A., Sayour, E. J., Reap, E., Schmittling, R., de Leon, G., Norberg, P., Desjardins, A., Friedman, A. H., Friedman, H. S., Archer, G., & Sampson, J. H. (2015). Severe adverse immunologic reaction in a patient with glioblastoma receiving autologous dendritic cell vaccines combined with GM-CSF and dose-intensified temozolomide. *Cancer Immunology Research*, *3*(4), 320–325. https://doi.org/10.1158/2326-6066.CIR-14-0100.

Monach, P. A., Arnold, L. M., & Merkel, P. A. (2010). Incidence and prevention of bladder toxicity from cyclophosphamide in the treatment of rheumatic diseases: A data-driven review. *Arthritis and Rheumatism*, *62*(1), 9–21. https://doi.org/10.1002/art.25061.

Murphy, M. A., O'Leary, J. J., & Cahill, D. J. (2012). Assessment of the humoral immune response to cancer. *Journal of Proteomics*, *75*(15), 4573–4579. https://doi.org/10.1016/j.jprot.2012.01.021.

Murray, A., Chapman, C. J., Healey, G., Peek, L. J., Parsons, G., Baldwin, D., Barnes, A., Sewell, H. F., Fritsche, H. A., & Robertson, J. F. R. (2010). Technical validation of an autoantibody test for lung cancer. *Annals of Oncology*, *21*(8), 1687–1693. https://doi.org/10.1093/annonc/mdp606.

Nakanishi, S., & Hatayama, T. (2006). Adenocarcinoma of the prostate associated with anti Jo-1 antibody positive polymyositis. *Acta Urologica Japonica*, *52*(4), 289–291.

Neller, M. A., López, J. A., & Schmidt, C. W. (2008). Antigens for cancer immunotherapy. *Seminars in Immunology*, *20*(5), 286–295. https://doi.org/10.1016/j.smim.2008.09.006.

Ohtake, H., Kawamura, H., Matsuzaki, M., Yokoyama, E., Kitajima, M., Onizuka, S., & Yamakawa, M. (2010). Oncocytic adrenocortical carcinoma. *Annals of Diagnostic Pathology*, *14*(3), 204–208. https://doi.org/10.1016/j.anndiagpath.2009.06.006.

Olsen, A. H., Parkin, D. M., & Sasieni, P. (2008). Cancer mortality in the United Kingdom: Projections to the year 2025. *British Journal of Cancer*, *99*(9), 1549–1554. https://doi.org/10.1038/sj.bjc.6604710.

Parkin, D. M., Bray, F., Ferlay, J., & Pisani, P. (2005). Global cancer statistics, 2002. *CA: A Cancer Journal for Clinicians*, *55*(2), 74–108. https://doi.org/10.3322/canjclin.55.2.74.

Pereira-Faca, S. R., Kuick, R., Puravs, E., Zhang, Q., Krasnoselsky, A. L., Phanstiel, D., Qiu, J., Misek, D. E., Hinderer, R., Tammemagi, M., Landi, M. T., Caporaso, N., Pfeiffer, R., Edelstein, C., Goodman, G., Barnett, M., Thornquist, M., Brenner, D., & Hanash, S. M. (2007). Identification of 14-3-3θ as an antigen that induces a humoral response in lung cancer. *Cancer Research*, *67*(24), 12000–12006. https://doi.org/10.1158/0008-5472.CAN-07-2913.

Polesie, S., Gillstedt, M., Sönnergren, H. H., Osmancevic, A., & Paoli, J. (2017). Methotrexate treatment and risk for cutaneous malignant melanoma: a retrospective comparative registry-based cohort study. *British Journal of Dermatology*, *176*(6), 1492–1499. https://doi.org/10.1111/bjd.15170.

Prasad, P. D., Stanton, J. A. L., & Assinder, S. J. (2010). Expression of the actin-associated protein transgelin (SM22) is decreased in prostate cancer. *Cell and Tissue Research*, *339*(2), 337–347. https://doi.org/10.1007/s00441-009-0902-y.

Quartuccio, L., Baldini, C., Bartoloni, E., Priori, R., Carubbi, F., Corazza, L., Alunno, A., Colafrancesco, S., Luciano, N., Giacomelli, R., Gerli, R., Valesini, G., Bombardieri, S., & de Vita, S. (2015). Anti-SSA/SSB-negative Sjögren's syndrome shows a lower prevalence of lymphoproliferative manifestations, and a lower risk of lymphoma evolution. *Autoimmunity Reviews*, *14*(11), 1019–1022. https://doi.org/10.1016/j.autrev.2015.07.002.

Ran, Y., Hu, H., Zhou, Z., Yu, L., Sun, L., Pan, J., Liu, J., & Yang, Z. (2008). Profiling tumor-associated autoantibodies for the detection of colon cancer. *Clinical Cancer Research*, *14*(9), 2696–2700. https://doi.org/10.1158/1078-0432.CCR-07-2021.

Rao, J. Y., Seligson, D., Visapaa, H., Horvath, S., Eeva, M., Michel, K., Pantuck, A., Belldegrun, A., & Palotie, A. (2002). Tissue microarray analysis of cytoskeletal actin-associated biomarkers Gelsolin and E-cadherin in urothelial carcinoma. *Cancer*, *95*(6), 1247–1257. https://doi.org/10.1002/cncr.10823.

Rattner, J. B., Rees, J., Whitehead, C. M., Casiano, C. A., Tan, E. M., Humbel, R. L., Conrad, K., & Fritzler, M. J. (1997). High frequency of neoplasia in patients with autoantibodies to centromere protein CENP-F. *Clinical and Investigative Medicine*, *20*(5), 308–319.

Roberts, J., Ennis, D., Hudson, M., Ye, C., Saltman, A., Himmel, M., Rottapel, R., Pope, J., Hoa, S., Tisseverasinghe, A., Fifi-Mah, A., Maltez, N., & Jamal, S. (2020). Rheumatic immune-related adverse events associated with cancer immunotherapy: A nationwide multi-center cohort. *Autoimmunity Reviews*, *19*(8), 1–7. https://doi.org/10.1016/j.autrev.2020.102595.

Ruiz de Morales, J. M. G., Puig, L., Daudén, E., Cañete, J. D., Pablos, J. L., Martín, A. O., Juanatey, C. G., Adán, A., Montalbán, X., Borruel, N., Ortí, G., Holgado-Martín, E., García-Vidal, C., Vizcaya-Morales, C., Martín-Vázquez, V., & González-Gay, M. Á. (2020). Critical role of interleukin (IL)-17 in inflammatory and immune disorders: An updated review of the evidence focusing in controversies. *Autoimmunity Reviews*, *19*(1), 1–15. https://doi.org/10.1016/j.autrev.2019.102429.

Sakamoto, J., Fujiya, M., Okamoto, K., Nata, T., Inaba, Y., Moriichi, K., Tanabe, H., Mizukami, Y., Watari, J., Ashida, T., & Kohgo, Y. (2010). Immunoprecipitation of nucleosomal DNA is a novel procedure to improve the sensitivity of serum screening for the p16 hypermethylation associated with colon cancer. *Cancer Epidemiology*, *34*(2), 194–199. https://doi.org/10.1016/j.canep.2010.01.004.

Salavoura, K., Kolialexi, A., Tsangaris, G., & Mavrou, A. (2008). Development of cancer in patients with primary immunodeficiencies. *Anticancer Research*, *28*(2 B), 1263–1269.

Shah, A. A., Casciola-Rosen, L., & Rosen, A. (2015). Review: Cancer-induced autoimmunity in the rheumatic diseases. *Arthritis and Rheumatology*, *67*(2), 317–326. https://doi.org/10.1002/art.38928.

Sidari, L., Tirelli, G., Papanikolla, L., Sasso, F., Russolo, M., & Melato, M. (2003). Flow cytometry expression of p53 and PCNA in oral/oropharynx carcinomas and their lymph node metastases. *Anticancer Research*, *23*(5 B), 4127–4132.

Slovin, S. F., Ragupathi, G., Fernandez, C., Diani, M., Jefferson, M. P., Wilton, A., Kelly, W. K., Morris, M., Solit, D., Clausen, H., Livingston, P., & Scher, H. I. (2007). A polyvalent vaccine for high-risk prostate patients: "Are more antigens better?" *Cancer Immunology, Immunotherapy*, *56*(12), 1921–1930. https://doi.org/10.1007/s00262-007-0335-y.

Solomon, D. H., Mercer, E., & Kavanaugh, A. (2012). Observational studies on the risk of cancer associated with tumor necrosis factor inhibitors in rheumatoid arthritis: A review of their methodologies and results. *Arthritis and Rheumatism*, *64*(1), 21–32. https://doi.org/10.1002/art.30653.

Sotiriou, C., & Pusztai, L. (2009). Gene-expression signatures in breast cancer. *New England Journal of Medicine*, *360*(8), 790–800. https://doi.org/10.1056/nejmra0801289.

Swaak, A. J. G., Groenwold, J., & Bronsveld, W. (1986). Predictive value of complement profiles and anti-dsDNA in systemic lupus erythematosus. *Annals of the Rheumatic Diseases*, *45*(5), 359–366. https://doi.org/10.1136/ard.45.5.359.

Syrigos, K. N., Charalambopoulos, A., Pliarchopoulou, K., Varsamidakis, N., Machairas, A., & Mandrekas, D. (2000). The prognostic significance of autoantibodies against dsDNA in patients with colorectal adenocarcinoma. *Anticancer Research*, *20*(6 B), 4351–4353.

Szekanecz, Z., Gomez, I., Soós, B., Bodoki, L., Szamosi, S., András, C., Juhász, B., Váróczy, L., Antal-Szalmás, P., Szodoray, P., Bittner, N., Árkosy, P., Illés, Á., Szűcs, G., Dankó, K., Bender, T., Tamási, L., & Szekanecz, É. (2020). Eight pillars of oncorheumatology: Crossroads between malignancies and musculoskeletal diseases. *Autoimmunity Reviews*, *19*(11), 1–12. https://doi.org/10.1016/j.autrev.2020.102658.

Tan, E. M., & Zhang, J. (2008). Autoantibodies to tumor-associated antigens: Reporters from the immune system. *Immunological Reviews*, *222*(1), 328–340. https://doi.org/10.1111/j.1600-065X.2008.00611.x.

Tan, H. T., Low, J., Lim, S. G., & Chung, M. C. M. (2009). Serum autoantibodies as biomarkers for early cancer detection. *FEBS Journal*, *276*(23), 6880–6904. https://doi.org/10.1111/j.1742-4658.2009.07396.x.

Targoff, I. N., Mamyrova, G., Trieu, E. P., Perurena, O., Koneru, B., O'Hanlon, T. P., Miller, F. W., & Rider, L. G. (2006). A novel autoantibody to a 155-kd protein is associated with dermatomyositis. *Arthritis and Rheumatism*, *54*(11), 3682–3689. https://doi.org/10.1002/art.22164.

Taylora, B. S., Pale, M., Yu, J., Laxman, B., Kalyana-Sundaram, S., Zhao, R., Menon, A., Wei, J. T., Nesvizhskii, A. I., Ghosh, D., Omenn, G. S., Lubman, D. M., Chinnaiyan, A. M., & Sreekumar, A. (2008). Humoral response profiling reveals pathways to prostate cancer progression. *Molecular and Cellular Proteomics*, *7*(3), 600–611. https://doi.org/10.1074/mcp.M700263-MCP200.

Tschernatsch, M., Gross, O., Kneifel, N., Kaps, M., & Blaes, F. (2009). SOX-1 autoantibodies in patients with paraneoplastic neurological syndromes. *Autoimmunity Reviews*, *8*(7), 549–551. https://doi.org/10.1016/j.autrev.2009.01.015.

Tsou, P., Katayama, H., Ostrin, E. J., & Hanash, S. M. (2016). The emerging role of b cells in tumor immunity. *Cancer Research*, *76*(19), 5597–5601. https://doi.org/10.1158/0008-5472.CAN-16-0431.

van den Reek, J. M. P. A., van Lümig, P. P. M., Janssen, M., Schers, H. J., Hendriks, J. C. M., van de Kerkhof, P. C. M., Seyger, M. M. B., & de Jong, E. M. G. J. (2014). Increased incidence of squamous cell carcinoma of the skin after long-term treatment with azathioprine in patients with autoimmune inflammatory rheumatic diseases. *Journal of the European Academy of Dermatology and Venereology*, *28*(1), 27–33. https://doi.org/10.1111/jdv.12041.

Vera-Sempere, F., & Vera-Sirera, B. (2011). Usefulness of antimitochondrial antibody 113-1 in diagnosis and classification of salivary gland tumours with oncocytic differentiation. *Acta Otorrinolaringologica (English Edition)*, *62*(1), 1–9. https://doi.org/10.1016/s2173-5735(11)70001-1.

Vlagea, A., Falagan, S., Gutiérrez-Gutiérrez, G., Moreno-Rubio, J., Merino, M., Zambrana, F., Casado, E., & Sereno, M. (2018). Antinuclear antibodies and cancer: A literature review. *Critical Reviews in Oncology/Hematology*, *127*, 42–49. https://doi.org/10.1016/j.critrevonc.2018.05.002.

Waldhauer, I., & Steinle, A. (2008). NK cells and cancer immunosurveillance. *Oncogene*, *27*(45), 5932–5943. https://doi.org/10.1038/onc.2008.267.

Whiteside, T. L. (2008). The tumor microenvironment and its role in promoting tumor growth. *Oncogene*, *27*(45), 5904–5912. https://doi.org/10.1038/onc.2008.271.

Wolfe, F., & Michaud, K. (2004). Lymphoma in rheumatoid arthritis: The effect of methotrexate and anti-tumor necrosis factor therapy in 18,572 patients. *Arthritis and Rheumatism*, *50*(6), 1740–1751. https://doi.org/10.1002/art.20311.

Wu, C. Y., Chen, D. Y., Shen, J. L., Ho, H. J., Chen, C. C., Kuo, K. N., Liu, H. N., Chang, Y. T., & Chen, Y. J. (2014). The risk of cancer in patients with rheumatoid arthritis taking tumor necrosis factor antagonists: A nationwide cohort study. *Arthritis Research and Therapy*, *16*(5), 1–12. https://doi.org/10.1186/s13075-014-0449-5.

Xie, W., Huang, H., Xiao, S., Fan, Y., Deng, X., & Zhang, Z. (2020). Immune checkpoint inhibitors therapies in patients with cancer and pre-existing autoimmune diseases: A meta-analysis of observational studies. *Autoimmunity Reviews*, *19*(12), 1–8. https://doi.org/10.1016/j.autrev.2020.102687.

Yach, D., Hawkes, C., Gould, C. L., & Hofman, K. J. (2004). The global burden of chronic diseases: Overcoming impediments to prevention and control. *Journal of the American Medical Association*, *291*(21), 2616–2622. https://doi.org/10.1001/jama.291.21.2616.

Yang, Z., Lin, F., Qin, B., Yan, L., & Renqian, Z. (2015). Polymyositis/dermatomyositis and malignancy risk: A metaanalysis study. *Journal of Rheumatology*, *42*(2), 281–291. https://doi.org/10.3899/jrheum.140566.

Yigit, R., Massuger, L. F. A. G., Figdor, C. G., & Torensma, R. (2010). Ovarian cancer creates a suppressive microenvironment to escape immune elimination. *Gynecologic Oncology*, *117*(2), 366–372. https://doi.org/10.1016/j.ygyno.2010.01.019.

Zaenker, P., & Ziman, M. R. (2013). Serologic autoantibodies as diagnostic cancer biomarkers - A review. *Cancer Epidemiology Biomarkers and Prevention*, *22*(12), 2161–2181. https://doi.org/10.1158/1055-9965.EPI-13-0621.

Zhang, J. Y., Casiano, C. A., Peng, X. X., Koziol, J. A., Chan, E. K. L., & Tan, E. M. (2003). Enhancement of antibody detection in cancer using panel of recombinant tumor-associated antigens. *Cancer Epidemiology Biomarkers and Prevention*, *12*(2), 136–143.

Zitvogel, L., Tesniere, A., & Kroemer, G. (2006). Cancer despite immunosurveillance: Immunoselection and immunosubversion. *Nature Reviews Immunology*, *6*(10), 715–727. https://doi.org/10.1038/nri1936.

Zou, H. Y., Gu, X., Yu, W. Z., Wang, Z., & Jiao, M. (2015). Detection of serum antinuclear antibodies in lymphoma patients. *Genetics and Molecular Research*, *14*(4), 16546–16552. https://doi.org/10.4238/2015.December.11.1.

Chapter 13

Cytokines and Cancer

Melike Bayindir Bilgic,
Gizem Inetas Yengin
and Omer Faruk Bayrak*, PhD
Department of Medical Genetics,
Yeditepe University School of Medicine, Istanbul, Turkey

Abstract

Cancer is a global disease with an increasing incidence each year, and recently ranked first among the causes of death according to cancer statistics around the world. Cytokines play a critical role in cancer development, progression, and control. Many cells are included in the tumor microenvironment, which has a great impact on the defense of the immune system, directing the defense through the cytokines they secrete. The defense interaction between immune system cells and invading cells is directed to a certain direction by changing the balance of cytokines in the environment. Therefore, the role of cytokines is very important in determining the fate of cancer. In this chapter, you will find information about the relationship of cancer with cytokines and cell groups that secrete them, and the dynamics of these relationships. In addition, you will be able to find the effects of cancer stem cells (CSCs), which are located in the tumor microenvironment and give direction to cancer, on this microenvironment through cytokines.

Keywords: Tumor Microenvironment (TME), inflammation, CSC, JAK, STAT

---

* Corresponding Author's Email: ofbayrak@yeditepe.edu.tr.

In: Autoimmunity and Cancer
Editors: Soner Şahin and Kenan Demir
ISBN: 978-1-68507-937-6

Introduction

Cytokines are very critical elements of the defense of the immune system. They are polypeptides that make important connections in the cell by providing growth, differentiation, and inflammatory or anti-inflammatory signals. Cytokines are released for a short time, usually in response to a stimulus, to bind to high affinity receptors on target cells and are degraded at the end of their half-life. The cytokine-receptor relationship activates downstream pathways, triggering a series of signals (Melero et al., 2015). Thus, they are effective in the proliferation and differentiation mechanisms in the cell. The relationship between cancer and cytokines is critical at this point (Chen & Mellman, 2013). Immune cells in the tumor microenvironment aim for the cytokines they call to the region with the inflammatory stimuli they create to take part in defeating cancer. However, cytokines that can directly affect pathways such as cell growth and differentiation can turn this balance in favor of cancer cells (Chen & Mellman, 2017). The structure, mechanism of action, and related cell groups of cytokines, which affect the fate of cancer and have a critical target potential in cancer treatment, should be examined in detail. In the following sections, detailed information about the structure, mechanism of action, and functioning of cytokines and their relations with other cells is given.

Signal Transduction Process

Intercellular communication is critical for cells to manage their complex signaling networks. Cells need this complex communication for their systemic response to stimuli, their response to infection, embryonic development, and differentiation. Thanks to these signal networks, the orientations of the cell such as survival, differentiation, and apoptosis can be affected. Growth factors are the precursor molecules that initiate this signaling. The growth factor-specific receptor binding interaction required for this signaling triggers a series of biochemical reactions, enabling biological responses to occur (O'Shea et al., 2002). There are several classes of receptors involved in the transmission of these extracellular signals. The most important of these are G-protein coupled receptors, receptor tyrosine kinases, and cytokine receptors. In addition to the ligand-receptor interaction, there are also cytoplasmic molecules that support and mediate this interaction. Basically, the transmission of signaling to the nucleus as a result of this interaction leads to altered expression of various genes that can affect the fate of the cell (Roskoski, 2019; Watanabe et al., 2018).

Some protein groups are involved in the regulation and coordination of the signal chain that occurs through the interaction between the ligand and its specific receptor. Scaffold proteins and adapter proteins are among these groups and play very important roles in intracellular signaling by holding certain proteins together or forming various molecular networks in the cell (Ortega et al., 2020). Adapter proteins are of great importance for receptor tyrosine kinases. Because these molecules can increase the efficiency of signaling by providing multiple binding sites to which effector molecules can bind through protein-protein interaction. Scaffold proteins, on the other hand, allow the formation of multienzyme structures by mediating the formation of signal cascades and the close/appropriate positioning of related molecules (Roskoski, 2019; Siveen et al., 2018).

Receptor Protein-Tyrosine Kinases

Protein-tyrosine kinases are part of enzyme-linked receptors. These kinases phosphorylate substrate proteins on tyrosine domains. Since the receptors of many mammalian cell growth factors are members of this protein family, this topic has been well studied to explore signaling (Hunter & Sefton, 1980).

The first step of signaling for receptor protein-tyrosine kinases is ligand-mediated dimerization of the receptor. In this way, dimerized polypeptides cross-phosphorylate each other and autophosphorylate the receptor. Such phosphorylation is highly efficient as it creates increased kinase activity and specific binding sites for additional intracellular signal transducing proteins. The association of signaling molecules with the receptor is mediated by protein domains that bind to peptides such as SH2 (for SRC homology 2) and PTB (for phosphotyrosine binding) (Bhanumathy et al., 2021; Sevillano et al., 2021).

Cytokine Receptors and Nonreceptor Protein-Tyrosine Kinases

Similar to receptor protein-tyrosine kinases, cytokine receptors contain an extracellular ligand binding domain at the N-terminal, single transmembrane-α helices, and a C-terminal cytosolic binding domain. Unlike receptor protein-tyrosine kinases, cytokine receptors work together with "non-receptor protein-tyrosine kinases" that are activated by ligand binding. In other words, cytokine receptors are activated by stimulating intracellular protein-tyrosine kinases with which they are non-covalently linked, rather than by intrinsic enzymatic activity (Giraldez et al., 2021; Masjedi et al., 2021).

The first step in cytokine receptor signaling is dimerization of the receptor that occurs after ligand binding. Subsequently, cross-phosphorylation of non-receptor protein-tyrosine kinases occurs (Figure 1). The cytokine receptor homodimerizes by binding of the ligand molecule or consists of two different subunits that heterodimerize in response to the receptor-ligand interaction. The heterodimerized group consists of a ligand-specific chain called gp130 shared by different cytokines (interleukin-6 (IL-6), IL-11, oncostatin M, LIF, cardiotrophin-1 and ciliary neurotrophic factors) (Chauhan et al., 2021; Giraldez et al., 2021; Masjedi et al., 2021). Activation of downstream pathways occurs when activated kinases at this stage phosphorylate the receptor and provide phosphotyrosine binding sites. The activity of non-receptor tyrosine kinases instead of receptor tyrosine kinases in the intracellular domain distinguishes cytokine receptors from RTKs. The Janus kinase (JAK) family consists of four non-receptor protein-tyrosine kinases (JAK-1, JAK-2, JAK-3 and Tyk-2). The JAK family is indispensable for signaling transmission with cytokine receptors. JAKs are receptor-associated molecules and carry both a catalytic and pseudokinase domain. When receptor-ligand interaction occurs, activated JAKs cause phosphorylation of the receptor and molecules containing a phosphotyrosine binding site (STATs) (Babon et al., 2014; M. Chen et al., 1997). Structure of STAT molecules; consisting of a DNA binding domain, an SH2 domain, and some domains for protein-protein interaction. The tyrosine residue is phosphorylated upon coupling of the ligand-receptor and STATs form homodimer-heterodimer complexes through SH2 domains. Thus, STATs ensure that target genes are activated in the nucleus (Babon et al., 2014; Chauhan et al., 2021).

There are some studies in which some components of the cytokine pathway are associated with cancer. These components are related to uncontrolled cell proliferation and invasion. E.g; Drosophila-Hop kinase is a member of the JAK family and exhibits a leukemia-like phenotype with its mutation. The TEL-JAK2 mutation (Lacronique et al., 1997), identified in 2005 for human leukemia, has been detected in a large proportion of patients with different types of neoplasms. Protein-function studies have shown that this mutation blocks the autoinhibitory activity of JAK, greatly increasing its sensitivity to cytokines. In this way, cells gained the ability to grow cytokine independent (Pilati et al., 2011). In addition, there are studies in the literature showing that proliferative pathways are activated in JAK2 mutant cells (Quintás-Cardama et al., 2011). Mutations in the STAT3 molecule, which is one of the components of the cytokine pathway, have been determined to be activated by cancer cells using alternative mechanisms (Yu et al., 2007). Mutation-bearing components of the cytokine pathway have been determined to contribute to cancer by activating genes associated with uncontrolled division, proliferation, and resistance in the cell (Lee et al., 2009; Pilati et al., 2011; Wang et al., 2009).

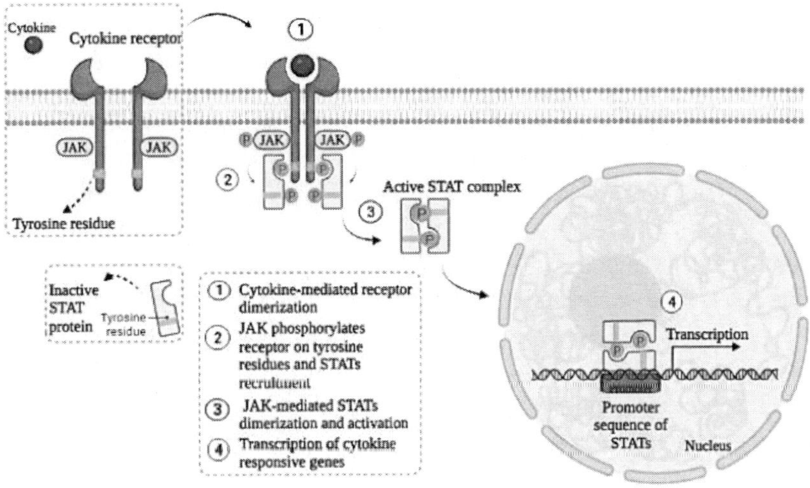

Figure 1. Cytokine receptor signalization processes (*BioRender*, n.d.).

Cytokines

Cytokines are a group of low molecular weight proteins (~5–25 kDa (Murphy & Weaver, 2016)) that are secreted to effect intercellular communication and a specific interaction. It has subgroups such as interleukins (ILs), interferons (IFNs), tumor necrosis factors (TNFs), and growth factors (GF). They can be secreted from many cell types, especially immune system cells. Cytokines are pleiotropic molecules, which means that they can act on more than one cell type. In addition, a cell type may contain more than one cytokine receptor (Arango Duque & Descoteaux, 2014). They can initiate signals to increase the effectiveness of the immune system, affecting the increase of all blood cells and other cells that support the inflammatory and immune responses of the body. Cytokines have a wide range of functions; they also regulate many important processes such as metabolism, proliferation, tissue repair, inflammation, and chemotaxis. In addition, they may aid in anticancer activity, while at the same time supporting the development of cancer. Briefly, these proteins, which play a dominant role on immune system cells, are very critical as they can determine the fate of cancer (*ASCO Annual Meeting 2019*, 2019; *Understanding Immunotherapy*, 2013).

Cytokine signaling begins when the cytokine molecule binds to a specific cell surface receptor, forming a signaling cascade of the receptor. This signaling influences the regulation of target genes in the nucleus. This positive/negative regulation may cause suppression of the cytokine's own effect. Cytokines, which can act on the cell with synergistic, agonist, or antagonist functions, can control many functions. Cytokines have short-term effects at the autocrine and paracrine positions. Some cytokines (TGF-β, M-CSF, EPO) are found in the blood and can act over a long distance (Ievins & Moritz, 2017; Unanue et al., 1976).

Although cytokines can be produced from many cell types (poly-morphonuclear leukocytes (PMN), endothelial and epithelial cells, mast cells, adipocytes, and connective tissue), they are vital for macrophages and lymphocytes (helper T cells (Th)) to function. They provide the micro-environment necessary for the recruitment of macrophages to the inflammatory site and mediate the activation of the immune response. In addition, they play a role as the intersection element of innate and adaptive immunity.

Proinflammatory and Anti-inflammatory Cytokines

Activated macrophages release pro-inflammatory cytokines, which are involved in up-regulation of inflammatory processes. Examples of pro-inflammatory cytokines are IL-1, IL-6, and TNF-α, IL-8, and IL-12. Pro-inflammatory cytokines can induce local inflammation as well as produce fever or acute inflammation proteins that produce systemic effects. If these cytokines are produced at a sufficient level and show their activities in harmony, they will contribute to the inflammatory response (Beutler, 1999; Zhang & An, 2007). Although cytokines are grouped pro/anti in terms of their response to inflammation, these two groups actually work together. Because it works in harmony with specific cytokine inhibitors and soluble cytokine receptors. Anti-inflammatory cytokines (TGF-β, IL-4, IL-10, IL-13) control the immune response of pro-inflammatory cytokines. Disruption in this intertwined trend is an important research topic, as it may predispose to autoimmune disorders (Opal & DePalo, 2000; Vlahopoulos et al., 1999).

The inflammatory system plays an important role in the defense of the body against many pathogens, especially viruses and bacteria. Inflammatory cells also play a critical role in the initiation and maintenance of the tumor and the vascularization and metastasis that occur with its location (Vickers, 2017). Inflammatory cells are diversified and called into the environment by cytokine-chemokine orientation in the environment. Therefore, cytokines are of great importance in the success of inflammatory cells and their environment in attacking cancer or pathogenic molecules (Baumgarten & Frasor, 2012; Marotta & Polyak, 2011). The association of inflammation with cancer began with the discovery of inflammatory cells infiltrating the tumor stroma by Rudolf Virchow in 1863 (Balkwill & Mantovani, 2001).

Just as inflammatory cells and infiltrating cells work in concert in the microenvironment to eliminate the pathogen in the body's defenses, promote healing, and restore homeostasis, tumor cells work in similar harmony with infiltrating cells and inflammatory agents in their microenvironment (Coussens & Werb, 2002). However, there are some differences with respect to the balance that is tried to establish for normal tissue homeostasis in the cancer microenvironment. Because cancer cells have gained the ability to bypass healing-normalization signals from healthy adult tissue, they will use the microenvironment/infiltrating cells involved in it to their advantage (Medzhitov, 2008). The onset of tumorigenesis is supported by the accumulation of immune cells in the tumor microenvironment, the disruption of homeostasis balances, and the formation of a pro-tumorigenic niche by these accumulating cells secreting critical growth factors and cytokines (Coussens & Werb, 2002). To give an example of this situation, the discovery of the src, which is the first oncogene, can be given. In chickens infected with Rous sarcoma virus (RSV) (Murphy & Rous, 1912), a tumor virus that develops in chickens, tumor growth was observed only at the first injection and the site of inflammation, proving that unregulated inflammation is associated with tumor formation (Dolberg et al., 1985; Martins-Green et al., 1994; Rous, 1910). Similarly, the chronic inflammation-tumor relationship caused by Hepatitis B and C virus, which increases the probability of hepatocellular carcinoma, can be given as an example (Bruix & Llovet, 2003).

Cancer Stem Cells and the Microenvironment

Significant evidence has consistently demonstrated the presence of cancer stem cells (CSCs, also known as tumor-initiating cells TICs) as a small subpopulation in malignancies, leading to higher abnormally of cellular heterogeneity within the tumor throughout the last few decades. CSCs contribute to tumor growth and recurrence by prolonged proliferation and invasion into normal tissue, stimulation of angiogenesis, immune system evasion, and resistance to traditional anticancer therapy. Being resistant to classical cancer treatment methods such as chemotherapy, radiotherapy or surgery, CSCs are responsible for tumor metastasis and ultimately leading to tumor relapse (Batlle & Clevers, 2017). The capacities of CSCs to self-renew and differentiate, typically in response to cues from their microenvironment, are functionally defined. Therefore, targeting different intracellular signal transduction pathways in cancer progenitor cells and developing more effective therapeutic treatments for recurrent aggressive cancers may be possible with microenvironment-focused research (Korkaya et al., 2011). Understanding the crosstalk between CSCs and the niche may thus help to create novel therapeutic techniques and pave the path for the creation of newer cancer-treatment strategies.

A small number of stem cells have the capacity to self-renew as well as to differentiate into different lineages of normal tissues. CSCs are regulated in the tumor microenvironment, like regular stem cells are regulated via their niche. Cells attracted to the microenvironment, such as mesenchymal stem cells (MSCs), tissue-associated fibroblasts, and endothelial cells, interact with CSCs via cytokine and growth factor networks. The tumor microenvironment (TME) contains extracellular matrix (ECM), MSCs, tumor-associated macrophages (TAMs), cancer-associated fibroblasts (CAFs), endothelial cells (ECs), immune system cells, and a complex network of cytokines and growth factors (Figure 2). TME cells are known to be resistant to cancer therapies. The secreted factors from TME including transforming growth factor β (TGF-β), interleukin-6 (IL-6), hepatocyte growth factor (HGF), fibroblast growth factor (FGF) and some ECM adhesion proteins are related to signaling pathways (Wu & Dai, 2017). Major signaling pathways related to CSCs are Wnt, Notch, Janus kinase/signal transducers and activators of transcription (JAK-STAT), Sonic Hedgehog (SHH), nuclear factor-κB (NF-κB), transforming growth factor (TGF/SMAD), phosphoinositide 3-kinase/AKT/mammalian target of rapamycin (PI3K/AKT/mTOR), Peroxisome proliferator-activated receptors (PPARs), thus far (Yang et al., 2020).

Genetic polymorphisms in the genes of chronic inflammatory-associated cytokines such as IL-1β, IL-6, and IL-8 may cause cancer. These inflammatory cytokines encourage CSC self-renewal, which can lead to tumor development and metastasis. IL-6 has been demonstrated to enhance tumorigenicity, angiogenesis, and metastasis and a direct regulator of breast CSC self-renewal, a process mediated by the IL-6 receptor/gp130 complex via STAT3 activation (Chang et al., 2013). IL-6 is a critical component of a positive feedback loop that includes these MSCs and CSCs. Sethi *et al.* found that IL-6–mediated Jagged1/Notch signaling enhances bone metastasis in breast cancer (Sethi et al., 2011). These data point to IL-6 and its receptor as promising treatment targets for CSC depletion. NFκB regulates the transcription of many cytokines, including IL-6 and IL-8. Furthermore, a positive feedback loop in tumor cells maintains a persistent inflammatory state. This loop includes a component implicated in embryonic stem cell self-renewal. This feedback loop is maintained by IL-6 by activating STAT3, which in turn activates and targets Lin28 and let7 (Iliopoulos et al., 2009; Kaltschmidt et al., 2019). ECM remodeling is also important for cancer research. ECM is primarily mediated by the activity of matrix metalloproteinase-10 (MMP10), which promotes EMT, metastasis, and the CSC state. CSCs have been observed to overexpress MMP-9, which facilitates the activation of dormant TGF-b in ECM, MMP-2, and MMP-13, all of which are associated with a greater metastatic and angiogenic capability. CSCs overexpress CCL5 and its CCR5, CCR3, and CCR1 receptors in ovarian cancer cell lines, increasing MMP-9 secretion and activation of NF-kB (Long et al., 2012).

Interactions between CSCs and TME Associated Cells

Mesenchymal Stem Cells (MSCs)

MSCs are an important population of stem cell-like cells which have self-renewal and differentiation capacities and can be derived from bone marrow, peripheral blood, umbilical cord, placenta, and adipose tissue (Hass et al., 2011). With the ability to differentiate, MSCs can be transformed into CSCs with the support of aberrant alterations of intrinsic and extrinsic microenvironments. MSCs also play a critical role in cancer formation, including modulation of inflammatory processes, angiogenesis, metastasis, maintenance of CSCs, and tumor growth. The migration capabilities of MSCs allow them to be used in clinical applications; however, the homing of MSCs is related to chemokines and receptors, which also stimulates the transfer of various accessory cells to the tumors. These contain growth factors such as SCF, HGF, GF, PDGF and IGF-1E; cytokines and inflammatory factors such as TGFβ, TNFα, IL-8 and IL-1β; angiogenic factors such as VEGF, β-FGF and HIF1-α; chemokines such as CCL5, CCL2, CXCL12 and CCL22. As a result, MSCs are drawn into the tumor niche by CSCs and communicate with one another via a complex structure of cytokines. IL-6, IL-8, BMP, CXC6, and CXCL5 are responsible for the proliferation of CSCs and increase their invasive features between MSCs and cancer stem cells (Liang et al., 2021). Liu et al. demonstrated a cytokine network that mediates the interaction between mesenchymal cells and cancer cells. Cancer cells that are generated by IL-6 interact with IL6R/GP130 expressed on MSCs, which then releases CXCL7 in response to IL-6 stimulation. CXCL7 causes breast cancer cells and mesenchymal cells to secrete a variety of cytokines, including IL6, IL8, CXCL6, and CXCL5 (Liu et al., 2011).

Cancer Associated Fibroblasts (CAFs)

CAFs are also known as an important group of cells in TME, assisting with tumor growth, angiogenesis, EMT, and metastasis, as well as producing ECM components. CAFs can be produced by smooth muscle cells, pericytes, adipocytes, or immune cells. The origin of CAFs in the stroma is not clear yet; however, researchers presume that they can be originated from EMT, differentiation of MSCs derived from bone marrow, transdifferentiation of perivascular cells, and transference of fibroblasts in the host stroma (Yang et al., 2020). CSCs, on the other hand, can stimulate MSC development into CAFs by secreting TGF-β and activating the TGFβ1/SMAD pathway. Tan et al. demonstrated the critical function of the TGFβ-1/CXCR4 axis in the change of the tumor microenvironment by driving the differentiation of MSCs into CAFs, promoting the growth and metastasis of colorectal carcinoma (Tan et al., 2020). CAFs and CSCs are both engaged in TME-mediated signaling to remodel cancer cells. CAFs express high levels of extracellular factors such as the chemokine CC motif ligand CCL2, CCL8, the CXC motif ligand CXCL12 and the insulin-like growth factor binding protein 7 (IGFBP7), forming an inflammatory niche (Chen et al., 2015). Valenti et al. showed that Sonic Hedgehog is secreted by CSCs, which induces paracrine activation of Hedgehog signaling in CAFs. CAFs secrete soluble substances such as ACTIVIN A, IGF-1, and LIF that promote CSC proliferation, self-renewal, and possibly invasive activity (Valenti et al., 2017). Also, CAFs integrate cancer cell signals to regulate macrophage differentiation, with IL6 and GM-CSF acting as CAF-derived inducible factors to enhance this process. TAM production and infiltration are supported by CAF-derived IL6, which promotes tumor growth (Cho et al., 2018).

Tumor-Associated Macrophages (TAMs)

Macrophages are heterogeneous subpopulations of immune cells and can be found in almost every organ. They can be classified as either pro-inflammatory classical (M1) or suppressive alternatively activated (M2) macrophages. In aggressive cancers, tumor-infiltrating immune cells can enhance chemo-resistance and metastatic development. Tumor-associated macrophages (TAMs), a separate alternatively activated M2 polarized population, have been found to enhance tumor angiogenesis, invasion, and metastasis in addition to their immunosuppressive effect (Solinas et al., 2010). TAMs have angiostatic activities and are related to growth factors and inflammatory cytokines which induce EMT and increase cancer cell stemness., e.g., TGF-β, IL-6, IL-10, IL-8, macrophage migration inhibition factor (MIF), tumor necrosis factor (TNF)-α, VEGF (Vascular endothelial growth factor), basic fibroblast growth factor (bFGF), macrophage-inhibitory factor (MIF), platelet activating factor (PAF), matrix metalloproteinase-9 (MMP-9), Platelet-derived growth factor (PDGF) etc. (Y. Chen et al., 2018; Dirkx et al., 2006). Furthermore, TAMs enhance tumor invasiveness and metastatic progression. They produce proteolytic proteins, for example, MMPs, which are involved in ECM breakdown and remodeling, thus promoting invasion to tumor cells (Allavena & Mantovani, 2012).

Immune System Components That Contribute to the Tumor Microenvironment

Tumor-Infiltrating Lymphocytes (TILs)

TILs are basically white blood cells; however, these cells tend to leave the vasculature and are located in the peritumoral space (stromal) or inside the tumor mass (intraepithelial). Macrophages, B and T lymphocytes, NK cells are immune system cells belonging to the TILs cell group. It has been determined that cell group plays an important role in tumor growth and development (Berghuis et al., 2011; Eggermont et al., 2014). The tumor that develops and starts to grow in the tissue is noticed by the immune system and an inflammatory stimulus is created in this region. Immune system elements such as macrophages, lymphocytes, and cytokines in the region act to eliminate tumor cells. At this point, the TILs give directions to which side the balance will be disturbed. Because tumor cells that survived the attack of immune cells and gained the ability to do so, rendered the lymphocytes infiltrating the tumor dysfunctional (Eggermont et al., 2014; Yigit et al., 2010).

Tumor-Associated Endothelial Cells (TAEs)

TAEs enhance invasion, metastasis, and drug resistance by providing vasculature. Vascular endothelial cells regulate blood flow and nutrient delivery in tissues and control the balance of leukocytes in the region. Endothelial cells form the dynamic structure of blood vessels (Nagl et al., 2020; Potente et al., 2011). Normally, endothelial cells play a major role in angiogenesis and immune system control. They can provide new vessel formations under appropriate signals and eliminate old vessels. Abnormalities in tumor endothelial cells play a critical role in tumor growth and metastasis. Besides exhibiting a stem-cell-like (CSC) phenotype, they are the main control elements of the cell population that infiltrate the TME and determine the fate of the tumor (Buckanovich et al., 2008; Goveia et al., 2020; Nagl et al., 2020). Mutations and chromosomal abnormalities are frequently encountered in TAEs compared to normal epithelial cells. Therefore, investigation of their structures may be important in terms of determining prognostic targets in cancer (Baudino et al., 2002; Goveia et al., 2020; Maishi et al., 2019).

Tumor-Associated Neutrophils (TANs)

TANs are precursor cells that are called to the site after an inflammatory stimulus in the tissue. They take part in protecting the host organisms from pathogenic microorganisms and in repair of the tissue (ECK et al., 2003; Sparmann & Bar-Sagi, 2004). Because of the different roles they play against tumors, neutrophils are also classified with N1 and N2 phenotypes, similar to macrophages. TGF-β plays a major role in the transition to the N2/tumor-associated neutrophil (TAN) phenotype (Fridlender et al., 2009). They perform this function by secreting cytokines and chemokines into the environment, thus destroying the invading microorganism by engulfing it with cytotoxic agents. During these functions, neutrophils cause some damage to the ECM of host tissue with the proteinases that they secrete into the environment. The cytokines, chemokines, ECM-degrading proteinases and reactive oxygen species (ROS) that neutrophils use to destroy the invading microorganism also modify tumor growth and invasion (Pekarek et al., 1995; Shojaei et al., 2008; Tazawa et al., 2003). This process, which is followed in the inflammation process, also takes place in the tumor microenvironment.

However, TANs often act in favor of tumor cells in this battle (ECK et al., 2003; Ji et al., 2006).

T-Regulatory Cells (Tregs)

Treg cells act as T cells that play an active role in homeostasis and suppress autoimmunity. Characterization studies have shown that CD25 is a Treg marker and Foxp3 is an important and conserved gene for Treg. Although Tregs play an active role in homeostasis, they suppress antitumor immunity in the malignant environment and facilitate tumor progression. In many types of cancer, low CD8+ levels accompanying high Treg levels have been detected (Ormandy et al., 2005; Sasada et al., 2003; Schaefer et al., 2005; Wolf et al., 2003). Immune system suppression by Tregs occurs with metabolic arrest, suppressive cytokines (IL-10, IL-35, TGF-β) and suppression of dendritic cells (DC). The contribution of Tregs to tumor development is also accomplished by suppression of CD8+ T cells. Through suppressed CD8+ T cells, tumor cells can escape from immune system checkpoints (Adeegbe & Nishikawa, 2013; Garín et al., 2006; Vignali et al., 2008).

Myeloid-Derived Suppressor Cells (MDSCs)

MDSCs are heterogeneous populations derived from myeloid origin, which are seen in tumors that have low HLA-DR and high CD33 and CD14 levels. The expansion of MDSCs is promoted by many factors, e.g., granulocyte/macrophage colony stimulating factor (GM-CSF), macrophage colony stimulating factor (M-CSF), stem cell factor (SCF), prostaglandins, vascular endothelial growth factor (VEGF), and IL-6. Many of these factors have a relationship with the JAKSTAT3 pathway. Thus, while survival and proliferation increase, differentiation and apoptosis decrease (Gabrilovich & Nagaraj, 2009). MDSCs are affected by CSCs in a reciprocal manner. CSCs were shown to release macrophage migration inhibitory factor (MIF) in a mouse model of GBM, which boosted the suppressive efficiency of MDSC by increasing Arg1 levels via a CXCR2-dependent pathway (Otvos et al., 2016). MDSCs have a relationship with TAMs as well as with CSCs, they have characteristics and gene expression patterns in common with M2-polarized TAMs. In breast cancer, IL-6 promotes the accumulation and immune-suppressive capacity of MDSCs. The IL6-dependent suppressor of cytokine signaling 3 (SOCS3) promoted the phosphorylation of the STAT1, STAT3, JAK1, JAK2, and TYK2 proteins, which was associated with the suppression of MDSC T cells *in vitro* (Jiang et al., 2017). In another study, Peng et al. indicated that MDSCs enhance tumor initiation by enriching breast cancer cell stemness and suppressing T cell activation, which depend on the interaction between the NOTCH and STAT3 pathways in cancer cells (Peng et al., 2016).

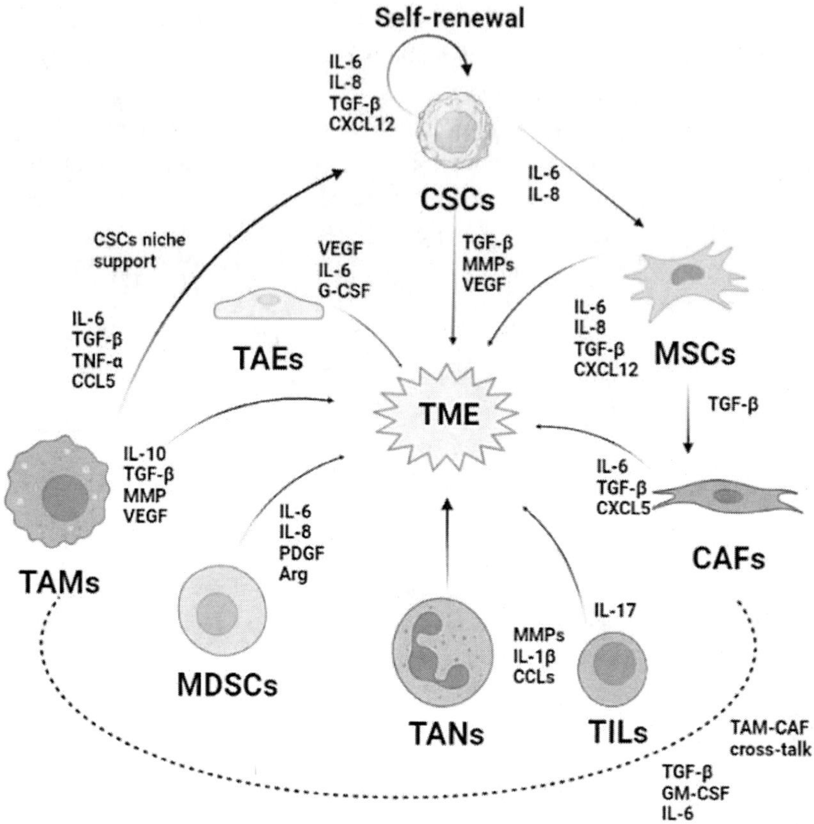

Figure 2. Cytokines and their relationship with CSC-TME (*BioRender*, n.d.).

Conclusion

The immune system can play both encouraging and suppressive roles on tumors. Immune system components can destroy tumor cells, but not always CSCs. Cytokines have many functions, including proliferation, tissue repair, inflammation, and chemotaxis. They can play an anti-inflammatory and pro-inflammatory role in the cell microenvironment, because of the fact that they are associated with many pathways. Immune system cells located in the tumor microenvironment and fighting the invader/cancer cells direct this system by secreting cytokines. Cytokines play a critical role in guiding the fate of this war. Cytokines can eliminate cancer cells or promote their growth with their ability to have a dual effect. Therefore, the potential power of immune system cells is related to their ability to cytokine trafficking. Considering this situation, cytokine-focused treatment alternatives that can be developed in cancer treatment are very important. For further studies, researchers can lead studies to reduce the pro-inflammatory effects of cytokines on TME and neutralize the immunosuppressive effects of cytokines, understanding the CSCs and CSC-TME-related components on metastasis. In addition, instead of depleting immune cell populations or changing their balance, treatment alternatives that aim to "retrain" the defense mechanisms of these immune cells in the cancer microenvironment on the basis of cytokines will be more advantageous.

In future developments, some considerations should be considered for cytokine-based cancer therapy. It will be an important detail not to expose the whole system to changes in order to avoid a systemic response by limiting the effect site of cytokines to the tumor microenvironment, and thus to correct the disturbed cytokine balance. In addition, a cytokine treatment that will be combined with the main treatment method to be used in cancer treatment will make the main treatment method even stronger and provide synergistic success.

References

Adeegbe, D., & Nishikawa, H. (2013). Natural and induced T regulatory cells in cancer. *Frontiers in Immunology*, *4*. https://www.frontiersin.org/article/10.3389/fimmu.2013.00190.

Allavena, P., & Mantovani, A. (2012). Immunology in the clinic review series; focus on cancer: Tumour-associated macrophages: undisputed stars of the inflammatory tumour microenvironment. *Clinical and Experimental Immunology*, *167*(2), 195–205. https://doi.org/10.1111/j.1365-2249.2011.04515.x.

Arango Duque, G., & Descoteaux, A. (2014). Macrophage cytokines: involvement in immunity and infectious diseases. *Frontiers in Immunology*, *5*. https://www.frontiersin.org/article/10.3389/fimmu.2014.00491.

Babon, J. J., Lucet, I. S., Murphy, J. M., Nicola, N. A., & Varghese, L. N. (2014). The molecular regulation of Janus kinase (JAK) activation. *Biochemical Journal*, *462*(1), 1–13. https://doi.org/10.1042/BJ20140712.

Balkwill, F., & Mantovani, A. (2001). Inflammation and cancer: Back to Virchow? *The Lancet*, *357*(9255), 539–545. https://doi.org/10.1016/S0140-6736(00)04046-0.

Batlle, E., & Clevers, H. (2017). Cancer stem cells revisited. *Nature Medicine*, *23*(10), 1124–1134. https://doi.org/10.1038/nm.4409.

Baudino, T. A., McKay, C., Pendeville-Samain, H., Nilsson, J. A., Maclean, K. H., White, E. L., Davis, A. C., Ihle, J. N., & Cleveland, J. L. (2002). C-Myc is essential for vasculogenesis and angiogenesis during development and tumor progression. *Genes & Development*, *16*(19), 2530–2543. https://doi.org/10.1101/gad.1024602.

Baumgarten, S. C., & Frasor, J. (2012). Minireview: Inflammation: An instigator of more aggressive Estrogen Receptor (ER) positive breast cancers. *Molecular Endocrinology*, *26*(3), 360–371. https://doi.org/10.1210/me.2011-1302.

Berghuis, D., Santos, S. J., Baelde, H. J., Taminiau, A. H., Maarten Egeler, R., Schilham, M. W., Hogendoorn, P. C., & Lankester, A. C. (2011). Pro-inflammatory chemokine–chemokine receptor interactions within the Ewing sarcoma microenvironment determine CD8+ T-lymphocyte infiltration and affect tumour progression. *The Journal of Pathology*, *223*(3), 347–357. https://doi.org/10.1002/path.2819.

Beutler, B. A. (1999). The role of tumor necrosis factor in health and disease. *The Journal of Rheumatology Supplement*, *57*, 16–21.

Bhanumathy, K., K., Balagopal, A., Vizeacoumar, F. S., Vizeacoumar, F. J., Freywald, A., & Giambra, V. (2021). Protein tyrosine kinases: their roles and their targeting in leukemia. *Cancers*, *13*(2), 184. https://doi.org/10.3390/cancers13020184.

BioRender. (n.d.). *BioRender*. Retrieved 17 February 2022, from https://biorender.com/.

Bruix, J., & Llovet, J. M. (2003). Hepatitis B virus and hepatocellular carcinoma. *Journal of Hepatology*, *39*, 59–63. https://doi.org/10.1016/S0168-8278(03)00140-5.

Buckanovich, R. J., Facciabene, A., Kim, S., Benencia, F., Sasaroli, D., Balint, K., Katsaros, D., O'Brien-Jenkins, A., Gimotty, P. A., & Coukos, G. (2008). Endothelin B receptor mediates the endothelial barrier to T cell homing to tumors and disables immune therapy. *Nature Medicine*, *14*(1), 28–36. https://doi.org/10.1038/nm1699.

Cancer.net. *ASCO Annual Meeting 2019: Immunotherapy for Lung Cancer, Gastro-intestinal Cancers and Targeted Therapy for Breast Cancer*. (2019, June 1). https://www.cancer.net/blog/2019-06/asco-annual-meeting-2019-immunotherapy-lung-cancer-gastrointestinal-cancers-and-targeted-therapy.

Cancer.net. *Understanding Immunotherapy*. (2013, March 25). https://www.cancer.net/navigating-cancer-care/how-cancer-treated/immunotherapy-and-vaccines/understanding-immunotherapy.

Chang, Q., Bournazou, E., Sansone, P., Berishaj, M., Gao, S. P., Daly, L., Wels, J., Theilen, T., Granitto, S., Zhang, X., Cotari, J., Alpaugh, M. L., de Stanchina, E., Manova, K., Li, M., Bonafe, M., Ceccarelli, C., Taffurelli, M., Santini, D., Bromberg, J. (2013). The IL-6/JAK/Stat3 feed-forward loop drives tumorigenesis and metastasis. *Neoplasia*, *15*(7), 848-IN45. https://doi.org/10.1593/neo.13706.

Chauhan, P., Nair, A., Patidar, A., Dandapat, J., Sarkar, A., & Saha, B. (2021). A primer on cytokines. *Cytokine*, *145*, 155458. https://doi.org/10.1016/j.cyto.2021.155458.

Chen, D. S., & Mellman, I. (2013). Oncology meets immunology: the cancer-immunity cycle. *Immunity*, 39(1), 1–10. https://doi.org/10.1016/j.immuni.2013.07.012.

Chen, D. S., & Mellman, I. (2017). Elements of cancer immunity and the cancer–immune set point. *Nature*, 541(7637), 321–330. https://doi.org/10.1038/nature21349.

Chen, F., Zhuang, X., Lin, L., Yu, P., Wang, Y., Shi, Y., & Sun, Y. (2015). New horizons in tumor microenvironment biology: challenges and opportunities. *BMC Medicine*, 13(1), 1-14.

Chen, M., Cheng, A., Chen, Y. Q., Hymel, A., Hanson, E. P., Kimmel, L., Minami, Y., Taniguchi, T., Changelian, P. S., & O'Shea, J. J. (1997). The amino terminus of JAK3 is necessary and sufficient for binding to the common γ chain and confers the ability to transmit interleukin 2-mediated signals. *Proceedings of the National Academy of Sciences*, *94*(13), 6910–6915. https://doi.org/10.1073/pnas.94.13.6910.

Chen, Y., Tan, W., & Wang, C. (2018). Tumor-associated macrophage-derived cytokines enhance cancer stem-like characteristics through epithelial–mesenchymal transition. *OncoTargets and Therapy*, *11*, 3817. https://doi.org/10.2147/OTT.S168317.

Cho, H., Seo, Y., Loke, K. M., Kim, S. W., Oh, S. M., Kim, J. H., Soh, J., Kim, H. S., Lee, H., Kim, J., Min, J. J., Jung, D. W., & Williams, D. R. (2018). Cancer-stimulated CAFs enhance monocyte differentiation and protumoral TAM activation via IL6 and GM-CSF secretion. *Clinical Cancer Research*, *24*(21), 5407–5421. https://doi.org/10.1158/1078-0432.CCR-18-0125.

Coussens, L. M., & Werb, Z. (2002). Inflammation and cancer. *Nature*, *420*(6917), 860–867. https://doi.org/10.1038/nature01322.

Dirkx, A. E. M., oude Egbrink, M. G. A., Wagstaff, J., & Griffioen, A. W. (2006). Monocyte/macrophage infiltration in tumors: Modulators of angiogenesis. *Journal of Leukocyte Biology*, *80*(6), 1183–1196. https://doi.org/10.1189/jlb.0905495.

Dolberg, D. S., Hollingsworth, R., Hertle, M., & Bissell, M. J. (1985). Wounding and its role in RSV-mediated tumor formation. *Science*, *230*(4726), 676–678. https://doi.org/10.1126/science.2996144.

Eck, M., Schmaußer, B., Scheller, K., Brändlein, S., & Müller-Hermelink, H. K. (2003). Pleiotropic effects of CXC chemokines in gastric carcinoma: Differences in CXCL8 and CXCL1 expression between diffuse and intestinal types of gastric carcinoma. *Clinical and Experimental Immunology*, *134*(3), 508–515. https://doi.org/10.1111/j.1365-2249.2003.02305.x.

Eggermont, A., Robert, C., Soria, J. C., & Zitvogel, L. (2014). Harnessing the immune system to provide long-term survival in patients with melanoma and other solid tumors. *OncoImmunology*, *3*(1), e27560. https://doi.org/10.4161/onci.27560.

Fridlender, Z. G., Sun, J., Kim, S., Kapoor, V., Cheng, G., Ling, L., Worthen, G. S., & Albelda, S. M. (2009). Polarization of tumor-associated neutrophil phenotype by TGF-β: "N1" versus "N2" TAN. *Cancer Cell*, *16*(3), 183–194. https://doi.org/10.1016/j.ccr.2009.06.017.

Gabrilovich, D. I., & Nagaraj, S. (2009). Myeloid-derived suppressor cells as regulators of the immune system. *Nature Reviews Immunology*, *9*(3), 162–174. https://doi.org/10.1038/nri2506.

Garín, M. I., Chu, C. C., Golshayan, D., Cernuda-Morollón, E., Wait, R., & Lechler, R. I. (2006). Galectin-1: A key effector of regulation mediated by CD4+CD25+ T cells. *Blood*, *109*(5), 2058–2065. https://doi.org/10.1182/blood-2006-04-016451.

Giraldez, M. D., Carneros, D., Garbers, C., Rose-John, S., & Bustos, M. (2021). New insights into IL-6 family cytokines in metabolism, hepatology and gastroenterology.

Nature Reviews Gastroenterology & Hepatology, *18*(11), 787–803. https://doi.org/10.1038/s41575-021-00473-x.

Goveia, J., Rohlenova, K., Taverna, F., Treps, L., Conradi, L. C., Pircher, A., Geldhof, V., de Rooij, L. P. M. H., Kalucka, J., Sokol, L., García-Caballero, M., Zheng, Y., Qian, J., Teuwen, L. A., Khan, S., Boeckx, B., Wauters, E., Decaluwé, H., De Leyn, P., … Carmeliet, P. (2020). An integrated gene expression landscape profiling approach to identify lung tumor endothelial cell heterogeneity and angiogenic candidates. *Cancer Cell*, *37*(1), 21-36.e13. https://doi.org/10.1016/j.ccell.2019.12.001.

Hass, R., Kasper, C., Böhm, S., & Jacobs, R. (2011). Different populations and sources of human mesenchymal stem cells (MSC): A comparison of adult and neonatal tissue-derived MSC. *Cell Communication and Signaling*, *9*(1), 12. https://doi.org/10.1186/1478-811X-9-12.

Hunter, T., & Sefton, B. M. (1980). Transforming gene product of Rous sarcoma virus phosphorylates tyrosine. *Proceedings of the National Academy of Sciences*, *77*(3), 1311–1315. https://doi.org/10.1073/pnas.77.3.1311.

Ievins, A., & Moritz, C. T. (2017). Therapeutic stimulation for restoration of function after spinal cord injury. *Physiology*, *32*(5), 391–398. https://doi.org/10.1152/physiol.00010.2017.

Iliopoulos, D., Hirsch, H. A., & Struhl, K. (2009). An epigenetic switch involving NF-κB, Lin28, Let-7 MicroRNA, and IL6 links inflammation to cell transformation. *Cell*, *139*(4), 693–706. https://doi.org/10.1016/j.cell.2009.10.014.

Ji, H., Houghton, A. M., Mariani, T. J., Perera, S., Kim, C. B., Padera, R., Tonon, G., McNamara, K., Marconcini, L. A., Hezel, A., El-Bardeesy, N., Bronson, R. T., Sugarbaker, D., Maser, R. S., Shapiro, S. D., & Wong, K. K. (2006). K-ras activation generates an inflammatory response in lung tumors. *Oncogene*, *25*(14), 2105–2112. https://doi.org/10.1038/sj.onc.1209237.

Kaltschmidt, C., Banz-Jansen, C., Benhidjeb, T., Beshay, M., Förster, C., Greiner, J., Hamelmann, E., Jorch, N., Mertzlufft, F., Pfitzenmaier, J., Simon, M., Schulte am Esch, J., Vordemvenne, T., Wähnert, D., Weissinger, F., Wilkens, L., & Kaltschmidt, B. (2019). A role for NF-κB in organ specific cancer and cancer stem cells. *Cancers*, *11*(5), 655. https://doi.org/10.3390/cancers11050655.

Korkaya, H., Liu, S., & Wicha, M. S. (2011). Regulation of cancer stem cells by cytokine networks: attacking cancer's inflammatory roots. *Clinical Cancer Research*, *17*(19), 6125–6129. https://doi.org/10.1158/1078-0432.CCR-10-2743.

Lacronique, V., Boureux, A., Della Valle, V., Poirel, H., Quang, C. T., Mauchauffé, M., Berthou, C., Lessard, M., Berger, R., Ghysdael, J., & Bernard, O. A. (1997). A TEL-JAK2 fusion protein with constitutive kinase activity in human leukemia. *Science*, *278*(5341), 1309–1312. https://doi.org/10.1126/science.278.5341.1309.

Lee, H., Herrmann, A., Deng, J. H., Kujawski, M., Niu, G., Li, Z., Forman, S., Jove, R., Pardoll, D. M., & Yu, H. (2009). Persistently activated stat3 maintains constitutive NF-κB activity in tumors. *Cancer Cell*, *15*(4), 283–293. https://doi.org/10.1016/j.ccr.2009.02.015.

Liang, W., Chen, X., Zhang, S., Fang, J., Chen, M., Xu, Y., & Chen, X. (2021). Mesenchymal stem cells as a double-edged sword in tumor growth: Focusing on MSC-derived cytokines. *Cellular & Molecular Biology Letters*, *26*(1), 3. https://doi.org/10.1186/s11658-020-00246-5.

Liu, S., Ginestier, C., Ou, S. J., Clouthier, S. G., Patel, S. H., Monville, F., Korkaya, H., Heath, A., Dutcher, J., Kleer, C. G., Jung, Y., Dontu, G., Taichman, R., & Wicha, M. S. (2011). Breast cancer stem cells are regulated by mesenchymal stem cells through cytokine networks. *Cancer Research*, *71*(2), 614–624. https://doi.org/ 10.1158/0008-5472.CAN-10-0538.

Long, H., Xie, R., Xiang, T., Zhao, Z., Lin, S., Liang, Z., Chen, Z., & Zhu, B. (2012). Autocrine CCL5 signaling promotes invasion and migration of CD133+ ovarian cancer stem-like cells via NF-κB-mediated MMP-9 upregulation. *Stem Cells*, *30*(10), 2309–2319. https://doi.org/10.1002/stem.1194.

Maishi, N., Annan, D. A., Kikuchi, H., Hida, Y., & Hida, K. (2019). Tumor endothelial heterogeneity in cancer progression. *Cancers*, *11*(10), 1511. https://doi.org/10.3390/cancers11101511.

Marotta, L. L. C., & Polyak, K. (2011). Unraveling the complexity of basal-like breast cancer. *Oncotarget*, *2*(8), 588–589.

Martins-Green, M., Boudreau, N., & Bissell, M. J. (1994). Inflammation is responsible for the development of wound-induced tumors in chickens infected with Rous Sarcoma Virus. *Cancer Research*, *54*(16), 4334–4341.

Masjedi, A., Hajizadeh, F., Beigi Dargani, F., Beyzai, B., Aksoun, M., Hojjat-Farsangi, M., Zekiy, A., & Jadidi-Niaragh, F. (2021). Oncostatin M: A mysterious cytokine in cancers. *International Immunopharmacology*, *90*, 107158. https://doi.org/10.1016/j.intimp.2020.107158.

Medzhitov, R. (2008). Origin and physiological roles of inflammation. *Nature*, *454*(7203), 428–435. https://doi.org/10.1038/nature07201.

Melero, I., Berman, D. M., Aznar, M. A., Korman, A. J., Gracia, J. L. P., & Haanen, J. (2015). Evolving synergistic combinations of targeted immunotherapies to combat cancer. Nature Reviews Cancer, 15(8), 457–472. https://doi.org/10.1038/nrc3973.

Murphy, J. B., & Rous, P. (1912). The behavior of chicken sarcoma implanted in the developing embryo. *Journal of Experimental Medicine*, *15*(2), 119–132. https://doi.org/10.1084/jem.15.2.119.

Murphy, K., & Weaver, C. (2016). *Janeway's Immunobiology*. Garland Science.

Nagl, L., Horvath, L., Pircher, A., & Wolf, D. (2020). Tumor Endothelial Cells (TECs) as potential immune directors of the tumor microenvironment – new findings and future perspectives. *Frontiers in Cell and Developmental Biology*, *8*. https://www.frontiersin.org/article/10.3389/fcell.2020.00766.

O'Shea, J. J., Gadina, M., & Schreiber, R. D. (2002). Cytokine signaling in 2002: new surprises in the Jak/Stat pathway. *Cell*, *109*(2, Supplement 1), S121–S131. https://doi.org/10.1016/S0092-8674(02)00701-8.

Opal, S. M., & DePalo, V. A. (2000). Anti-inflammatory cytokines. *Chest*, *117*(4), 1162–1172. https://doi.org/10.1378/chest.117.4.1162.

Ormandy, L. A., Hillemann, T., Wedemeyer, H., Manns, M. P., Greten, T. F., & Korangy, F. (2005). Increased populations of regulatory T cells in peripheral blood of patients with hepatocellular carcinoma. *Cancer Research*, *65*(6), 2457–2464. https://doi.org/10.1158/0008-5472.CAN-04-3232.

Ortega, M. A., Fraile-Martínez, O., Asúnsolo, Á., Buján, J., García-Honduvilla, N., & Coca, S. (2020). Signal transduction pathways in breast cancer: the important role of PI3K/Akt/mTOR. *Journal of Oncology*, *2020*, e9258396. https://doi.org/10.1155/2020/9258396.

Otvos, B., Silver, D. J., Mulkearns-Hubert, E. E., Alvarado, A. G., Turaga, S. M., Sorensen, M. D., Rayman, P., Flavahan, W. A., Hale, J. S., Stoltz, K., Sinyuk, M., Wu, Q., Jarrar, A., Kim, S. H., Fox, P. L., Nakano, I., Rich, J. N., Ransohoff, R. M., Finke, J., Lathia, J. D. (2016). Cancer stem cell-secreted macrophage migration inhibitory factor stimulates myeloid derived suppressor cell function and facilitates glioblastoma immune evasion. *Stem Cells*, *34*(8), 2026–2039. https://doi.org/10.1002/stem.2393.

Pekarek, L. A., Starr, B. A., Toledano, A. Y., & Schreiber, H. (1995). Inhibition of tumor growth by elimination of granulocytes. *Journal of Experimental Medicine*, *181*(1), 435–440. https://doi.org/10.1084/jem.181.1.435.

Pilati, C., Amessou, M., Bihl, M. P., Balabaud, C., Van Nhieu, J. T., Paradis, V., Nault, J. C., Izard, T., Bioulac-Sage, P., Couchy, G., Poussin, K., & Zucman-Rossi, J. (2011). Somatic mutations activating STAT3 in human inflammatory hepatocellular adenomas. *Journal of Experimental Medicine*, *208*(7), 1359–1366. https://doi.org/10.1084/jem.20110283.

Potente, M., Gerhardt, H., & Carmeliet, P. (2011). Basic and therapeutic aspects of angiogenesis. *Cell*, *146*(6), 873–887. https://doi.org/10.1016/j.cell.2011.08.039.

Quintás-Cardama, A., Kantarjian, H., Cortes, J., & Verstovsek, S. (2011). Janus kinase inhibitors for the treatment of myeloproliferative neoplasias and beyond. *Nature Reviews Drug Discovery*, *10*(2), 127–140. https://doi.org/10.1038/nrd3264.

Roskoski, R. (2019). Targeting ERK1/2 protein-serine/threonine kinases in human cancers. *Pharmacological Research*, *142*, 151–168. https://doi.org/10.1016/j.phrs.2019.01.039.

Rous, P. (1910). A transmissible avian neoplasm. (sarcoma of the common fowl.). *Journal of Experimental Medicine*, *12*(5), 696–705. https://doi.org/10.1084/jem.12.5.696.

Sasada, T., Kimura, M., Yoshida, Y., Kanai, M., & Takabayashi, A. (2003). CD4+CD25+ regulatory T cells in patients with gastrointestinal malignancies. *Cancer*, *98*(5), 1089–1099. https://doi.org/10.1002/cncr.11618.

Schaefer, C., Kim, G. G., Albers, A., Hoermann, K., Myers, E. N., & Whiteside, T. L. (2005). Characteristics of CD4+CD25+ regulatory T cells in the peripheral circulation of patients with head and neck cancer. *British Journal of Cancer*, *92*(5), 913–920. https://doi.org/10.1038/sj.bjc.6602407.

Sethi, N., Dai, X., Winter, C. G., & Kang, Y. (2011). Tumor-derived Jagged1 promotes osteolytic bone metastasis of breast cancer by engaging notch signaling in bone cells. *Cancer Cell*, *19*(2), 192–205. https://doi.org/10.1016/j.ccr.2010.12.022.

Sevillano, J., Sánchez-Alonso, M. G., Pizarro-Delgado, J., & Ramos-Álvarez, M. del P. (2021). Role of Receptor Protein Tyrosine Phosphatases (RPTPs) in insulin signaling and secretion. *International Journal of Molecular Sciences*, *22*(11), 5812. https://doi.org/10.3390/ijms22115812.

Shojaei, F., Singh, M., Thompson, J. D., & Ferrara, N. (2008). Role of Bv8 in neutrophil-dependent angiogenesis in a transgenic model of cancer progression. *Proceedings of the National Academy of Sciences*, *105*(7), 2640–2645. https://doi.org/10.1073/pnas.0712185105.

Siveen, K. S., Prabhu, K. S., Achkar, I. W., Kuttikrishnan, S., Shyam, S., Khan, A. Q., Merhi, M., Dermime, S., & Uddin, S. (2018). Role of non receptor tyrosine kinases in hematological malignances and its targeting by natural products. *Molecular Cancer*, *17*(1), 31. https://doi.org/10.1186/s12943-018-0788-y.

Solinas, G., Schiarea, S., Liguori, M., Fabbri, M., Pesce, S., Zammataro, L., Pasqualini, F., Nebuloni, M., Chiabrando, C., Mantovani, A., & Allavena, P. (2010). Tumor-conditioned macrophages secrete migration-stimulating factor: a new marker for M2-polarization, influencing tumor cell motility. *The Journal of Immunology*, *185*(1), 642–652. https://doi.org/10.4049/jimmunol.1000413.

Sparmann, A., & Bar-Sagi, D. (2004). Ras-induced interleukin-8 expression plays a critical role in tumor growth and angiogenesis. *Cancer Cell*, *6*(5), 447–458. https://doi.org/10.1016/j.ccr.2004.09.028.

Tan, H. X., Xiao, Z. G., Huang, T., Fang, Z. X., Liu, Y., & Huang, Z. C. (2020). CXCR4/TGF-β1 mediated self-differentiation of human mesenchymal stem cells to carcinoma-associated fibroblasts and promoted colorectal carcinoma development. *Cancer Biology & Therapy*, *21*(3), 248–257. https://doi.org/10.1080/15384047.2019.1685156.

Tazawa, H., Okada, F., Kobayashi, T., Tada, M., Mori, Y., Une, Y., Sendo, F., Kobayashi, M., & Hosokawa, M. (2003). Infiltration of neutrophils is required for acquisition of metastatic phenotype of benign murine fibrosarcoma cells: implication of inflammation-associated carcinogenesis and tumor progression. *The American Journal of Pathology*, *163*(6), 2221–2232. https://doi.org/10.1016/S0002-9440(10) 63580-8.

Unanue, E. R., Beller, D. I., Calderon, J., Kiely, J. M., & Stadecker, M. J. (1976). Regulation of immunity and inflammation by mediators from macrophages. *The American Journal of Pathology*, *85*(2), 465–478.

Valenti, G., Quinn, H. M., Heynen, G. J. J. E., Lan, L., Holland, J. D., Vogel, R., Wulf-Goldenberg, A., & Birchmeier, W. (2017). Cancer stem cells regulate cancer-associated fibroblasts via activation of hedgehog signaling in mammary gland tumors. *Cancer Research*, *77*(8), 2134–2147. https://doi.org/10.1158/0008-5472.CA N-15-3490.

Vickers, N. J. (2017). Animal communication: when I'm calling you, will you answer too? *Current Biology*, *27*(14), R713–R715. https://doi.org/10.1016/j.cub.2017.05.064.

Vignali, D. A. A., Collison, L. W., & Workman, C. J. (2008). How regulatory T cells work. *Nature Reviews Immunology*, *8*(7), 523–532. https://doi.org/10.1038/nri2343.

Vlahopoulos, S., Boldogh, I., Casola, A., & Brasier, A. R. (1999). Nuclear factor-κB–dependent induction of interleukin-8 gene expression by tumor necrosis factor: evidence for an antioxidant sensitive activating pathway distinct from nuclear translocation. *Blood*, *94*(6), 1878–1889. https://doi.org/10.1182/blood.V94.6.1878.

Wang, L., Yi, T., Kortylewski, M., Pardoll, D. M., Zeng, D., & Yu, H. (2009). IL-17 can promote tumor growth through an IL-6–Stat3 signaling pathway. *Journal of Experimental Medicine*, *206*(7), 1457–1464. https://doi.org/10.1084/jem.20090207.

Watanabe, T., Imamura, T., & Hiasa, Y. (2018). Roles of protein kinase R in cancer: Potential as a therapeutic target. *Cancer Science*, *109*(4), 919–925. https://doi.org/10.1111/cas.13551.

Wolf, A. M., Wolf, D., Steurer, M., Gastl, G., Gunsilius, E., & Grubeck-Loebenstein, B. (2003). Increase of regulatory T cells in the peripheral blood of cancer Patients1. *Clinical Cancer Research*, *9*(2), 606–612.

Wu, T., & Dai, Y. (2017). Tumor microenvironment and therapeutic response. *Cancer Letters*, *387*, 61–68. https://doi.org/10.1016/j.canlet.2016.01.043.

Yang, L., Shi, P., Zhao, G., Xu, J., Peng, W., Zhang, J., Zhang, G., Wang, X., Dong, Z., Chen, F., & Cui, H. (2020). Targeting cancer stem cell pathways for cancer therapy. *Signal Transduction and Targeted Therapy*, *5*(1), 1–35. https://doi.org/10.1038/s41392-020-0110-5.

Yigit, R., Massuger, L. F. A. G., Figdor, C. G., & Torensma, R. (2010). Ovarian cancer creates a suppressive microenvironment to escape immune elimination. *Gynecologic Oncology*, *117*(2), 366–372. https://doi.org/10.1016/j.ygyno.2010.01.019.

Yu, H., Kortylewski, M., & Pardoll, D. (2007). Crosstalk between cancer and immune cells: Role of STAT3 in the tumour microenvironment. *Nature Reviews Immunology*, *7*(1), 41–51. https://doi.org/10.1038/nri1995.

Zhang, J. M., & An, J. (2007). Cytokines, inflammation and pain. *International Anesthesiology Clinics*, *45*(2), 27–37. https://doi.org/10.1097/AIA.0b013e318034194e.

Chapter 14

The Effect of the Occupational Environment by Autoimmunity on Cancer Development

Selim Görgün[1,*], MD
and Aydan Çevik Varol[2]
[1]Department of Microbiology and Clinical Microbiology,
Health Science University,
Samsun Training and Research Hospital,
Samsun, Turkey
[2]Department of Family Physician,
Namık Kemal University,
Tekirdag, Turkey

Abstract

Millions of people around the world are diagnosed with cancer every year. Taking into account the increased morbidity and mortality due to the long and difficult treatment process and the loss of production in society, this picture can be considered a serious threat. However, despite the fact that it is a preventable disease, considering the impact of the individual exposed to the family and society, occupation-related diseases appear as a major problem in many countries of the world. To solve this complex problem, preventing health risks and identifying possible actionable solutions should be our top priority. In particular, to eliminate occupational cancers, the control of carcinogenic agents, the environment, and the time to which we are exposed, in other words, related processes, and legal regulations, is necessary. Workplace exposures, the cause of which is not clear, but where immunological

---

* Corresponding Author's Email: selimgorgun55@gmail.com.

In: Autoimmunity and Cancer
Editors: Soner Şahin and Kenan Demir
ISBN: 978-1-68507-937-6

reactions are observed and different parts of the body are affected, must be controlled.

As a result, we have to implement evidence-based policies and cooperate with all stakeholders in the new world order, which is globalized and industrial waste is increasing.

Keywords: cancer, environmental effect, occupational health

Introduction

History

About 500 years ago, Paracelsus argued that exposure of workers in mines to arsenic salts and sulfur deposits caused cancer. In fact, the first interaction between cancer and environmental factors has been demonstrated. In the next period, exposure to flue soot was investigated by Percival Pott, exposure to snuff by John Hill, and exposure to aniline dyes by Ludwig Rehn (Senga and Grose, 2021).

Nowadays, according to annual data from the International Labor Organization (ILO), workplace-related cancer deaths are estimated to be more than half a million per year and nearly twice as many as deaths from occupational accidents. The ten carcinogenic substances that cause the most frequent cancer formation with exposure to environmental effects in the workplace are responsible for 85% of all occupational cancer mortality (Takala, 2015).

Environmental Effect

The processing of industrial intermediates and much human-made waste affects natural life and ecosystems and causes every individual in the society to be exposed to carcinogenic risk factors in some way (Dujon et al., 2021). The emphasis is placed on differentiation, epigenetic dysregulation, altered microbiome, and altered neuronal signaling in cancer development (Senga and Grose, 2021). In addition, considering the process of cancer that extends over the years, the definition of environmental risk is made and it partially sheds light on the complex nature of the picture (Dujon et al., 2021).

Cancerogens in the Workplace Area

When exposed to silica, asbestos and coal dust, particles less than 5 microns inhaled into the lungs reach the terminal bronchioles and alveoli. The small ones are phagocytosed by alveolar macrophages. In addition, IL-1 and TNF-alpha and lysosomal enzymes are released into the area of inflammation. Cellular interactions occur to clean up the accumulated particles. Phagocytosing macrophages migrate to the interstitium along the perivascular and peribronchiolar regions. At this stage, the fibrotic process begins with the stimulation of growth factors. The immune response results in the release of various chemokines. These changes continue for years and pneumoconiosis is observed clinically (Wang and Christiani, 2000; DeLight and Sachs, 2021).

Environmental exposure to crystalline silica has been reported to increase the risk of silicosis, tuberculosis, cancer, and pulmonary fibrosis (Peruzzi et al., 2022). As an example, studies based on RNA sequences have been conducted to show that coal dust is a trigger for lung cancer development, and PHLDB2 has been identified as the main differentially expressed gene, highlighting its role in cancer development (Ge et al., 2021). In addition, asbestos fibers have been used in construction, transportation, mining, and aerospace for many years due to their high electrical and thermal resistance and low operating costs. It produces asbestosis, progressive interstitial lung disease, and fibrosis. It is a clinical picture with a poor prognosis resulting from the inhalation of asbestos fibers in the environment of the person. Asbestos fibers activate C5a. This complement is a chemotactic mediator for macrophages. The disease process is irreversible and may predispose to progressive lung cancer (Bhandari et al., 2021). In different studies, the risk of mesothelioma has been determined to increase with asbestosis in workers who are known or suspected to be exposed to asbestos at work (DeBono et al., 2021). Interestingly, smoking in the workplace is also reported in the literature to increase the risk of lung cancer in asbestos workers. This is important in terms of emphasizing the necessity of considering carcinogenic environmental factors together during exposure (Lordi and Reichman, 1993). A different publication investigated the relationship between occupational exposure to asbestos and ovarian cancer (Rajput et al., 2019).

With the heavy use of hard woods, wood dust can create an allergic asthma-like picture for those working in the furniture industry. Causes to nasal and nasal cavity cancers. It is thought to increase the risk of lung cancer (Socko, 2021; Scarabelli et al., 2021).

Diesel engine exhaust emissions and particulate matter emitted from diesel engines can be defined as a mixture of gases, vapors, and submicron in varying proportions. Diesel engine exhaust emissions have been classified among carcinogenic factors for humans after 2012 by the International Agency for Research on Cancer. Especially on this subject, many articles have been published on miners and transport sector transport workers. Various legal regulations have been made for safety limit values to protect employees in professional environments (Silverman, 2018). It has been reported to be associated with lung cancer, especially in mine workers (Möhner, 2019). Interestingly, diesel exhaust particles are also environmental pollutants thought to be stimulating in the development of asthma and exacerbation of asthma attacks. In this regard, the ingestion of soybean hull extract and/or diesel exhaust particles from the respiratory tract by workers may trigger different reactions. For example, these polluting factors increase the levels of H2O2 in the bronchoalveolar lavage and IgE in the serum. Furthermore, studies have found different immunological results from inhalation of the two agents alone. Inhalation of soybean hull extract alone increases the number of eosinophils, B cells, and monocytes and decreases the ratio of natural cellar cells. Inhalation of diesel exhaust particles increases neutrophils and decreases the total monocyte ratio (de Homdedeu et al., 2021). Along with these data, it is vital for workers' health to emphasize the risk of lung cancer in workers who have immunological changes and allergic reactions to environmental factors. It also shows the value of restrictions and regulations to be taken.

For workers working in industrial workshops, oil mists and metalworking fluids used in the workplace pose serious health risks to workers, especially if they are inhaled for long periods of time and their exposure is to high oil vapor concentrations (Zhang et al., 2021). In recent years, studies on oxidative potential have evaluated the oxidation function of a chemical/biological probe of pollutants in the workplace environment. When the results are examined, processes associated with inflammatory-based pathologies are also observed in those who have been exposed. Furthermore, diseases such as asthma, rhinitis, and cancer have been reported to occur in those working in the metal industry and are exposed to metalworking fluids, aerosols, and oil mists (Sauvain et al., 2021). Workers in the metal industry have to work every day in metal-rich welding fumes on a regular basis. During the welding process, the fumes produced cause acute and chronic effects in affected patients when inhaled. This factor has also been shown as a cancer factor by the International Agency for Research on Cancer since 2017 (Zeidler-Erdely et al., 2019). In recent years, animal model studies investigating the effect of mild steel and mild steel welding fumes on lung toxicity markers and tumor development associated with welding fumes have also been conducted to support these findings (Zeidler-Erdely et al., 2019).

Changes, which are investigated by epigenetic science and include various gene modifications, may shed light on the pathogenesis of different diseases involving various systems in humans. In different studies in the literature, DNA methylation changes in the inducible nitric oxide synthase gene, which is involved in nitric oxide production and is believed to be effective in the development of various cardiopulmonary diseases, are considered important by scientists. The chronic metal richness of different particles in workplace breathing air leads to various immunological changes and is associated with this problem (Leso et al., 2019).

Rosin is a readily available, inexpensive, natural product with potential for chemical modification. Although the reson is not considered toxic, its derivatives are considered allergens (Kugler et al., 2019). The crude methanolic extract derived from rosin was found to exhibit significant and selective cytotoxicity against the two breast cancer cells tested (MCF-7 and MDA-MB231) (El-Hallouty et al., 2020).

Conclusion

The development of inflammation is accepted as a process that promotes tumor formation and increases cancer development in living organisms. During this formation, cancer cells interact with stromal and inflammatory cells surrounding this foreign structure in the organism. Various chemical, biological, and organic factors in the workplace and our environment can cause deterioration of our health. In particular, they can come to the fore in the development of cancer with their contribution to inflammation and even to chronic immunological reaction processes. Although some of these changes and responses have been elucidated in the pathogenesis and proven in the literature, more detailed studies are still needed.

For this reason, it should be accepted as a necessity to carry out preventive activities in occupational health. It is lifesaving to monitor occupational exposures that are considered harmful and pose a risk to workers' health, and to carry out adequate medical inspections. It is important in terms of risk management to increase our awareness by accepting that occupational carcinogens are in our lives and to improve ourselves in this regard.

References

Bhandari J, Thada PK and Sedhai YR. (2021). *Asbestosis*. In StatPearls. StatPearls Publishing.

DeBono NL, Warden H, Logar-Henderson C, Shakik S, Dakouo M, MacLeod J and Demers PA. (2021). Incidence of mesothelioma and asbestosis by occupation in a diverse workforce. *American Journal of Industrial Medicine* 64(6), 476-487. https://doi.org/10.1002/ajim.23245.

de Homdedeu M, Cruz MJ, Sánchez-Díez S, Gómez-Ollés S, Ojanguren I, Ma D and Muñoz X. (2021). Role of diesel exhaust particles in the induction of allergic asthma to low doses of soybean. *Environmental Research* 196, 110337. https://doi.org/10.1016/j.envres.2020.110337.

DeLight N and Sachs H. (2021). *Pneumoconiosis*. In StatPearls. StatPearls Publishing.

Dujon AM, Ujvari B and Thomas F. (2021). Cancer risk landscapes: A framework to study cancer in ecosystems. *The Science of the Total Environment* 763, 142955. https://doi.org/10.1016/j.scitotenv.2020.142955.

El-Hallouty SM, Soliman A, Nassrallah A, Salamatullah A, Alkaltham MS, Kamal KY, Hanafy EA, Gaballa HS and Aboul-Soud M. (2020). Crude methanol extract of rosin gum exhibits specific cytotoxicity against human breast cancer cells via apoptosis induction. *Anti-Cancer Agents in Medicinal Chemistry* 20(8), 1028-1036. https://doi.org/10.2174/1871520620666200423074826.

Ge D, Shao Y, Wang M, Tao H, Mu M and Tao X. (2021). RNA-seq-based screening in coal dust-treated cells identified PHLDB2 as a novel lung cancer-related molecular marker. *BioMed Research International* 2021, 1978434. https://doi.org/10.1155/2021/1978434.

Kugler S, Ossowicz P, Malarczyk-Matusiak K and Wierzbicka E. (2019). Advances in rosin-based chemicals: the latest recipes, applications and future trends. *Molecules* (Basel, Switzerland), 24(9), 1651. https://doi.org/10.3390/molecules 24091651.

Leso V, Vetrani I, Della Volpe I, Nocera C and Iavicoli I. (2019). Welding fume exposure and epigenetic alterations: a systematic review. *International Journal of Environmental Research and Public Health* 16(10), 1745. https://doi.org/10.3390/ijerph16 101745.

Lordi GM and Reichman LB. (1993). Pulmonary complications of asbestos exposure. *American Family Physician*, 48(8), 1471-1477.

Möhner M. (2019). Re: "Reanalysıs of dıesel engıne exhaust and lung cancer mortalıty in the dıesel exhaust in mıners study cohort usıng alternatıve exposure estımates and radon adjustment" and "Dıesel exhaust and lung cancer-aftermath of becomıng an iarc group 1 carcınogen". *American Journal of Epidemiology* 188(2), 484-485. https://doi.org/10.1093/aje/kwy166.

Peruzzi CP, Brucker N, Bubols G, Cestonaro L, Moreira R, Domingues D, Arbo M, Olivo Neto P, Knorst MM and Garcia SC. (2022). Occupational exposure to crystalline silica and peripheral biomarkers: An update. *Journal of Applied Toxicology: JAT* 42(1), 87-102. https://doi.org/10.1002/jat.4212.

Rajput Z, Hering KG, Kraus T, Tannapfel A, Sonnenschein G, Centmayer A, Radon K, Nowak D and Weinmann T. (2019). Investigating the association between occupational exposure to asbestos and ovarian carcinoma: Results from a pilot study in Germany. *BMC Public Health*, 19(1), 1341. https://doi.org/10.1186/s12889-019-7590-7.

Sauvain JJ, Suarez G, Hopf NB, Batsungnoen K, Charriere N, Andre F, Levilly R and Wild P. (2021). Oxidative potential of aerosolized metalworking fluids in occupational settings. *International Journal of Hygiene and Environmental Health,* 235, 113775. https://doi.org/10.1016/j.ijheh.2021.113775.

Scarabelli TM, Corsetti G, Chen-Scarabelli C and Saravolatz LD. (2021). Follicular B-cell lymphoma and particulate matter associated with environmental exposure to wood dust. *The American Journal of Case Reports,* 22, e929396. https://doi.org/10.12659/AJCR.929396.

Senga SS and Grose RP. (2021). Hallmarks of cancer-the New Testament. *Open Biology*, 11(1), 200358. https://doi.org/10.1098/rsob.200358.

Silverman DT. (2018). Diesel exhaust and lung cancer-aftermath of becoming an IARC group 1 carcinogen. *American Journal of Epidemiology*, 187(6), 1149-1152. https://doi.org/10.1093/aje/kwy036.

Soćko R. (2021). A quantitative risk assessment of sinonasal cancer as a function of time in workers occupationally exposed to wood dust. *International Journal of Occupational Medicine and Environmental Health,* 34(4), 541-549. https://doi.org/10.13075/ijomeh.1896.01673.

Takala J. (2015). Eliminating occupational cancer. *Industrial Health*, 53(4), 307-309. https://doi.org/10.2486/indhealth.53-307.

Wang XR and Christiani DC. (2000). Respiratory symptoms and functional status in workers exposed to silica, asbestos, and coal mine dusts. *Journal of Occupational and Environmental Medicine,* 42(11), 1076-1084. https://doi.org/10.1097/00043764-200011000-00009.

Zeidler-Erdely PC, Falcone LM and Antonini JM. (2019). Influence of welding fume metal composition on lung toxicity and tumor formation in experimental animal models. *Journal of Occupational and Environmental Hygiene*, 16(6), 372-377. https://doi.org/10.1080/15459624.2019.1587172.

Zhang H, Zhang S, Pan W and Long Z. (2021). Low-cost sensor system for monitoring the oil mist concentration in a workshop. *Environmental Science and Pollution Research International,* 28(12), 14943-14956. https://doi.org/10.1007/s11356-020-11709-9.

Chapter 15

mRNA Vaccines

Didem Seven, PhD, Didem Tecimel, BSc and Ömer Faruk Bayrak*, PhD
Department of Medical Genetics,
School of Medicine, Yeditepe University, Istanbul, Turkey

Abstract

mRNA vaccines offer enormous promise in the fight against cancer and viral diseases, due to their superiority in terms of efficacy, safety, and industrial manufacturing. In the last few decades, sequence optimization has resulted in the development of several types of mRNAs to solve the disadvantages of high mRNA immunogenicity, instability, and inefficiency. mRNA vaccines are combined with immunological adjuvants and various delivery techniques based on immunological studies. By using mRNA-delivery techniques, mRNA efficiency and stabilization can be increased aside from sequence optimization. Increased antigen reactivity provides an understanding of mRNA-induced immunity, both innate and adaptive, without the need for antibody-dependent enhancing activity. Therefore, scientists have turned to carrier-based mRNA vaccines, dendritic cell-based mRNA vaccines, and naked mRNA vaccines to solve the problem. The molecular mechanism of mRNA vaccines and the underlying process will be discussed in this chapter, delivery strategies, and relevance to Corona Virus Disease 2019 (COVID-19).

Keywords: mRNA vaccine, vaccine design, delivery methods, COVID-19 vaccine

* Corresponding Author's Email: ofbayrak@yeditepe.edu.tr.

In: Autoimmunity and Cancer
Editors: Soner Şahin and Kenan Demir
ISBN: 978-1-68507-937-6

Introduction

Messenger RNA (mRNA) vaccination has lately emerged as a viable alternative to traditional DNA vaccines for viral disease prevention and anticancer treatment. mRNAs can be translated into both nondividing and dividing cells, and RNA just has to be imported into the cytoplasm and then translated into the antigen(s) of interest in a single movement, which is one of the advantages of employing mRNA rather than DNA as a cancer vaccination method. mRNA vaccines typically have a higher quantity of protein expression than DNA vaccines. Unlike DNA vaccines, mRNA-based vaccines do not integrate into the genome sequence and are therefore not subject to insertional mutagenesis (Pardi et al., 2018).

Major technological innovations during the last few decades have made mRNA a more viable vaccine candidate. IVT mRNA has completed considerable preclinical testing and is now in Phase III clinical trials for therapeutic cancer vaccination. Various alterations to the mRNA untranslated regions and backbone render mRNA more reliable, less RNase sensitive, and high capability of translation. mRNA products now lack double-stranded contaminations, reducing nonspecific activation of innate immunity as a result of the improved purification methods. By incorporating mRNA into delivery vehicles, researchers were able to achieve more efficient in vivo delivery of mRNA. Due to their quick, low-cost production and large-scale installation, mRNA vaccines offer a significant advantage over other vaccine approaches now that scale-up manufacturing has matured. Non-replicating mRNAs have been studied largely in cancer clinical trials thus far. However, owing to their long-lasting efficacy and lower necessary dosages, self-amplifying mRNAs (SAM) have received much interest and are being studied in infectious disease and cancer (Bloom et al., 2021). More than twenty mRNA-based immunotherapies have been tested in clinical trials so far, with encouraging results in tumor treatments. mRNA vaccines, in addition to anticancer immunotherapies, offer a significant advantage in responding quickly to the global outbreak of the coronavirus disease in 2019 (COVID-19). Pfizer-BioNTech and Moderna just received emergency approval for two mRNA-based vaccines for COVID-19 prophylaxis by the US Food and Drug Administration, the mRNA vaccine field will see a dramatic increase in market value and draw wide attention in cancer and infectious disease applications (L. A. Jackson et al., 2020; Sahin et al., 2020).

In this chapter, we review current mRNA vaccine design, delivery methods, emphasize problems, and recent accomplishments, and estimate the next improvements in mRNA vaccines.

mRNA Vaccine Structures

The basic idea behind using mRNA for vaccination is to transfer the desired transcript, which encodes one or more immunogens, to the cytoplasm of the host cell, where expression results in translated protein(s) that are either released or cytosolically located (N. A. C. Jackson et al., 2020). The generation of cDNA templates by in vitro transcription, commonly plasmid DNA (pDNA), using a bacteriophage RNA polymerase can yield functional synthetic mRNA (Krieg & Melton, 1984). IVT mRNA is generated from a linear DNA template, using certain enzymes such as T7, T3, or Sp6 phage RNA polymerase (Pardi et al., 2013). The final product should have an open reading frame that encodes the desired protein, flanking UTRs, a 5'cap, and a poly(A) tail. As a result, mRNA is designed to look like fully processed mature mRNA molecules seen in the cytoplasm of eukaryotic cells (Pardi et al., 2018).

Nonreplicating mRNA (NRM) and self-amplifying mRNA (SAM) constructs are the two main types of mRNAs currently being studied. Nonreplicating mRNA structures are short, basic, and lack extra encoded proteins that could trigger undesirable immune responses (Schlake et al., 2012). NRM structures encode the coding sequence (CDS) and are flanked by 5' and 3'untranslated regions (UTRs), a 5'cap structure that includes 7-methylguanosine (m7G) attached to the first nucleotide by a triphosphate bridge and a 3'poly (A) tail (Ulmer & Geall, 2016). The 5′ m7G cap prevents the identification of the cytoplasmic RNA sensor, the retinoic acid-inducible gene I (RIG-I) of RNA helicases, inhibits destruction mediated by exonuclease 5′-3′, invites translation initiation factors, and stimulates efficient translation (Devarkar et al., 2016). The poly(A) tail and its size are essential for translation and to prevent degrading of the mRNA vaccine construct (Lima et al., 2017). The sequence design process (codon optimization) and nucleoside modification (i.e., uridine substitution with pseudouridine) also improve translation performance by suppressing Toll-like receptor (TLR) recognition and the innate immunological response to mRNA structures (Kariko et al., 2005) (Figure 1).

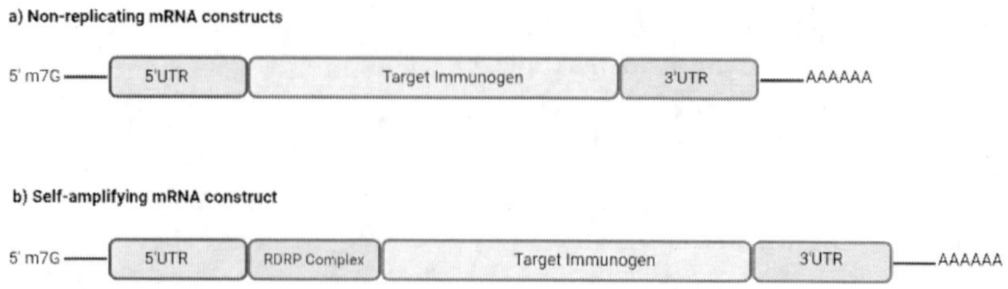

Figure 1. Composition of mRNA vaccine constructs (*BioRender*, n.d.).

The majority of currently employed self-amplifying mRNA (SAM or self-replicating mRNA) vaccines are based on a positive stranded alphavirus such as the Sindbis and Semliki-Forest viruses genome, with the RNA replication organizer genes intact but the structural protein genes substituted with the antigen of interest. Positive-strand RNA viruses serve as an mRNA template for extremely rapid RNA-dependent RNA polymerase (RDRP) translation as well as a genomic template for replication by the corresponding RDRP. The negative-strand RNA of the first replication acts as a template for the continuation of the positive-strand viral genome's production. Behind infection, RNA polymerase moves to a downstream promoter along the RNA molecule and begins to transcribe capped mRNA encoding structural viral proteins (Cheng et al., 2001; Perri et al., 2003; Ljungberg & Liljestrom, 2015). The structural genes of the RNA virus are substituted by heterologous coding sequences regulated by a subgenomic promoter (Ljungberg & Liljestrom, 2015; Lundstrom, 2015). By amplification of the transgene, high levels of protein can be produced from small quantities of transfected recombinant replicon RNA while avoiding the formation of infective viruses. Intracellular replication is transitory, and double-stranded RNA (dsRNA) activates interferon-mediated host defense mechanisms by activating pattern recognition receptors (PRRs). As a result, the encoded target molecules elicit strong antigen-specific immune responses. So, self-amplifying mRNA vector products are suitable for vaccine improvement due to their short-term transgene expression and inherent adjuvant effects (Sahin et al., 2014).

Compared to a nonreplicating mRNA vaccine, vaccination with a self-amplifying mRNA structure caused extra protein synthesis for a longer period of time and a stronger immune response in mice (Brito et al., 2014). Another power of self-replicating mRNA constructs is the act of combining multiple genetic codes into the same replicon, resulting in the expression of both target antigen and immunomodulatory molecules such as CD70, OX40L, CD40L, and GM-CSF in efficacy (Kowalski et al., 2019; Vogel et al., 2018). Self-replicating mRNA structures (9.3kb) are significantly larger than non-replicating mRNA structures (2.2 kb) making construction and stability more difficult and potentially restricting internalization of vaccines (Kowalzik et al., 2021). They can withstand only a few nucleotide or sequence changes without losing their self-amplifying ability. Traditional designs of nonreplicating mRNA vaccines are effective in eliciting immunological responses, but their half-lives are short. Self-replicating mRNA vaccination designs show comparable gains in message expression magnitude and duration, as well as immunogen synthesis (N. A. C. Jackson et al., 2020).

mRNA Vaccine Design & Optimization

Significant progress has been made in enhancing the efficacy of mRNA vaccines during the previous decade. Some ways used to improve RNA stability and gene expression, as well as vaccination effectiveness, include changes to the 5 cap, poly (A) tail, coding and UTRs, and nucleoside bases.

Cap

Eukaryotic mRNAs, containing viral RNAs like those from alphaviruses, have a methylguanosine cap with two forms of methylation at the 5'position. The m7G cap (cap 0), which is inserted through a triphosphate bridge during transcription, prevents premature destruction of the RNA and is required for the maturity, exporting, and translation initiation of mRNA (Ziemniak et al., 2013). To assist ribosome recognition and translation initiation, the 5′ cap interacts with the eukaryotic translation initiation factor 4E (eIF4E). For mRNA 5′ capping, enzymatic and chemical methods or cap analogs are used. The Vaccinia capping system, which is derived from Vaccinia virus Capping Enzyme (VCE), is the most extensively used in vitro post-translational capping enzymatic technique (Muttach et al., 2017). The VCE is divided into two subunits D1 and D12. The D1 subgroup has the guanylyltransferase, triphosphatase, and methyltransferase action, all of which are required for the formation of a full Cap 0 structure, whereas D12 has an important function in D1 activation. The Vaccinia capping system achieves about 100% capping capability with correct position; on the other hand, large-scale capped RNA production requires efficient VCE expression and purification (Fuchs et al., 2016). In addition to chemical and enzymatic post-translational capping techniques, add cap analogs co-transcriptionally; nevertheless, this may result in reversely integrating into the mRNA sequence, resulting in reduced downstream mRNA translation efficiency. Antireverse cap analogs (ARCA) have been designed to inhibit reverse incorporation. In order to ensure the insertion of a nucleotide exclusively at the non-methylated guanosine during IVT, soon after ARCA adds a methyl group at the C3 location (closer to m7G) (Rydzik et al., 2012). Enzymatically capped mRNA can be boosted more by enzymatic 2'-O-methylation of the first transcribed nucleotide, protein expression from in vitro transcribed, ensuing in protein expression in comparison with that from mRNA co-transcribed with ARCA (Zhao et al., 2010).

Poly A(tail)

The poly(A) sequence can decelerate RNA exonuclease degradation, enhance RNA stability, and improve translation efficiency. Poly(A) must be of an appropriate length. Poly(A) is commonly utilized and has a length of 250 units, but various cells may have different priorities. For instance, Poly(A) should be 120–150 nucleotides long in human monocyte-derived Dendritic Cells and 300 nucleotides long in human primary T cells. The translational initiation factors eiF4G and eiF4E are intimately connected with the adjacent poly-A-binding protein (PABP) at the 30 UTR in stable mRNAs, favoring a closed-loop structure and effective translation (Linares-Fernandez et al., 2020). The many protein–protein and protein–RNA interactions of the closed-loop structure prevent the transcript from further deadenylation and mRNA from being degraded (Lima et al., 2017). As a result, future research should look into the role of poly-A size in IVT-mRNA antigen kinetic expression.

UTRs

The replication and translation of mRNA genes can be affected by mRNA UTRs. Multiple sequence regions that can alter mRNA stability and expression have been discovered inside the two of 5' and 3' UTRs are cellular and viral mRNAs. Humans or Xenopus laevis have great stability in the UTR region of α-globin or β-globin and that has been the common strategy in mRNA vaccination in the past (Weissman, 2015). As a consequence, any mRNA vaccination must identify which UTR sequences in the targeted cells are most important for high expression. To begin, the existence of start codons (AUG) and noncanonical start codons (CUG) in the 5′ UTR should be avoided, since these codons can disrupt the ORF's regular translation process (Miao et al., 2021). The existence of highly persistent secondary structures, which inhibit scanning, ribosome recruitment, and start codon recognition, is another factor that hinders mRNA translation. Shorter 5'UTRs may be used, as past research has pointed out that this type of 5'UTR is more usable for mRNA translation. Finally, based on the 5'UTR sequence, a bioinformatics technique can be utilized to predict the efficiency of mRNA translation. Protein expression could also be increased by adding 3' UTR sequences twice in tandem, in addition to using stable mRNA sequences (Holtkamp et al., 2006). In mRNA vaccination and genetic reprogramming investigations, the novel 3' UTR motifs were found to have more potent therapeutic effects than mRNA with the β-globin 3' UTR. The performance of UTRs is influenced by species, cell type, and cell state. To improve the design of therapeutic mRNA vaccine UTRs, one must first understand the pharmacology of the targeted cells.

Codon Optimization of Open Reading Frame (ORF)

The most important component of the mRNA vaccine is the open reading frame, which includes the coding sequence that is translated into protein. The viral RNA-dependent RNA polymerase is preserved to control cytoplasmic amplification of the replicon structure, and the ORF encoding viral structural proteins is replaced with the chosen target transcript. Although not as flexible as non-coding areas, the open reading frame can be adjusted to boost translation without changing the protein sequence by replacing rarely used codons with more commonly take place codons that encode the same amino acid residue (Chaudhary et al., 2021). A number of codon optimization schemes have been devised in order to improve the translational process. Codon optimization is usually accomplished by selecting the best amino acid codes based on the occurrence rates of various species. CureVac AG, a biopharmaceutical organization, identified that human mRNA codons infrequently carry A or U in the third position and patented an approach to substitute A or U with G or C in the open reading frame (Class & USPC, 2016). Although rare codon replacement is a tempting optimization method, it must be utilized with caution due to the slower translation rate of rare codons that are required for correct protein folding in some cases. This is why more consideration must be given after screening for secondary structure and increasing the GC content of the sequence (Spencer et al., 2012).

Modified Nucleotides

Some nucleotides in mRNA (ATP, CTP, GTP, and UTP) are post-transcriptionally changed during maturation. In the generation of IVT mRNA, pseudouridine and 5-methylcytidine are examples of typically occurring modified nucleotides that can be used (Kariko & Weissman, 2007). The use of these modified nucleotides can prevent the innate immune system from recognizing IVT mRNA, preventing unwanted immunological reactions. For example, the replacement of uridine with pseudouridine in IVT mRNA lowers innate immunological responses to mRNA, such as TLRs and Protein Kinase R, while also increasing protein translation. Furthermore, as substitutes for basic nucleotides, 5-methylcytidine, 2-thiouridine, and N1-methyl-pseudouridine were investigated and shown that combinations of modified nucleotides outperformed their unmodified counterparts. On the other hand, in mice, counterarguments indicated that unmodified mRNA produces more protein and induces less cytokine stimulation than pseudouridine-substituted mRNA. When delivered intravenously via Lipid Nanoparticles (LNPs), pseudouridine substitution of mRNA had no effect on in vivo protein expression or levels of different cytokines versus to unmodified mRNA (Kauffman et al., 2016). Although modified nucleotides reduced immune responses to a less extent than unmodified nucleotides, HPLC purification had a greater impact on cytokine levels. Overall, the effects of the changed nucleotides appear to be inconsistent and may vary depending on the experimental conditions, such as cell type, delivery vector, and administration route. However, with approximately 143 essential nucleotide modifications, it is difficult to argue that changed nucleotides are major elements in RNA activity regulation in cells (McCown et al., 2020). At the same time, additional data reveal that abnormal RNA modifications, present or absent, can cause diseases in humans, highlighting the need to complete the assessment of the advantage of changed nucleotides (Yu et al., 2019).

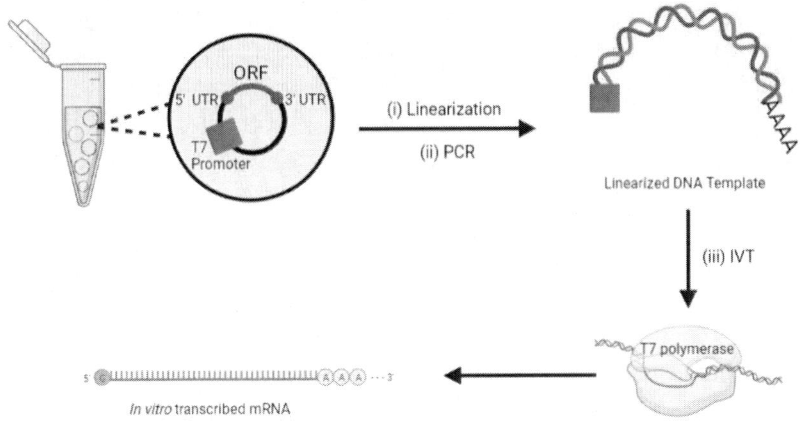

Figure 2. IVT process from template DNA (*BioRender*, n.d.).

mRNA Purification

mRNA vaccines must meet purity requirements as pharmaceutical items. Efficient protein expression and immunogenicity is achieved by transcript purification following the IVT which is a crucial and standard procedure in mRNA vaccine production. The IVT by-product, dsRNA, is removed by HPLC purification, increasing protein expression (Kariko et al., 2011). However, there are some limitations to ion-paired reversed-phase HPLC purification. The drawbacks are related to both cost and production. The biotechnology industry not only considers the utility of a product, but also deals with it to be cost- and time-effective. The ion-paired reversed-phase HPLC purification restricts both the cost and time effectiveness. The required equipment and consumables, as well as the batch size expansion, are difficult to sustain in a cost-effective manner. The handling of acetonitrile waste production from the HPLC procedure requires additional cost and an appropriate plant design. Additionally, the yield is reduced by about 50% during the procedure, and the purification time is long. A new purification approach, *fast protein liquid chromatography (FPLC)*, was lately described that could solve the major drawbacks of HPLC while yet offering comparable dsRNA purification. This approach utilizes cellulose powder as an adsorbent to bind dsRNA with the aid of a buffer containing ethanol and allows for the removal of up to 90% of dsRNA. FPLC is cost-effective, rapid, and scalable and enables the purification of large amounts of IVT mRNA without the production of hazardous waste (Baiersdorfer et al., 2019). FPLC purification enabled the protein expression to be boosted from IVT mRNA in primary human DCs by up to 1,000-fold. If Good Manufacturing Practices (GMPs), *sterility, integrity, purity, and activity testing* are employed to the purified mRNA transcript, then the product is manufactured into a drug product (mRNA vaccine).

Delivery Systems

One of the main reasons why mRNA vaccines are emerging is their capacity to be produced rapidly. On the basis of the sequencing information from a target virus, mRNA vaccines can be produced in a short period of time (days or months). Furthermore, in vitro transcription reactions are not only rapid but also provide a high yield, making the procedure affordable and scalable. Another benefit of mRNA vaccines is that they do not contain any viral elements that can cause infection or insertional mutagenesis (Cao & Gao, 2021). mRNA vaccines, on the other hand, have certain intrinsic restrictions. While allergic reactions, infarction, and heart/renal failure are still possible, the mRNA vaccine can break down shortly after injection or trigger cytokine storms. Therefore, effective administration of the mRNA vaccine to human cells is a major challenge. As foreign mRNA is easily recognized by the immune system of recipient patients, it can rapidly degrade by nucleases (Rauch et al., 2018). Consequently, relying solely on mRNA delivery is insufficient, and pharmaceutical action remains inadequate. Protection of mRNA from degradation and improvement of immune efficiency are achievable by optimizing delivery systems. Appropriate carriers of mRNA are not only able to prevent degradation but also enhance immune responses, provide a better effector presentation, and present improved biocompatibility, and biosafety (Liang et al., 2021).

mRNA vaccines need to pass through the phospholipid bilayer of the cell membrane, which is negatively charged, and reach into the cytoplasm to be translated into protein. The cell membrane is only permissive to molecules smaller than 1000 Da by passive diffusion. Nonphagocytic eukaryotic cells, such as basophiles, can directly internalize a particle that is smaller than 1 μm (e.g., liposomes and pathogens). Microspheres less than 200 nm need protein coating for diffusion, whereas intracellular entry particles that are 500 nm and larger are mediated by caveole-dependent internalization (REJMAN et al., 2004). Regardless of its relatively large size, naked mRNA can be delivered without the use of a special carrier. The proof of concept demonstrating the feasibility of injection of naked intramuscular mRNA into the mouse was introduced in 1990 (Wolff et al., 1990). Since then, the efficiency of intramuscular, subcutaneous, and intradermal injections of naked mRNA has been further verified (Pardi et al., 2015, 2017; Zhang et al., 2019). For mRNA delivered subcutaneously, efficient translation of the encoded protein has been reported (Probst et al., 2007; Van Lint et al., 2012). Additionally, subcutaneous delivery of mRNA enables its expression by both nonimmune cells and skin-resident dendritic cells. This provides stimulation for both cellular and humoral immune responses (McNamara et al., 2015; Selmi et al., 2016; De Beuckelaer et al., 2017). However, naked mRNA cannot diffuse through the membrane passively; it is controversial how it is transported intracellularly. Though, studies suggest that the internalization mechanism could be relying on micropinocytosis, a vesicle-mediated endocytosis mechanism seen in dendritic cells. (Diken et al., 2011; Selmi et al., 2016). Even naked mRNA delivery is conceivable, facilitation of intracellular delivery enhances both cell entry and prevents degradation by RNases. Delivery methods can be classified as nonviral and viral vectors. Nonviral vectors can also be classified as ex vivo loading of dendritic cells, peptide-based, lipid- based nanoparticles, polymers, nanomaterials, and lipid-polymer hybrid systems (Wadhwa et al., 2020; Cao & Gao, 2021). In this section, we will evaluate both viral and non-viral delivery systems.

Viral Delivery Methods

Viral delivery methods have been widely investigated for both DNA and RNA delivery. Depending on the need for genomic integration or transient expression, the viral packaging could utilize retroviruses, lentiviruses, adenoviruses, and adeno-associated viruses. However, the packaging capacity of viral vectors is limited by the size of the nucleic acid. Severe side effects, immunological reactions, and off-target effects constrain the clinical application of viral vectors (Hecker, 2016).

Recently, VLPs, or viral-like particles, have been introduced as a novel type of mRNA delivery method. PEG10, a gag homolog protein, has been found to bind its own mRNA and release VLPs once the capsid has been produced. Thus, Segel et. al. suggested that PEG10 can only be used as an mRNA delivery tool if it can bind mRNAs other than its own while still allowing the creation of capsid-like structures that construct VLPs (Segel et al., 2021). Despite the potential use of PEG10, the study is still in its early stages; therefore, the efficiency as a delivery method cannot be claimed. The extracellular vesicle-like structure originating from humans enhances the biocompatibility and might be useful for surpassing the immunological reactions such as allergies, cytokine storms, etc. The nonimmunogenic property might be beneficial for repeated administration of mRNA vaccines. VLPs are expected to emerge in the future, but it is also assumed to be challenging progress based on the experiences gained in *in vivo* gene therapies (Riecken et al., 2021; Segel et al., 2021).

Non-Viral Delivery Methods

Ex Vivo Loading of Dendritic Cells

Dendritic cells (DCs) are antigen-presenting cells. Autologous DCs of origin are loaded with antigens and subjected to maturation under *ex vivo* conditions. The subsequent DCs are then injected back into the patient. Therefore, it initiates a protective immune response (Gu et al., 2020).

Dendritic cells are found in two stages: immature and mature. The majority of dendritic cells are immature and present in nonlymphoid tissues. They are specialized in antigen presentation in their immature stage, express low levels of costimulatory molecules and large numbers of receptors related to phagocytosis, and have limited antigen presentation capacity, making them relatively ineffective in activating T cells (Collin & Bigley, 2018). Immature DCs migrate to peripheral lymphoid organs (e.g., lymph nodes) after antigen uptake and stimulation by inflammatory factors. During this migration process, dendritic cells mature, resulting in a phenotype in which they display high quantities of major histocompatibility complex (MHC) and costimulatory molecules and begin to secrete inflammatory cytokines including interleukin 6. One of the most important characteristics of mature dendritic cells is that they upregulated C-C chemokine receptor type 7 expression, which is involved in lymph node homing and crucial for T cell activation (Anguille et al., 2015). In the lymph nodes, a peptide-MHC complex is presented to naive T cells. The CD3 complex initiates the transduction of antigen recognition signals into T cells. During the T cell activation process, cytokines, as well as proliferation and differentiation, influence T cell memory and cytotoxicity. Cytotoxic T cells leave the lymphoid organs after activation and migrate to the site of action where they exert their killer function (Tai et al., 2018). The production of cytokines including IL-15, IL-12 and IL-18, and the interaction of NK cell-expressed CX3CR1 with DC-expressed CX3CL1 has recently been discovered to enhance NK cell proliferation, activation, and cytotoxicity (Thomas & Yang, 2016).

The use of dendritic cells for vaccination involves two principal steps: preparation of DCs and pulsing of the antigens into DCs.

Preparation

The mature DCs only compromise ~1% of the peripheral blood mononuclear cell population. DC expansion is required to obtain the number of cells required for antigen loading and administration back to the patient. DC cells can be produced by transdifferentiation, differentiation, or indirect dedifferentiation followed by redifferentiation from CD14+ monocytes and CD34+ precursor cells or various cell types (Unal et al., 2016; Plantinga et al., 2019; Rosa et al., 2020).

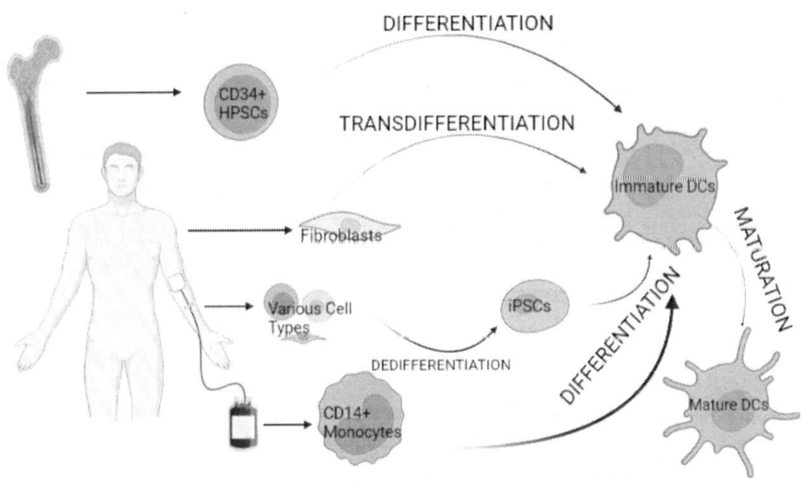

Figure 3. Schema of DCs generation from various source (*BioRender*, n.d.).

Pulsing the Antigens into DCs

Boczkowski et al. pioneered the idea of pulsing DCs with mRNAs expressing cancer antigens in the late 1990s (Boczkowski et al., 1996). In their study, the DCs received the mRNA by micropinocytosis. However, mRNA triggers the pattern recognition receptor pathway, causing rapid restriction of mRNA ingestion by DCs (Diebold et al., 2004; Diken et al., 2011; Kranz et al., 2016). Also, the efficiency of mRNA delivery by endosomal delivery was very low. Therefore, only a small fraction of mRNAs reached the cytosol and translated into proteins (Boczkowski et al., 1996). Considering those challenges of endosome mediated transfer of mRNA, the pulse has started to be done widely by electroporation. The advantage is that mRNA was only needed to gain access to the cytosol, not the nucleus. Therefore, a weak electrical pulse is adequate to prevent cell damage (Van Nuffel et al., 2010; Gerer et al., 2017). By electroporation, the activation of the demonstrated pattern recognition receptor pathway and the consequent destruction of foreign mRNA in endosomal delivery are surpassed (Figure 4). In addition, sonoporation, inducing mRNA impulsion by ultrasound, and nanofection, a delivery method that combines nanomaterial and mRNA, are other options (McCullough et al., 2014; Harizaj et al., 2021).

Dendritic cell vaccination is emerging, especially in cancer treatment. In clinical trials, they have already proven to be safe in terms of both short and long-term side effects. Even though many clinical trials are continuing, data show that 781 patients with cancer and HIV have been successfully treated using DCs loaded with mRNA (Dörrie et al., 2020).

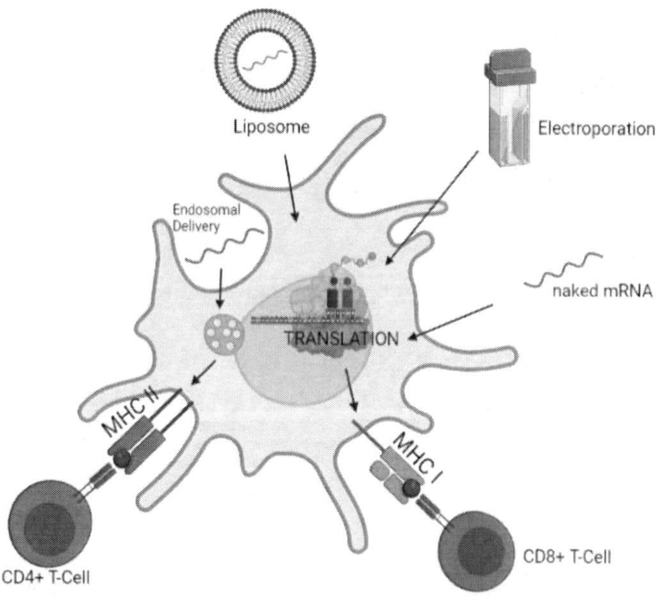

Figure 4. Pulsed dendritic cell vaccination (*BioRender*, n.d.).

Peptide Based Vectors

Peptides are a type of vaccination strategy that can also act as a carrier molecule. Peptides must be cationic for carrier purposes so that amino acids with positively charged amino groups (such as lysine and arginine) can facilitate electrostatic interactions between the peptide and the nucleic acid, resulting in the formation of a complex (Grau et al., 2018). Encapsulation efficiency depends on the ratio of the positively charged amino group (of the peptide) ratio to the negatively charged phosphate groups (on the mRNA) (Udhayakumar et al., 2017). It was recently shown that boosting positively charged amino groups by tenfold in comparison to phosphate groups increased electrostatic repulsion, zeta potential, and allowed for smaller particle size (Udhayakumar et al., 2017).

Anionic peptides are utilized as well. However, they cannot form complexes with mRNA as a result of their negative charges; rather, they conjugated with a positively charged polymer, which functions as a scaffold for RNA encapsulation. This conjugation provides both efficiency (as high as lipofectamine 2000 based transfections) and low cytotoxicity (Lou et al., 2019).

Protamine is a cationic peptide that is tested primarily for mRNA delivery and is the only peptide that is being evaluated in clinical trials of mRNA vaccines (Zeng et al., n.d.). Protamine improves the stability of mRNA not only by providing resistance to RNases but also by protecting it from damage caused by storage conditions. (Hoerr et al., 2000; Stitz et al., 2017). Protamine-mRNA complex exerts an adjuvant activity due to triggering the immunogenic reaction through activation of TLR7 (Scheel et al., 2005; Fotin-Mleczek et al., 2011). Clinical studies, on the other hand, revealed a favorable safety profile, however immunological responses were limited considering the translation of mRNA remains insufficient (Scheel et al., 2004, 2005; Fotin-Mleczek et al., 2011; Kallen et al., 2013). The use of protamine needs to be further evaluated, and optimizations are required to increase the efficiency of the immunological response.

Cell-penetrating peptides (CPPs) are 4- to 40-amino-acid peptides that have been designed to deliver membrane-impermeable medications, proteins, nucleic acids and peptides to cells and tissues (Yokoo et al., 2021). Phagocytosis and clathrin-dependent endocytosis, followed by endosomal escape, are thought to be the intracellular uptake mechanisms (Coolen et al., 2019). CPPs may provide enhanced uptake efficiency, targeted direction to DCs, and prolonged protein expression by stabilizing mRNA (Yokoo et al., 2021). A study using CPP that derived from EBV ZEBRA protein is conjugated with OVA derived peptide containing a CD8 specific OVA epitope. The conjugation is administered to mice at very low doses and an OVA-specific CD8 T-cell response is observed. However, when the OVA peptide was injected solely, the immune response was not significant (Derouazi et al., 2015). The lack of cell or tissue selectivity is the fundamental disadvantage of CPP-based technology. As a result, systemic injection of CPP causes integration in a variety of cell types (epithelial cells, fibroblasts, and leukocytes) in numerous organs (Grau et al., 2018). The design of a CPP composition that specifically targets immune cells is promising and needs to be investigated promptly.

Polymer Based Vectors

Polymeric materials for the delivery of mRNA therapeutics are an effective alternative. The polymer-based vector is particularly beneficial for extrahepatic delivery applications. Delivery efficiency, loading capacity, and lower immunogenicity could be achieved by changing the physiochemical characteristics. The conformational structure or the bonding properties may regulate immunological stimuli. Adjusting the physiochemical characteristics may enhance transfection efficiency and biocompatibility enabling a specialized and programmed delivery (Ulkoski et al., 2019). Common characteristics of polymers include cationic charge, amphicity, and fusogenicity. The most common polymers that are used include polyethyleneimine (PEI), poly(acrylates), polyesters, poly (β-amino esters), poly (amido amine)s, and poly(aspartamides).

PEI contains a vast amount of amine groups within its structure whether it is in linear or branched structure. The interaction between PEI-mRNA complex and the extracellular matrix is enhanced when the amine from PEI/phosphate (from mRNA) ratio is larger than 10. Therefore, the mRNA administration into the cell is improved (Boussif et al., 1995; Godbey et al., 1999). The amine groups are separated by small alkyl fragments, preventing charge repulsion. Buffering mechanisms and acidity strength (pKa value) are important determinants of PEI protonation and aggregation state. Thus, adjusting its binding capacity to mRNA and its stability within solution (Demeneix & Behr, 2005; Curtis et al., 2016). *In vivo* cytotoxicity is a limiting factor for the use of PEI in clinical applications. The high cationic density improves mRNA binding, but it also induces intra- and extracellular proteins to bind once supplied to the patient, resulting in cytotoxicity or other side effects. This drawback could be avoided by making changes in its chemistry such as lowering the cationic charge density or using a PEI derivative, which has a lower molecular weight. Even though these changes result in reduced cytotoxicity, they also limit transfection efficiency. The promising strategy to compensate for the drawbacks of PEI is to use hybrid systems. Hybrid systems can be designed by combining PEI with lipid materials. Hybrid designs not only improve the physicochemical properties of PEI, but also increase its biocompatibility, biodegradability, and transfection efficiency (Godbey et al., 1999; Boeckle et al., 2004; Lv et al., 2006; Zhong et al., 2013).

Polyacrylates require side chain modifications to interact with mRNA due to the lack of electrostatic interactions. The transfection efficiency and cargo release are further improved by combining polyacrylates with endosomolytic and lipophilic modules. Modifications to the polymer backbone could also increase its stability.

Polyesters can be hydrolyzed under physiological conditions and the by-products can be eliminated through renal filtration. This biodegradable property of polyesters exerts a better safety profile, eliminating the possibility of polymer or residual by-product accumulation within tissues. The biodegradable nature of polyesters enables multiple dose administration without any concern of toxicity and adverse effects. Therefore, investigations using polyesters are warranted and hold promise (Vert et al., 1992; Yan et al., 2016, 2017).

Polymers can also be designed as smart carriers. These smart carriers could sense changes in environmental conditions such as pH changes and enzymatic activations (Ulkoski et al., 2019). Stimuli-responsive polymer-based design was widely discussed by Ulkoski et al. previously.

Lipid Based Vectors

Lipid or lipid-like compounds are widely used as non-viral gene delivery systems. Lipids can form liposomal structures and lipid nanoparticles (LNPs) when combined with nucleic acids, and both have been demonstrated to be an efficient delivery method for mRNA vaccines as well (Wadhwa et al., 2020). An aqueous pocket is surrounded by lipid bilayer rings in liposomes, but it is not a necessary surrounding for LNPs. They could encapsulate the mRNA in a nonaqueous core (Tenchov et al., 2021).

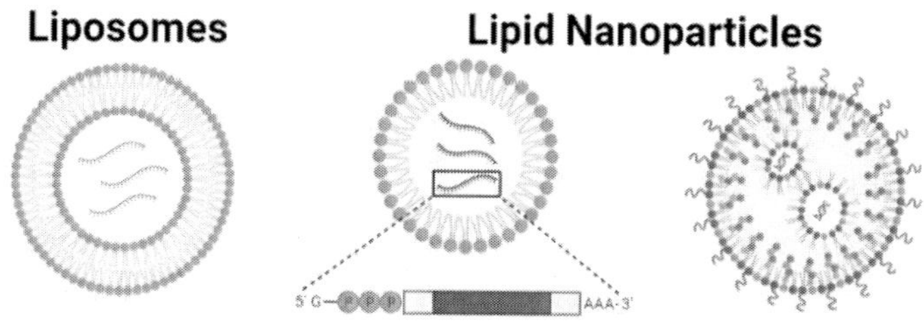

Figure 5. Schema of mRNA loaded liposomes and LNPs (*BioRender*, n.d.).

The encapsulation strategy of cationic lipids is like peptide and polymer-based vectors being facilitated by electrostatic and hydrophobic interactions. Cationic lipids that include tertiary or quaternary amine groups are used for the formulation of LNPs. The major drawback of cationic lipids is that they exert inflammatory responses and adverse effects. Combining with neutral lipids reduces *in vivo* toxicity while maintaining transfection efficiency (Granot & Peer, 2017). The same obstacle is valid for both LNPs and liposomes. It was demonstrated that intravenous injection induces hepatotoxicity and inflammation by triggering IFN-γ response (Ma et al., 2005; Platanias, 2005; Lv et al., 2006). The first formulated LNP for mRNA delivery consists of ionizable cationic lipid/phosphatidylcholine/cholesterol/PEG-lipid (Pardi et al., 2015). The exact mechanism of LNP-mediated delivery is not yet known, but it has been proposed to be via endocytosis. LNPs are suggested to be attached to cell membrane by electrostatic interactions and fused via inverted non-bilayer lipid phases (Yanez Arteta et al., 2018). Liposomes could also be conjugated with neutralizing proteins, causing a reduction in both toxicity and efficiency. Although toxicity is reduced by neutralization, several other challenges are introduced, such as colloidal instability and leakage from liposomes (Hecker, 2016).

Targeted Delivery

In the clinical aspect, regarding the cytotoxicity of repeated administration of mRNA vaccines, a reduction of the required dose is necessary. This might be accomplished by tailored delivery, which would also improve the immune response. Encapsulation techniques might be fine-tuned for site-specific delivery. Mannose-containing nanoparticles, for example, might aid endocytosis because the antigen-presenting cells, DCs and macrophages, produce antigen-presenting receptors that identify sugar groups, such as fucose-terminated glycans and mannose (Midoux & Pichon, 2015; Kranz et al., 2016; Hossain & Wall, 2019).

The route of administration of mRNA vaccines is just as crucial as the delivery mechanisms in terms of vaccination effectiveness (Eggert et al., 1999). The primary targets of mRNA vaccines are antigen-presenting immune cells and lymphoid organs. The safety and efficacy of the vaccine can be affected depending on whether it is injected directly into the skin, muscle, or lymphoid organ, or whether it is administered through the systemic circulation (Johansen & Kündig, 2015). The efficiency of the mRNA vaccine may vary depending on the route of injection. The efficiency of the administration route itself may differ depending on the type of mRNA and the delivery method (Zeng et al., n.d.).

A single optimized and valid delivery method is not rational when delivering mRNA. Carriers need to be tailored to individual target mRNA.

Immunological Activity of mRNA Vaccines

The main goal of any vaccine is to induce a long-lasting protective immune response over an antigen. This is accomplished with mRNA vaccines by transferring the antigenic sequence into vaccine cells, allowing them to express and present the encoded protein to the immune system. mRNA vaccination stimulates adaptive immunity via a few pathways, one of which is transfection of somatic cells like muscle and epidermal cells. The second way is transfection from the injection sites of tissue- resident immune cells, and thirdly, immune cells transfection from the secondary lymphoid tissues such as the spleen and lymph nodes (LNs). Nonimmune cells adjacent injection sites can be transfected by mRNA vaccines via main routes such as subcutaneous, intramuscular, and intradermal injections as mentioned above (Pardi et al., 2015).

mRNA vaccines are embodied by nonimmune cells typically at the injection site. After injection, muscle cells, fibroblasts, and keratinocytes were shown to internalize and express the protein (Probst et al., 2007). The cell type determines the expression and cellular location of PRRs that detect internalized RNA. Through cross-presentation, the expression of antigens in these unimmunized cells can lead to the activation of CD8+ T cell responses and the priming of antigen-specific antibodies. mRNA induces innate immunogenicity, and activates a range of different of cellular pathways, such as Toll-Like Receptors, functioning in the innate immune system, mainly TLR3, TLR7, and TLR8, as well as via various cytoplasmic proteins, most particularly MDA5 (Melanoma Differentiation-Associated protein 5), PKR (Protein Kinase R), OAS (20-50-Oligoadenylate synthetases), RIGI (Retinoic Acid-Inducible Gene I) (Chen et al., 2017). Furthermore, MHC class II pathway can help APCs receive antigen, mRNA transfection of APCs can result in the activation of CD4+ T-helper cells. Or else, the lymphatic system empties the mRNA vaccine and transfers it to the surrounding lymph nodes (Lindsay et al., 2019). LNs are secondary lymphoid organs that house a variety of immune cells, including naive T and B cells and monocytes, and the antigens found there trigger adaptive immune responses. There, LN-resident cells, like APCs and endothelial cells, are transfected by mRNA vaccines. Transfection of these cells can help to prepare T and B cells (Kim et al., 2021).

Endogenic translation is a crucial machinery for mRNA vaccines to be converted into antigens that activate adaptive immunity. Since the translated antigen originates in the cytoplasm, cells preferentially regard it as an endogenous antigen. It suggests that endogenous antigens from mRNA vaccines are displayed promptly in MHC class I molecules, stimulating CD8+ T lymphocytes. On the other hand, the priming of CD4 + T cells is required for the development of powerful and robust cellular immunity. Moreover, because T helper cells play a significant role in B cell priming, the capacity of mRNA vaccines to stimulate CD4+ T cells is particularly desirable for developing humoral immunity. As previously indicated, mRNA vaccination activates both CD8+ and CD4+ T lymphocytes, implying that transfected APCs have alternate routes for processing endogenous antigens prior to MHC class II presentation (Van Nuffel et al., 2012). Autophagy is one method of displaying endogenous antigens in class II MHC, which is related to the lysosomal breakdown of cytosolic antigens (Munz, 2012). Heat shock protein 90 and the transporter associated with the antigen processing (TAP) complex are also known to be non-autophagic routes to present endogenous antigen in MHC class II (Leung, 2015).

Endogenous antigen presentation on MHC class II can be enhanced further by modifying the mRNA sequence and also can be improved by encoding signal peptides that translocate proteins to specific intracellular compartments. Other signal peptides can be inserted into the mRNA coding area to prime antigen-specific CD4+ and CD8+ T lymphocytes, such as MHC class I and II and lysosome-associated membrane protein-1 (CD107a) (Su et al., 2005; Van Nuffel et al., 2012). Instead, an mRNA sequence can be engineered to express antigens outside of the cell, both in secreted and transmembrane forms (Corbett et al., 2020; Walsh et al., 2020). To enhance the safety and efficiency of vaccinations, mRNA sequences for antigen expression - secreted or membrane-anchored - can be customized for different virus strains. APCs can identify extracellularly produced antigens and use MHC class II presentation and cross-presenting to successfully elicit CD4+ and CD8+ T cell responses. Extracellular antigens produced from mRNA, in particular, aid in the development of antigen-specific humoral responses (Pardi et al., 2018).

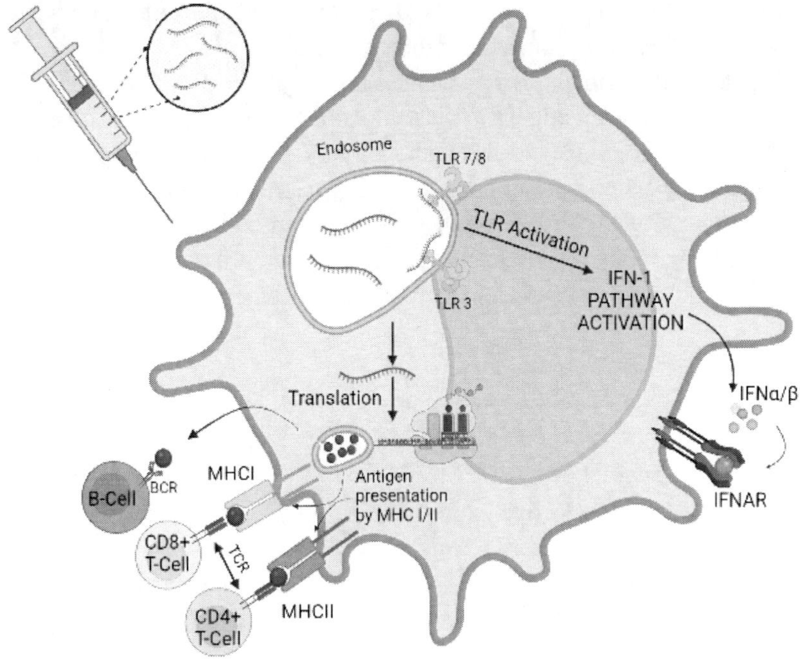

Figure 6. Immune activity of mRNA vaccines (*BioRender*, n.d.).

Antibodyant responses are an important mechanism of vaccination to neutralize foreign antigens. B cell activation through the mRNA vaccine is essential for antibody production to begin and continue. Once the B cell receptor encounters intact antigens in the extracellular space, the B cell is activated (BCR). B cell activation needs the transfer of antigens to LNs for an interaction since naive B cells dwell in LNs. Because blood flow rates are 100-500 times higher than lymph flow rates, soluble antigens reach drained LNs from the periphery; however, tiny proteins (less than 10 nm in size) prefer to penetrate the blood capillaries, restricting antigen availability in the LNs (Trevaskis et al., 2015). Antigens are carried to LNs by APCs such as monocytes and migrating DCs, which then deliver them to naive B cells; however, this method is inefficient compared to sending antigens directly to LNs (Irvine et al., 2020). Thus, mRNA vaccines that target cells within LNs could boost antibody responses by raising antigen concentrations in the LNs at a local level. While soluble antigens in LNs can be immediately identified by B cells, they can also be collected by other cells and used to activate B cells, resulting in more efficient antigen recognition by B cells (Carrasco & Batista, 2006). Subcapsular sinus macrophages or DCs can collect antigens and display them on their layers for B cell enactment depending on whether or not the antigen is opsonized (Gordon et al., 2014).

As a result, optimal mRNA vaccines not only activate CD4+ and CD8+ T cells, but also deliver antigens to LNs, allowing B cells to activate and produce antibody responses against the pathogen. By encoding signal peptides or extracellular versions of antigens, mRNA constructions can be designed to induce more powerful T cell priming. Additionally, given the role of the GC reaction in antibody responses, targeting LNs with effective delivery vectors could be one strategy to create potent mRNA vaccines (Schudel et al., 2019).

Cancer mRNA Vaccine

One of the potential treatments for the cancer patient is cancer vaccines. Antigens that have selective expression in cancer cells, such as antigens or growth factors that are specific to malignant cells due to somatic mutation, can be targeted by cancer vaccines (Vigneron, 2015). These neoantigens and neoepitopes within the mRNA vaccine have been used as targets for the cancer vaccine in humans (Tureci et al., 2016). Most cancer vaccines are not preventative, therapeutic instead, and aim to activate cell-mediated responses, including such Cytotoxic T Lymphocyte (CTL) responses, that can remove or reduce tumor burden. mRNA vaccines, which are administered intratumorally or intranodally to change the suppressive tumor microenvironment, have been shown to be effective in a number of preclinical and clinical studies to treat cancer. In addition, in certain preclinical investigations, combining mRNA vaccination with adjuvant treatments such standard chemotherapy, radiation, and immune checkpoint inhibitors improved the vaccines' favorable outcome (Miao et al., 2021). A number of immune regulatory proteins have been found that can improve the effectiveness of DC cancer vaccines. Several studies have shown that electroporating DCs with mRNAs encoding co-stimulatory molecules such as tumor necrosis factor receptor superfamily member 4 (TNFRSF4), CD83, and the 4-1BB ligand (4-1BBL) significantly increased DC immune stimulating activity in addition to the use of pro-inflammatory cytokines encoded with mRNA, such as trafficking-associated molecules, IL-12 (Bontkes et al., 2007). Numerous clinical studies have been conducted that employ DC vaccines to treat several types of cancer, including metastatic lung cancer, melanoma, and pancreatic cancer. metastatic prostate cancer, brain malignancies, acute myeloid leukemia, and renal cell carcinoma. Although DC-based mRNA vaccine continues to cover a broad range of mRNA cancer vaccines in clinical trials, CureVac, BioNTech, and Moderna are leading the charge in developing IVT mRNA-based immunotherapies administered by nonviral vectors, which have shown encouraging anticancer outcomes in preclinical investigations. mRNAs expressing immunostimulants (e.g., OX40L, IL-12, CD40L, IL32, CD70, etc.) that are administered intranodal or intratumoral routes to change the suppressive tumor microenvironment are one class of IVT mRNA-based immunotherapies that are being studied in clinical studies. These immunostimulants are not regarded as cancer vaccines, but are commonly used as adjuvants with cancer vaccines or immunotherapeutic treatments (e.g., checkpoint blockade regulators) to enhance the humoral and cellular response. Most current trials coupled mRNA cancer vaccines with checkpoint modulators or cytokine mixtures to boost antitumor effectiveness (Miao et al., 2021).

COVID-19 mRNA Vaccine

COVID-19 began to spread at the end of 2019 as a result of the Severe Acute Respiratory Syndrome Coronavirus 2 (SARS-CoV-2) virus. More than 100 million individuals have been infected and over 2 million people have died as a result of the COVID-19 epidemic. Several vaccine development studies have been achieved since then.

Pathophysiology of COVID-19

SARS-CoV-2, an enclosed virus with a positive strand and a single-stranded RNA genome that corresponds to the coronavirus subfamily, causes COVID-19. SARS-CoV-2 has a 30 kb RNA genome that encodes 14 open reading frames (Hu et al., 2021). A controlled -1 ribosomal frameshift at the 5'-proximal end of the genome generates two polypeptides, called pp1a and pp1b. Two polypeptides are divided into 16 nonstructural proteins (nsp1-16), which facilitate viral replication, transcription, and posttranscriptional activities by delivering viral replication units to subcellular domains (Bhatt et al., 2021). Spike (S) protein is a surface envelope glycoprotein that intermediates viral entry into the host and binds directly to angiotensin-converting enzyme 2 (ACE2) which is its functional receptor, abundantly expressed in epithelial cells of many other organs such as the heart, kidney, bladder, ileum, and also alveolar epithelial cells of the lung (Kim et al., 2020).

The most common symptoms of COVID-19 are shortness of breath, headache, fever, dry cough, nausea, muscular ache, dizziness, sore throat, rhinorrhea, chest pain, diarrhea, and vomiting. Infected people often develop acute respiratory syndrome and sepsis in a short period of time when the viral amount is significant or when the infection occurs in patients with underlying serious conditions (Yi et al., 2020).

Design of Target Immunogens for the SARSCoV2 mRNA Vaccine

All of the mRNA candidate vaccines were made in vitro from a DNA template encoding the full-length RBD (Receptor-Binding Domain) or S protein of SARS-CoV-2 by bacteriophage T7 RNA polymerase. The mRNA-1273, LNP-nCoVsaRNA, LUNAR-CoV19 and CVnCoV mRNA vaccines used a sequence expressing the full sequence S protein with 2P alterations at K986 and V987 locations to create the stable prefusion form of the S protein (Hsieh et al., 2020). Pfizer/BioNTech has created the RBD (BNT162b1) and the full-length S protein (BNT162b2). In a preliminary clinical experiment, BNT162b2 was demonstrated to be safer than BNT162b1, particularly in elderly persons, and was therefore selected for a phase 3 clinical trial (Walsh, et al., 2020). The RBD of SARS-CoV-2 is used in ARCoV vaccines. The 3'-UTR of the BNT162b mRNA vaccine was produced experimentally by screening naturally existing 3'-UTRs for maximum RNA stability, although the lengths of the 5' and 3'-UTR of the mRNA designs were not reported in the literature (Orlandini von Niessen et al., 2019). On the other hand, CVnCoV and LNP-nCoVsaRNA were created using the self-replicating vaccine derived from the Trinidad donkey Venezuelan equine encephalitis virus (VEEV). The replicon's viral protein-encoding gene is substituted with an altered SARS-CoV-2 S protein-encoding gene containing two proline mutations in the S2 subunit, K986P and V987P. A single dose of the SARS-CoV-2 vaccine engineered on self-transcribing and replicating RNA generates protective adaptive immunity in mice (McKay et al., 2020). The dose utilized for immunization was one to two orders of magnitude lower than standard mRNA vaccines, indicating that saRNA vaccines can self-amplify soon after transport to host cells (Park et al., 2021).

The Effectiveness of SARS-CoV-2 mRNA Vaccinations

The antigen-encoding mRNA vaccine was found to be effective and substantial after a successful preclinical and clinical examination. The delivery of mRNA expressing SARS-CoV-2 virus-like particles to mice elicited a significant antiviral-like immune response in the preclinical investigation (Laczko et al., 2020; Zhang et al., 2020). Zhang et al. effectively enclosed mRNA encoding the SARS-CoV-2 receptor binding domain (RBD) with a lipid nanoparticle. They used an intramuscular injection of such a vaccine to induce specific neutralizing antibodies and a Th1-biased cellular response in mice and nonhuman primates (Zhang et al., 2020). As a result, a vaccine for clinical testing was quickly created. BNT162b1, a lipid nanoparticle-formulated mRNA vaccine that expresses the SARS-CoV-2 spike glycoprotein RBD, is one of the most well-known vaccines. Targeted delivery of BNT162b1 is dose dependent. After a second injection, the RBD-specific IgG and SARS-CoV-2 neutralizing titers were enhanced (Mulligan et al., 2020). The phage I/II/III clinical trial enrolled a total of 29,481 patients based on curative benefits (NCT04368728).

The Benefits of mRNA Vaccines over Other Types of Vaccination against SARS-CoV-2

Compared to other types of vaccines such as synthetic peptide vaccines, inactivated vaccines, passive immunization-related vaccines, attenuated live vaccines, subunit vaccines, recombinant antigen vaccines, DNA vaccines, etc., mRNA vaccines are promising options against SARS-CoV-2. mRNA vaccines, unlike DNA vaccines, do not enter the nucleus and assist in DNA structural alteration. As a result, the process for expressing antigen is simpler and safer. Unlike standard immunizations, mRNA vaccines require virus gene sequences rather than virus strains. Since mRNA vaccines do not require cell culture or animal matrix, the manufacturing method is simpler and less expensive than protein vaccines. On the other hand, mRNAs are found in human sapiens cells. They can be spontaneously degraded without causing metabolic harm. Once SARS-CoV-2 mutates, changing the mRNA sequence is significantly easier than changing the protein structure. More critically, the outbreak pandemic necessitates a reduction in vaccine research timeframes. Inactivated vaccines, attenuated live vaccines, and subunit vaccines take longer to create than mRNA vaccines (Abbasi, 2020).

Current Challenges and Future Perspectives

mRNA vaccines have been shown to be an effective platform against cancer and viral diseases thanks to a growing body of preclinical and clinical research. Due to the lack of cell and animal components in the mRNA generation process, mRNA production carries significantly fewer dangers than recombinant protein manufacturing. All challenges that must be overcome for optimum treatment are purification, scale-up, and source, as well as processing of the reagents used for in vitro transcription. When mRNA is employed to deliver patient-specific neoantigens in the context of customized immunization, process automation may be required. The time it takes to make mRNA would be reduced if the synthetic genes needed for the DNA template could be assembled quickly. In terms of stability, the use of specific buffers in an alkaline environment can improve mRNA stability. Furthermore, the impact of mRNA sequence length and coding and regulatory region sequence on mRNA production and stability must be thoroughly investigated (Diken et al., 2017).

As COVID-19 mRNA vaccines are on the market, mRNA technology platforms hit a record high in 2020. After this breakout of mRNA technologies, market competition gathers speed. Trends include prophylactic and therapeutic vaccines, as well as therapeutics. Prophylactic vaccines are estimated to dominate the field within the next 15 years due to the higher probability of success, accessibility, and availability of many pipeline assets and the advantages of mRNA over other vaccine modalities. Currently, at least one prophylactic vaccine is in manufacturing by 77% of mRNA companies. Estimates predict that Covid-19 vaccines will be the source of revenues in the short term, but other diseases such as influenza are expected to contribute to income by 2028. A decline in revenue is expected due to a decrease in demand for COVID-19 vaccines by 2025. Though, booster shots and wider global vaccination are still predicted to occupy approximately $20 billion. By the introduction of other prophylactic and therapeutic vaccines, the market is expected to grow from 2028 to 2035, reaching a revenue of $23 billion. The share between trends in mRNA technology is expected to be more than 50% for prophylactic vaccines, ~30% for cancer mRNA vaccines, and less than 20% for therapeutics. The growing market size is inevitable for mRNA technologies, and it is an open field to become more competitive as the scope of applications expands while the mRNA delivery and stability improves (Xie et al., 2021).

Conclusion

Recent breakthroughs in understanding the impact of untranslated mRNA sequences, design and formulations, and injectable methods predict that mRNA vaccines will offer new and interesting developments in the coming years. Current technologies, like as machine learning and artificial intelligence, will bring new insights into the design of mRNA vaccines, resulting in better therapeutic compounds. COVID-19 is a major scientific, clinical, and social issue, and new vaccine formulations are crucial to achieve. In the next future, regulatory licensing of mRNA-based cancer vaccines will be facilitated by a better understanding of the complicated mRNA pharmacology paired with carefully conducted clinical investigations employing customized mRNA molecules.

References

Abbasi, J. (2020, Sep 22). COVID-19 and mRNA vaccines-first large test for a new approach. *JAMA, 324*(12), 1125-1127. https://doi.org/10.1001/jama.2020.16866.

Anguille, S., Smits, E. L., Bryant, C., Van Acker, H. H., Goossens, H., Lion, E., Fromm, P. D., Hart, D. N., Van Tendeloo, V. F., & Berneman, Z. N. (2015). Dendritic cells as pharmacological tools for cancer immunotherapy. *Pharmacological Reviews, 67*(4), 731–753. https://doi.org/10.1124/pr.114.009456.

Baiersdorfer, M., Boros, G., Muramatsu, H., Mahiny, A., Vlatkovic, I., Sahin, U., & Kariko, K. (2019, Apr 15). A facile method for the removal of dsRNA contaminant from in vitro-transcribed mRNA. *Mol Ther Nucleic Acids, 15*, 26-35. https://doi.org/10.1016/j.omtn.2019.02.018.

Bhatt, P. R., Scaiola, A., Loughran, G., Leibundgut, M., Kratzel, A., Meurs, R., Dreos, R., O'Connor, K. M., McMillan, A., Bode, J. W., Thiel, V., Gatfield, D., Atkins, J. F., & Ban, N. (2021, Jun 18). Structural basis of ribosomal frameshifting during translation of the SARS-CoV-2 RNA genome. *Science, 372*(6548), 1306-1313. https://doi.org/10.1126/science.abf3546.

BioRender. (n.d.). *BioRender*. Retrieved 14 February 2022, from https://biorender.com/.

Bloom, K., van den Berg, F., & Arbuthnot, P. (2021, Apr). Self-amplifying RNA vaccines for infectious diseases. *Gene Ther, 28*(3-4), 117-129. https://doi.org/10.1038/s41434-020-00204-y.

Boczkowski, D., Nair, S. K., Snyder, D., & Gilboa, E. (1996). Dendritic cells pulsed with RNA are potent antigen-presenting cells in vitro and in vivo. *The Journal of Experimental Medicine, 184*(2), 465–472. https://doi.org/10.1084/jem.184.2.465.

Boeckle, S., von Gersdorff, K., van der Piepen, S., Culmsee, C., Wagner, E., & Ogris, M. (2004). Purification of polyethylenimine polyplexes highlights the role of free polycations in gene transfer. *The Journal of Gene Medicine*, *6*(10), 1102–1111. https://doi.org/10.1002/jgm.598.

Bontkes, H. J., Kramer, D., Ruizendaal, J. J., Kueter, E. W., van Tendeloo, V. F., Meijer, C. J., & Hooijberg, E. (2007, Feb). Dendritic cells transfected with interleukin-12 and tumor-associated antigen messenger RNA induce high avidity cytotoxic T cells. *Gene Ther, 14*(4), 366-375. https://doi.org/10.1038/sj.gt.3302874.

Boussif, O., Lezoualc'h, F., Zanta, M. A., Mergny, M. D., Scherman, D., Demeneix, B., & Behr, J. P. (1995). A versatile vector for gene and oligonucleotide transfer into cells in culture and in vivo: Polyethylenimine. *Proceedings of the National Academy of Sciences of the United States of America*, *92*(16), 7297–7301.

Brito, L. A., Chan, M., Shaw, C. A., Hekele, A., Carsillo, T., Schaefer, M., Archer, J., Seubert, A., Otten, G. R., Beard, C. W., Dey, A. K., Lilja, A., Valiante, N. M., Mason, P. W., Mandl, C. W., Barnett, S. W., Dormitzer, P. R., Ulmer, J. B., Singh, M., O'Hagan, D. T., & Geall, A. J. (2014, Dec). A cationic nanoemulsion for the delivery of next-generation RNA vaccines. *Mol Ther, 22*(12), 2118-2129. https://doi.org/10.1038/mt.2014.133.

Cao, Y., & Gao, G. F. (2021). mRNA vaccines: A matter of delivery. *EClinicalMedicine*, *32*. https://doi.org/10.1016/j.eclinm.2021.100746.

Carrasco, Y. R., & Batista, F. D. (2006, Jun). B cell recognition of membrane-bound antigen: an exquisite way of sensing ligands. *Curr Opin Immunol, 18*(3), 286-291. https://doi.org/10.1016/j.coi.2006.03.013.

Chaudhary, N., Weissman, D., & Whitehead, K. A. (2021, Nov). mRNA vaccines for infectious diseases: principles, delivery and clinical translation. *Nat Rev Drug Discov, 20*(11), 817-838. https://doi.org/10.1038/s41573-021-00283-5.

Chen, N., Xia, P., Li, S., Zhang, T., Wang, T. T., & Zhu, J. (2017, May). RNA sensors of the innate immune system and their detection of pathogens. *IUBMB Life, 69*(5), 297-304. https://doi.org/10.1002/iub.1625.

Cheng, W. F., Hung, C. H., Chai, C. Y., Hsu, K. F., He, L., Ling, M., & Wu, T. C. (2001, Mar). Enhancement of sindbis virus self-replicating RNA vaccine potency by linkage of herpes simplex virus type 1 VP22 protein to antigen. *J Virol, 75*(5), 2368-2376. https://doi.org/10.1128/JVI.75.5.2368-2376.2001.

Class, I., & USPC, A. K. (2016). *Patent Application Title: Application oF mRNA for use as a therapeutic against tumour diseases inventors*: Ingmar Hoerr (Tubingen, DE) Florian Von Der MÜlbe (Stuttgart, DE) Florian Von Der MÜlbe (Stuttgart, DE) Steve Pascolo (Tubingen, DE) Steve Pascolo (Tubingen, DE) Assignees: CureVac AG.

Collin, M., & Bigley, V. (2018). Human dendritic cell subsets: An update. *Immunology*, *154*(1), 3–20. https://doi.org/10.1111/imm.12888.

Coolen, A.-L., Lacroix, C., Mercier-Gouy, P., Delaune, E., Monge, C., Exposito, J.-Y., & Verrier, B. (2019). Poly(lactic acid) nanoparticles and cell-penetrating peptide potentiate mRNA-based vaccine expression in dendritic cells triggering their activation. *Biomaterials*, *195*, 23–37. https://doi.org/10.1016/j.biomaterials.2018.12.019.

Corbett, K. S., Edwards, D. K., Leist, S. R., Abiona, O. M., Boyoglu-Barnum, S., Gillespie, R. A., Himansu, S., Schafer, A., Ziwawo, C. T., DiPiazza, A. T., Dinnon, K. H., Elbashir, S. M., Shaw, C. A., Woods, A., Fritch, E. J., Martinez, D. R., Bock, K. W.,

Minai, M., Nagata, B. M., Hutchinson, G. B., Wu, K., Henry, C., Bahl, K., Garcia-Dominguez, D., Ma, L., Renzi, I., Kong, W. P., Schmidt, S. D., Wang, L., Zhang, Y., Phung, E., Chang, L. A., Loomis, R. J., Altaras, N. E., Narayanan, E., Metkar, M., Presnyak, V., Liu, C., Louder, M. K., Shi, W., Leung, K., Yang, E. S., West, A., Gully, K. L., Stevens, L. J., Wang, N., Wrapp, D., Doria-Rose, N. A., Stewart-Jones, G., Bennett, H., Alvarado, G. S., Nason, M. C., Ruckwardt, T. J., McLellan, J. S., Denison, M. R., Chappell, J. D., Moore, I. N., Morabito, K. M., Mascola, J. R., Baric, R. S., Carfi, A., & Graham, B. S. (2020, Oct). SARS-CoV-2 mRNA vaccine design enabled by prototype pathogen preparedness. *Nature, 586*(7830), 567-571. https://doi.org/10.1038/s41586-020-2622-0.

Curtis, K. A., Miller, D., Millard, P., Basu, S., Horkay, F., & Chandran, P. L. (2016). Unusual salt and pH induced changes in polyethylenimine solutions. *PLoS ONE, 11*(9), e0158147. https://doi.org/10.1371/journal.pone.0158147.

De Beuckelaer, A., Grooten, J., & De Koker, S. (2017). Type I interferons modulate CD8+ T cell immunity to mRNA vaccines. *Trends in Molecular Medicine*, *23*(3), 216–226. https://doi.org/10.1016/j.molmed.2017.01.006.

Demeneix, B., & Behr, J.-P. (2005). Polyethylenimine (PEI). *Advances in Genetics*, *53PA*, 215–230. https://doi.org/10.1016/S0065-2660(05)53008-6.

Derouazi, M., Di Berardino-Besson, W., Belnoue, E., Hoepner, S., Walther, R., Benkhoucha, M., Teta, P., Dufour, Y., Yacoub Maroun, C., Salazar, A. M., Martinvalet, D., Dietrich, P.-Y., & Walker, P. R. (2015). Novel cell-penetrating peptide-based vaccine induces robust CD4+ and CD8+ T cell mediated antitumor immunity. *Cancer Research*, *75*(15), 3020–3031. https://doi.org/10.1158/0008-5472.CAN-14-3017.

Devarkar, S. C., Wang, C., Miller, M. T., Ramanathan, A., Jiang, F., Khan, A. G., Patel, S. S., & Marcotrigiano, J. (2016, Jan 19). Structural basis for m7G recognition and 2'-O-methyl discrimination in capped RNAs by the innate immune receptor RIG-I. *Proc Natl Acad Sci U S A, 113*(3), 596-601. https://doi.org/10.1073/pnas.15151521 13.

Diebold, S. S., Kaisho, T., Hemmi, H., Akira, S., & Reis e Sousa, C. (2004). Innate antiviral responses by means of TLR7-mediated recognition of single-stranded RNA. *Science (New York, N.Y.)*, *303*(5663), 1529–1531. https://doi.org/10.1126/science.1093616.

Diken, M., Kranz, L. M., Kreiter, S., & Sahin, U. (2017). mRNA: a versatile molecule for cancer vaccines. *Curr Issues Mol Biol, 22*, 113-128. https://doi.org/10.21775/cimb.022.113.

Diken, M., Kreiter, S., Selmi, A., Britten, C. M., Huber, C., Türeci, Ö., & Sahin, U. (2011). Selective uptake of naked vaccine RNA by dendritic cells is driven by macropinocytosis and abrogated upon DC maturation. *Gene Therapy*, *18*(7), 702–708. https://doi.org/10.1038/gt.2011.17.

Dörrie, J., Schaft, N., Schuler, G., & Schuler-Thurner, B. (2020). Therapeutic cancer vaccination with ex vivo RNA-transfected dendritic cells—an update. *Pharmaceutics*, *12*(2), 92. https://doi.org/10.3390/pharmaceutics12020092.

Eggert, A. A., Schreurs, M. W., Boerman, O. C., Oyen, W. J., de Boer, A. J., Punt, C. J., Figdor, C. G., & Adema, G. J. (1999). Biodistribution and vaccine efficiency of murine dendritic cells are dependent on the route of administration. *Cancer Research*, *59*(14), 3340–3345.

Fotin-Mleczek, M., Duchardt, K. M., Lorenz, C., Pfeiffer, R., Ojkic-Zrna, S., Probst, J., & Kallen, K.-J. (2011). Messenger RNA-based vaccines with dual activity induce balanced TLR-7 dependent adaptive immune responses and provide antitumor activity. *Journal of Immunotherapy*, *34*(1), 1–15. https://doi.org/10.1097/CJI.0b013e3181f7dbe8.

Fuchs, A. L., Neu, A., & Sprangers, R. (2016, Sep). A general method for rapid and cost-efficient large-scale production of 5' capped RNA. *RNA, 22*(9), 1454-1466. https://doi.org/10.1261/rna.056614.116.

Gerer, K. F., Hoyer, S., Dörrie, J., & Schaft, N. (2017). Electroporation of mRNA as universal technology platform to transfect a variety of primary cells with antigens and functional proteins. *Methods in Molecular Biology (Clifton, N.J.)*, *1499*, 165–178. https://doi.org/10.1007/978-1-4939-6481-9_10.

Godbey, W. T., Wu, K. K., & Mikos, A. G. (1999). Size matters: Molecular weight affects the efficiency of poly(ethylenimine) as a gene delivery vehicle. *Journal of Biomedical Materials Research*, *45*(3), 268–275. https://doi.org/10.1002/(sici)1097-4636(19990605)45:3<268::aid-jbm15>3.0.co;2-q.

Gordon, S., Pluddemann, A., & Mukhopadhyay, S. (2014, Dec 11). Sinusoidal immunity: macrophages at the lymphohematopoietic interface. *Cold Spring Harb Perspect Biol, 7*(4), a016378. https://doi.org/10.1101/cshperspect.a016378.

Granot, Y., & Peer, D. (2017). Delivering the right message: Challenges and opportunities in lipid nanoparticles-mediated modified mRNA therapeutics-An innate immune system standpoint. *Seminars in Immunology*, *34*, 68–77. https://doi.org/10.1016/j.smim.2017.08.015.

Grau, M., Walker, P. R., & Derouazi, M. (2018). Mechanistic insights into the efficacy of cell penetrating peptide-based cancer vaccines. *Cellular and Molecular Life Sciences*, *75*(16), 2887–2896. https://doi.org/10.1007/s00018-018-2785-0.

Gu, Y., Zhao, X., & Song, X. (2020). Ex vivo pulsed dendritic cell vaccination against cancer. *Acta Pharmacologica Sinica*, *41*(7), 959–969. https://doi.org/10.1038/s41401-020-0415-5.

Harizaj, A., De Smedt, S. C., Lentacker, I., & Braeckmans, K. (2021). Physical transfection technologies for macrophages and dendritic cells in immunotherapy. *Expert Opinion on Drug Delivery*, *18*(2), 229–247. https://doi.org/10.1080/17425247.2021.1828340.

Hecker, J. G. (2016). Non-Viral, Lipid-mediated DNA and mRNA gene therapy of the Central Nervous System (CNS): chemical-based transfection. *Methods in Molecular Biology (Clifton, N.J.)*, *1382*, 307–324. https://doi.org/10.1007/978-1-4939-3271-9_23.

Hoerr, I., Obst, R., Rammensee, H.-G., & Jung, G. (2000). In vivo application of RNA leads to induction of specific cytotoxic T lymphocytes and antibodies. *European Journal of Immunology*, *30*(1), 1–7. https://doi.org/10.1002/1521-4141(200001)30:1<1::AID-IMMU1>3.0.CO;2-#.

Holtkamp, S., Kreiter, S., Selmi, A., Simon, P., Koslowski, M., Huber, C., Tureci, O., & Sahin, U. (2006, Dec 15). Modification of antigen-encoding RNA increases stability, translational efficacy, and T-cell stimulatory capacity of dendritic cells. *Blood, 108*(13), 4009-4017. https://doi.org/10.1182/blood-2006-04-015024.

Hossain, M. K., & Wall, K. A. (2019). Use of dendritic cell receptors as targets for enhancing anti-cancer immune responses. *Cancers, 11*(3), E418. https://doi.org/10.3390/cancers11030418..

Hsieh, C. L., Goldsmith, J. A., Schaub, J. M., DiVenere, A. M., Kuo, H. C., Javanmardi, K., Le, K. C., Wrapp, D., Lee, A. G., Liu, Y., Chou, C. W., Byrne, P. O., Hjorth, C. K., Johnson, N. V., Ludes-Meyers, J., Nguyen, A. W., Park, J., Wang, N., Amengor, D., Lavinder, J. J., Ippolito, G. C., Maynard, J. A., Finkelstein, I. J., & McLellan, J. S. (2020, Sep 18). Structure-based design of prefusion-stabilized SARS-CoV-2 spikes. *Science, 369*(6510), 1501-1505. https://doi.org/10.1126/science.abd0826

Hu, B., Guo, H., Zhou, P., & Shi, Z. L. (2021, Mar). Characteristics of SARS-CoV-2 and COVID-19. *Nat Rev Microbiol, 19*(3), 141-154. https://doi.org/10.1038/s41579-020-00459-7.

Irvine, D. J., Aung, A., & Silva, M. (2020). Controlling timing and location in vaccines. *Adv Drug Deliv Rev, 158*, 91-115. https://doi.org/10.1016/j.addr.2020.06.019.

Johansen, P., & Kündig, T. M. (2015). Parenteral vaccine administration: tried and true. In C. Foged, T. Rades, Y. Perrie, & S. Hook (Eds.), *Subunit Vaccine Delivery* (pp. 261–286). Springer. https://doi.org/10.1007/978-1-4939-1417-3_14.

Jackson, L. A., Roberts, P. C., & Graham, B. S. (2020, Sep 17). A SARS-CoV-2 mRNA vaccine - preliminary report. Reply. *N Engl J Med, 383*(12), 1191-1192. https://doi.org/10.1056/NEJMc2026616.

Jackson, N. A. C., Kester, K. E., Casimiro, D., Gurunathan, S., & DeRosa, F. (2020). The promise of mRNA vaccines: a biotech and industrial perspective. *NPJ Vaccines, 5*, 11. https://doi.org/10.1038/s41541-020-0159-8.

Kallen, K.-J., Heidenreich, R., Schnee, M., Petsch, B., Schlake, T., Thess, A., Baumhof, P., Scheel, B., Koch, S. D., & Fotin-Mleczek, M. (2013). A novel, disruptive vaccination technology. *Human Vaccines & Immunotherapeutics, 9*(10), 2263–2276. https://doi.org/10.4161/hv.25181.

Kariko, K., & Weissman, D. (2007, Sep). Naturally occurring nucleoside modifications suppress the immunostimulatory activity of RNA: implication for therapeutic RNA development. *Curr Opin Drug Discov Devel, 10*(5), 523-532. https://www.ncbi.nlm.nih.gov/pubmed/17786850.

Kariko, K., Buckstein, M., Ni, H., & Weissman, D. (2005, Aug). Suppression of RNA recognition by Toll-like receptors: the impact of nucleoside modification and the evolutionary origin of RNA. *Immunity, 23*(2), 165-175. https://doi.org/10.1016/j.immuni.2005.06.008.

Kariko, K., Muramatsu, H., Ludwig, J., & Weissman, D. (2011, Nov). Generating the optimal mRNA for therapy: HPLC purification eliminates immune activation and improves translation of nucleoside-modified, protein-encoding mRNA. *Nucleic Acids Res, 39*(21), e142. https://doi.org/10.1093/nar/gkr695.

Kauffman, K. J., Mir, F. F., Jhunjhunwala, S., Kaczmarek, J. C., Hurtado, J. E., Yang, J. H., Webber, M. J., Kowalski, P. S., Heartlein, M. W., DeRosa, F., & Anderson, D. G. (2016, Dec). Efficacy and immunogenicity of unmodified and pseudouridine-modified mRNA delivered systemically with lipid nanoparticles in vivo. *Biomaterials, 109*, 78-87. https://doi.org/10.1016/j.biomaterials.2016.09.006.

Kim, D., Lee, J. Y., Yang, J. S., Kim, J. W., Kim, V. N., & Chang, H. (2020, May 14). The architecture of SARS-CoV-2 transcriptome. *Cell, 181*(4), 914-921 e910. https://doi.org/10.1016/j.cell.2020.04.011.

Kim, J., Eygeris, Y., Gupta, M., & Sahay, G. (2021, Mar). Self-assembled mRNA vaccines. *Adv Drug Deliv Rev, 170*, 83-112. https://doi.org/10.1016/j.addr.2020.12.014.

Kowalski, P. S., Rudra, A., Miao, L., & Anderson, D. G. (2019, Apr 10). Delivering the messenger: advances in technologies for therapeutic mRNA delivery. *Mol Ther, 27*(4), 710-728. https://doi.org/10.1016/j.ymthe.2019.02.012.

Kowalzik, F., Schreiner, D., Jensen, C., Teschner, D., Gehring, S., & Zepp, F. (2021, Apr 15). mRNA-based vaccines. *Vaccines (Basel), 9*(4). https://doi.org/10.3390/vaccines 9040390.

Kranz, L. M., Diken, M., Haas, H., Kreiter, S., Loquai, C., Reuter, K. C., Meng, M., Fritz, D., Vascotto, F., Hefesha, H., Grunwitz, C., Vormehr, M., Hüsemann, Y., Selmi, A., Kuhn, A. N., Buck, J., Derhovanessian, E., Rae, R., Attig, S., … Sahin, U. (2016). Systemic RNA delivery to dendritic cells exploits antiviral defence for cancer immunotherapy. *Nature*, *534*(7607), 396–401. https://doi.org/10.1038/nature18300.

Krieg, P. A., & Melton, D. A. (1984, Sep 25). Functional messenger RNAs are produced by SP6 in vitro transcription of cloned cDNAs. *Nucleic Acids Res, 12*(18), 7057-7070. https://doi.org/10.1093/nar/12.18.7057.

Laczko, D., Hogan, M. J., Toulmin, S. A., Hicks, P., Lederer, K., Gaudette, B. T., Castano, D., Amanat, F., Muramatsu, H., Oguin, T. H., 3rd, Ojha, A., Zhang, L., Mu, Z., Parks, R., Manzoni, T. B., Roper, B., Strohmeier, S., Tombacz, I., Arwood, L., Nachbagauer, R., Kariko, K., Greenhouse, J., Pessaint, L., Porto, M., Putman-Taylor, T., Strasbaugh, A., Campbell, T. A., Lin, P. J. C., Tam, Y. K., Sempowski, G. D., Farzan, M., Choe, H., Saunders, K. O., Haynes, B. F., Andersen, H., Eisenlohr, L. C., Weissman, D., Krammer, F., Bates, P., Allman, D., Locci, M., & Pardi, N. (2020, Oct 13). A single immunization with nucleoside-modified mRNA vaccines elicits strong cellular and humoral immune responses against SARS-CoV-2 in mice. *Immunity, 53*(4), 724-732 e727. https://doi.org/10.1016/j.immuni.2020.07.019.

Leung, C. S. (2015). Endogenous antigen presentation of MHC Class II epitopes through non-autophagic pathways. *Front Immunol, 6*, 464. https://doi.org/10.3389/fimmu. 2015.00464.

Liang, Y., Huang, L., & Liu, T. (2021). Development and delivery systems of mRNA vaccines. *Frontiers in Bioengineering and Biotechnology*, *9*. https://www.frontiers in.org/article/10.3389/fbioe.2021.718753.

Lima, S. A., Chipman, L. B., Nicholson, A. L., Chen, Y. H., Yee, B. A., Yeo, G. W., Coller, J., & Pasquinelli, A. E. (2017, Dec). Short poly(A) tails are a conserved feature of highly expressed genes. *Nat Struct Mol Biol, 24*(12), 1057-1063. https://doi.org/10.10 38/nsmb.3499.

Linares-Fernandez, S., Lacroix, C., Exposito, J. Y., & Verrier, B. (2020, Mar). Tailoring mRNA vaccine to balance innate/adaptive immune response. *Trends Mol Med, 26*(3), 311-323. https://doi.org/10.1016/j.molmed.2019.10.002

Lindsay, K. E., Bhosle, S. M., Zurla, C., Beyersdorf, J., Rogers, K. A., Vanover, D., Xiao, P., Arainga, M., Shirreff, L. M., Pitard, B., Baumhof, P., Villinger, F., & Santangelo, P. J. (2019, May). Visualization of early events in mRNA vaccine delivery in nonhuman primates via PET-CT and near-infrared imaging. *Nat Biomed Eng, 3*(5), 371-380. https://doi.org/10.1038/s41551-019-0378-3.

Ljungberg, K., & Liljestrom, P. (2015, Feb). Self-replicating alphavirus RNA vaccines. *Expert Rev Vaccines, 14*(2), 177-194. https://doi.org/10.1586/14760584.2015.965690.

Lou, B., De Koker, S., Lau, C. Y. J., Hennink, W. E., & Mastrobattista, E. (2019). MRNA polyplexes with post-conjugated GALA peptides efficiently target, transfect, and activate antigen presenting cells. *Bioconjugate Chemistry*, *30*(2), 461–475. https://doi.org/10.1021/acs.bioconjchem.8b00524.

Lundstrom, K. (2015, May 7). Alphaviruses in gene therapy. *Viruses, 7*(5), 2321-2333. https://doi.org/10.3390/v7052321.

Lv, H., Zhang, S., Wang, B., Cui, S., & Yan, J. (2006). Toxicity of cationic lipids and cationic polymers in gene delivery. *Journal of Controlled Release: Official Journal of the Controlled Release Society*, *114*(1), 100–109. https://doi.org/10.1016/j.jconrel.2006.04.014.

Ma, Z., Li, J., He, F., Wilson, A., Pitt, B., & Li, S. (2005). Cationic lipids enhance siRNA-mediated interferon response in mice. *Biochemical and Biophysical Research Communications*, *330*(3), 755–759. https://doi.org/10.1016/j.bbrc.2005.03.041.

McCown, P. J., Ruszkowska, A., Kunkler, C. N., Breger, K., Hulewicz, J. P., Wang, M. C., Springer, N. A., & Brown, J. A. (2020, Sep). Naturally occurring modified ribonucleosides. *Wiley Interdiscip Rev RNA, 11*(5), e1595. https://doi.org/10.1002/wrna.1595.

McCullough, K. C., Bassi, I., Milona, P., Suter, R., Thomann-Harwood, L., Englezou, P., Démoulins, T., & Ruggli, N. (2014). Self-replicating replicon-RNA delivery to dendritic cells by chitosan-nanoparticles for translation in vitro and in vivo. *Molecular Therapy. Nucleic Acids*, *3*(7), e173. https://doi.org/10.1038/mtna.2014.24.

McKay, P. F., Hu, K., Blakney, A. K., Samnuan, K., Brown, J. C., Penn, R., Zhou, J., Bouton, C. R., Rogers, P., Polra, K., Lin, P. J. C., Barbosa, C., Tam, Y. K., Barclay, W. S., & Shattock, R. J. (2020, Jul 9). Self-amplifying RNA SARS-CoV-2 lipid nanoparticle vaccine candidate induces high neutralizing antibody titers in mice. *Nat Commun, 11*(1), 3523. https://doi.org/10.1038/s41467-020-17409-9.

McNamara, M. A., Nair, S. K., & Holl, E. K. (2015). RNA-based vaccines in cancer Immunotherapy. *Journal of Immunology Research*, *2015*, 794528. https://doi.org/10.1155/2015/794528.

Miao, L., Zhang, Y., & Huang, L. (2021, Feb 25). mRNA vaccine for cancer immune-therapy. *Mol Cancer, 20*(1), 41. https://doi.org/10.1186/s12943-021-01335-5.

Midoux, P., & Pichon, C. (2015). Lipid-based mRNA vaccine delivery systems. *Expert Review of Vaccines*, *14*(2), 221–234. https://doi.org/10.1586/14760584.2015.986104.

Mulligan, M. J., Lyke, K. E., Kitchin, N., Absalon, J., Gurtman, A., Lockhart, S., Neuzil, K., Raabe, V., Bailey, R., Swanson, K. A., Li, P., Koury, K., Kalina, W., Cooper, D., Fontes-Garfias, C., Shi, P. Y., Tureci, O., Tompkins, K. R., Walsh, E. E., Frenck, R., Falsey, A. R., Dormitzer, P. R., Gruber, W. C., Sahin, U., & Jansen, K. U. (2020, Oct). Phase I/II study of COVID-19 RNA vaccine BNT162b1 in adults. *Nature, 586*(7830), 589-593. https://doi.org/10.1038/s41586-020-2639-4.

Munz, C. (2012). Antigen processing for MHC Class II presentation via autophagy. *Front Immunol, 3*, 9. https://doi.org/10.3389/fimmu.2012.00009

Muttach, F., Muthmann, N., & Rentmeister, A. (2017). Synthetic mRNA capping. *Beilstein J Org Chem, 13*, 2819-2832. https://doi.org/10.3762/bjoc.13.274.

Orlandini von Niessen, A. G., Poleganov, M. A., Rechner, C., Plaschke, A., Kranz, L. M., Fesser, S., Diken, M., Lower, M., Vallazza, B., Beissert, T., Bukur, V., Kuhn, A. N., Tureci, O., & Sahin, U. (2019, Apr 10). Improving mRNA-based therapeutic gene delivery by expression-augmenting 3' UTRs identified by cellular library screening. *Mol Ther, 27*(4), 824-836. https://doi.org/10.1016/j.ymthe.2018.12.011.

Pardi, N., Hogan, M. J., Naradikian, M. S., Parkhouse, K., Cain, D. W., Jones, L., Moody, M. A., Verkerke, H. P., Myles, A., Willis, E., LaBranche, C. C., Montefiori, D. C., Lobby, J. L., Saunders, K. O., Liao, H. X., Korber, B. T., Sutherland, L. L., Scearce, R. M., Hraber, P. T., Tombacz, I., Muramatsu, H., Ni, H., Balikov, D. A., Li, C., Mui, B. L., Tam, Y. K., Krammer, F., Kariko, K., Polacino, P., Eisenlohr, L. C., Madden, T. D., Hope, M. J., Lewis, M. G., Lee, K. K., Hu, S. L., Hensley, S. E., Cancro, M. P., Haynes, B. F., & Weissman, D. (2018, Jun 4). Nucleoside-modified mRNA vaccines induce potent T follicular helper and germinal center B cell responses. *J Exp Med, 215*(6), 1571-1588. https://doi.org/10.1084/jem.20171450.

Pardi, N., Hogan, M. J., Pelc, R. S., Muramatsu, H., Andersen, H., DeMaso, C. R., Dowd, K. A., Sutherland, L. L., Scearce, R. M., Parks, R., Wagner, W., Granados, A., Greenhouse, J., Walker, M., Willis, E., Yu, J.-S., McGee, C. E., Sempowski, G. D., Mui, B. L., Weissman, D. (2017). Zika virus protection by a single low-dose nucleoside-modified mRNA vaccination. *Nature, 543*(7644), 248–251. https://doi.org/10.1038/nature21428

Pardi, N., Hogan, M. J., Porter, F. W., & Weissman, D. (2018, Apr). mRNA vaccines - a new era in vaccinology. *Nat Rev Drug Discov, 17*(4), 261-279. https://doi.org/10.1038/nrd.2017.243

Pardi, N., Muramatsu, H., Weissman, D., & Kariko, K. (2013). In vitro transcription of long RNA containing modified nucleosides. *Methods Mol Biol, 969*, 29-42. https://doi.org/10.1007/978-1-62703-260-5_2

Pardi, N., Tuyishime, S., Muramatsu, H., Kariko, K., Mui, B. L., Tam, Y. K., Madden, T. D., Hope, M. J., & Weissman, D. (2015, Nov 10). Expression kinetics of nucleoside-modified mRNA delivered in lipid nanoparticles to mice by various routes. *J Control Release, 217*, 345-351. https://doi.org/10.1016/j.jconrel.2015.08.007.

Park, J. W., Lagniton, P. N. P., Liu, Y., & Xu, R. H. (2021). mRNA vaccines for COVID-19: what, why and how. *Int J Biol Sci, 17*(6), 1446-1460. https://doi.org/10.7150/ijbs.59233.

Perri, S., Greer, C. E., Thudium, K., Doe, B., Legg, H., Liu, H., Romero, R. E., Tang, Z., Bin, Q., Dubensky, T. W., Jr., Vajdy, M., Otten, G. R., & Polo, J. M. (2003, Oct). An alphavirus replicon particle chimera derived from venezuelan equine encephalitis and sindbis viruses is a potent gene-based vaccine delivery vector. *J Virol, 77*(19), 10394-10403. https://doi.org/10.1128/jvi.77.19.10394-10403.2003.

Plantinga, M., de Haar, C. G., Dünnebach, E., van den Beemt, D. A. M. H., Bloemenkamp, K. W. M., Mokry, M., Boelens, J. J., & Nierkens, S. (2019). Cord-blood-stem-cell-derived conventional dendritic cells specifically originate from CD115-Expressing Precursors. *Cancers, 11*(2), 181. https://doi.org/10.3390/cancers11020181.

Platanias, L. C. (2005). Mechanisms of type-I- and type-II-interferon-mediated signalling. *Nature Reviews. Immunology*, *5*(5), 375–386. https://doi.org/10.1038/nri1604.

Probst, J., Weide, B., Scheel, B., Pichler, B. J., Hoerr, I., Rammensee, H. G., & Pascolo, S. (2007, Aug). Spontaneous cellular uptake of exogenous messenger RNA in vivo is nucleic acid-specific, saturable and ion dependent. *Gene Ther, 14*(15), 1175-1180. https://doi.org/10.1038/sj.gt.3302964.

Rauch, S., Jasny, E., Schmidt, K. E., & Petsch, B. (2018). New vaccine technologies to combat outbreak situations. *Frontiers in Immunology*, *9*. https://www.frontiersin.org/article/10.3389/fimmu.2018.01963.

Rejman, J., Oberle, V., Zuhorn, I. S., & Hoekstra, D. (2004). Size-dependent internalization of particles via the pathways of clathrin- and caveolae-mediated endocytosis. *Biochemical Journal*, *377*(1), 159–169. https://doi.org/10.1042/bj20031253.

Riecken, K., Głów, D., & Fehse, B. (2021). How to package and SEND mRNA: A novel "humanized" vector system based on endogenous retroviruses. *Signal Transduction and Targeted Therapy*, *6*(1), 1–2. https://doi.org/10.1038/s41392-021-00803-0.

Rosa, F. F., Pires, C. F., Zimmermannova, O., & Pereira, C.-F. (2020). Direct reprogramming of mouse embryonic fibroblasts to conventional type 1 dendritic cells by enforced expression of transcription factors. *Bio-Protocol*, *10*(10), e3619. https://doi.org/10.21769/BioProtoc.3619.

Rydzik, A. M., Kulis, M., Lukaszewicz, M., Kowalska, J., Zuberek, J., Darzynkiewicz, Z. M., Darzynkiewicz, E., & Jemielity, J. (2012, Mar 1). Synthesis and properties of mRNA cap analogs containing imidodiphosphate moiety--fairly mimicking natural cap structure, yet resistant to enzymatic hydrolysis. *Bioorg Med Chem, 20*(5), 1699-1710. https://doi.org/10.1016/j.bmc.2012.01.013.

Sahin, U., Kariko, K., & Tureci, O. (2014, Oct). mRNA-based therapeutics--developing a new class of drugs. *Nat Rev Drug Discov, 13*(10), 759-780. https://doi.org/10.1038/nrd4278

Sahin, U., Muik, A., Derhovanessian, E., Vogler, I., Kranz, L. M., Vormehr, M., Baum, A., Pascal, K., Quandt, J., Maurus, D., Brachtendorf, S., Lorks, V., Sikorski, J., Hilker, R., Becker, D., Eller, A. K., Grutzner, J., Boesler, C., Rosenbaum, C., Kuhnle, M. C., Luxemburger, U., Kemmer-Bruck, A., Langer, D., Bexon, M., Bolte, S., Kariko, K., Palanche, T., Fischer, B., Schultz, A., Shi, P. Y., Fontes-Garfias, C., Perez, J. L., Swanson, K. A., Loschko, J., Scully, I. L., Cutler, M., Kalina, W., Kyratsous, C. A., Cooper, D., Dormitzer, P. R., Jansen, K. U., & Tureci, O. (2020, Oct). COVID-19 vaccine BNT162b1 elicits human antibody and TH1 T cell responses. *Nature, 586*(7830), 594-599. https://doi.org/10.1038/s41586-020-2814-7.

Scheel, B., Braedel, S., Probst, J., Carralot, J.-P., Wagner, H., Schild, H., Jung, G., Rammensee, H.-G., & Pascolo, S. (2004). Immunostimulating capacities of stabilized RNA molecules. *European Journal of Immunology*, *34*(2), 537–547. https://doi.org/10.1002/eji.200324198

Scheel, B., Teufel, R., Probst, J., Carralot, J.-P., Geginat, J., Radsak, M., Jarrossay, D., Wagner, H., Jung, G., Rammensee, H.-G., Hoerr, I., & Pascolo, S. (2005). Toll-like receptor-dependent activation of several human blood cell types by protamine-condensed mRNA. *European Journal of Immunology*, *35*(5), 1557–1566. https://doi.org/10.1002/eji.200425656

Schlake, T., Thess, A., Fotin-Mleczek, M., & Kallen, K. J. (2012, Nov). Developing mRNA-vaccine technologies. *RNA Biol, 9*(11), 1319-1330. https://doi.org/10.4161/rna.22269.

Schudel, A., Francis, D. M., & Thomas, S. N. (2019, Jun). Material design for lymph node drug delivery. *Nat Rev Mater, 4*(6), 415-428. https://doi.org/10.1038/s41578-019-0110-7.

Segel, M., Lash, B., Song, J., Ladha, A., Liu, C. C., Jin, X., Mekhedov, S. L., Macrae, R. K., Koonin, E. V., & Zhang, F. (2021). Mammalian retrovirus-like protein PEG10 packages its own mRNA and can be pseudotyped for mRNA delivery. *Science (New York, N.Y.), 373*(6557), 882–889. https://doi.org/10.1126/science.abg6155.

Selmi, A., Vascotto, F., Kautz-Neu, K., Türeci, Ö., Sahin, U., von Stebut, E., Diken, M., & Kreiter, S. (2016). Uptake of synthetic naked RNA by skin-resident dendritic cells via macropinocytosis allows antigen expression and induction of T-cell responses in mice. *Cancer Immunology, Immunotherapy*, *65*(9), 1075–1083. https://doi.org/10.1007/s00262-016-1869-7.

Spencer, P. S., Siller, E., Anderson, J. F., & Barral, J. M. (2012, Sep 21). Silent substitutions predictably alter translation elongation rates and protein folding efficiencies. *J Mol Biol, 422*(3), 328-335. https://doi.org/10.1016/j.jmb.2012.06.010.

Stitz, L., Vogel, A., Schnee, M., Voss, D., Rauch, S., Mutzke, T., Ketterer, T., Kramps, T., & Petsch, B. (2017). A thermostable messenger RNA based vaccine against rabies. *PLOS Neglected Tropical Diseases*, *11*(12), e0006108. https://doi.org/10.1371/journal.pntd.0006108

Su, Z., Dannull, J., Yang, B. K., Dahm, P., Coleman, D., Yancey, D., Sichi, S., Niedzwiecki, D., Boczkowski, D., Gilboa, E., & Vieweg, J. (2005, Mar 15). Telomerase mRNA-transfected dendritic cells stimulate antigen-specific CD8+ and CD4+ T cell responses in patients with metastatic prostate cancer. *J Immunol, 174*(6), 3798-3807. https://doi.org/10.4049/jimmunol.174.6.3798.

Tai, Y., Wang, Q., Korner, H., Zhang, L., & Wei, W. (2018). Molecular Mechanisms of T Cells activation by dendritic cells in autoimmune diseases. *Frontiers in Pharmacology*, *9*, 642. https://doi.org/10.3389/fphar.2018.00642.

Tenchov, R., Bird, R., Curtze, A. E., & Zhou, Q. (2021). Lipid nanoparticles─from liposomes to mRNA vaccine delivery, a landscape of research diversity and advancement. *ACS Nano*, *15*(11), 16982–17015. https://doi.org/10.1021/acsnano.1c04996.

Thomas, R., & Yang, X. (2016). NK-DC crosstalk in immunity to microbial infection. *Journal of Immunology Research*, *2016*, 6374379. https://doi.org/10.1155/2016/6374379.

Trevaskis, N. L., Kaminskas, L. M., & Porter, C. J. (2015, Nov). From sewer to saviour - targeting the lymphatic system to promote drug exposure and activity. *Nat Rev Drug Discov, 14*(11), 781-803. https://doi.org/10.1038/nrd4608.

Tureci, O., Vormehr, M., Diken, M., Kreiter, S., Huber, C., & Sahin, U. (2016, Apr 15). Targeting the heterogeneity of cancer with individualized neoepitope vaccines. *Clin Cancer Res, 22*(8), 1885-1896. https://doi.org/10.1158/1078-0432.CCR-15-1509.

Udhayakumar, V. K., De Beuckelaer, A., McCaffrey, J., McCrudden, C. M., Kirschman, J. L., Vanover, D., Van Hoecke, L., Roose, K., Deswarte, K., De Geest, B. G.,

Lienenklaus, S., Santangelo, P. J., Grooten, J., McCarthy, H. O., & De Koker, S. (2017). Arginine-rich peptide-based mRNA nanocomplexes efficiently instigate cytotoxic t cell immunity dependent on the amphipathic organization of the peptide. *Advanced Healthcare Materials*, *6*(13). https://doi.org/10.1002/adhm.201 601412.

Ulkoski, D., Bak, A., Wilson, J. T., & Krishnamurthy, V. R. (2019). Recent advances in polymeric materials for the delivery of RNA therapeutics. *Expert Opinion on Drug Delivery*, *16*(11), 1149–1167. https://doi.org/10.1080/17425247.2019.1663822.

Ulmer, J. B., & Geall, A. J. (2016, Aug). Recent innovations in mRNA vaccines. *Curr Opin Immunol, 41*, 18-22. https://doi.org/10.1016/j.coi.2016.05.008.

Unal, A., Birekul, A., Unal, M. C., Karakus, E., Köker, Y., Ozkul, Y., & Comu, F. M. (2016). Dendritic cell production from allogeneic donor Cd34+ stem cells and mononuclear cells; cancer vaccine. *Blood*, *128*(22), 5723. https://doi.org/10.1182/blood.V128.22.5723.5723.

Van Lint, S., Goyvaerts, C., Maenhout, S., Goethals, L., Disy, A., Benteyn, D., Pen, J., Bonehill, A., Heirman, C., Breckpot, K., & Thielemans, K. (2012). Preclinical evaluation of TriMix and antigen mRNA-based antitumor therapy. *Cancer Research*, *72*(7), 1661–1671. https://doi.org/10.1158/0008-5472.CAN-11-2957.

Van Nuffel, A. M., Benteyn, D., Wilgenhof, S., Pierret, L., Corthals, J., Heirman, C., van der Bruggen, P., Coulie, P. G., Neyns, B., Thielemans, K., & Bonehill, A. (2012, May). Dendritic cells loaded with mRNA encoding full-length tumor antigens prime CD4+ and CD8+ T cells in melanoma patients. *Mol Ther, 20*(5), 1063-1074. https://doi.org/10.1038/mt.2012.11.

Vert, M., Li, S. M., Spenlehauer, G., & Guerin, P. (1992). Bioresorbability and biocompatibility of aliphatic polyesters. *Journal of Materials Science: Materials in Medicine*, *3*(6), 432–446. https://doi.org/10.1007/BF00701240.

Vigneron, N. (2015). Human tumor antigens and cancer immunotherapy. *Biomed Res Int, 2015*, 948501. https://doi.org/10.1155/2015/948501.

Vogel, A. B., Lambert, L., Kinnear, E., Busse, D., Erbar, S., Reuter, K. C., Wicke, L., Perkovic, M., Beissert, T., Haas, H., Reece, S. T., Sahin, U., & Tregoning, J. S. (2018, Feb 7). Self-amplifying RNA vaccines give equivalent protection against influenza to mRNA vaccines but at much lower doses. *Mol Ther, 26*(2), 446-455. https://doi.org/10.1016/j.ymthe.2017.11.017.

Wadhwa, A., Aljabbari, A., Lokras, A., Foged, C., & Thakur, A. (2020). Opportunities and challenges in the delivery of mRNA-based vaccines. *Pharmaceutics*, *12*(2), 102. https://doi.org/10.3390/pharmaceutics12020102.

Walsh, E. E., Frenck, R. W., Jr., Falsey, A. R., Kitchin, N., Absalon, J., Gurtman, A., Lockhart, S., Neuzil, K., Mulligan, M. J., Bailey, R., Swanson, K. A., Li, P., Koury, K., Kalina, W., Cooper, D., Fontes-Garfias, C., Shi, P. Y., Tureci, O., Tompkins, K. R., Lyke, K. E., Raabe, V., Dormitzer, P. R., Jansen, K. U., Sahin, U., & Gruber, W. C. (2020, Dec 17). Safety and immunogenicity of two RNA-based Covid-19 vaccine candidates. *N Engl J Med, 383*(25), 2439-2450. https://doi.org/10.1056/NEJMoa2027906.

Walsh, E. E., Frenck, R., Falsey, A. R., Kitchin, N., Absalon, J., Gurtman, A., Lockhart, S., Neuzil, K., Mulligan, M. J., Bailey, R., Swanson, K. A., Li, P., Koury, K., Kalina, W., Cooper, D., Fontes-Garfias, C., Shi, P. Y., Tureci, O., Thompkins, K. R., Lyke, K. E.,

Raabe, V., Dormitzer, P. R., Jansen, K. U., Sahin, U., & Gruber, W. C. (2020, Aug 28). RNA-based COVID-19 vaccine BNT162b2 selected for a pivotal efficacy study. *medRxiv*. https://doi.org/10.1101/2020.08.17.20176651.

Weissman, D. (2015, Feb). mRNA transcript therapy. *Expert Rev Vaccines, 14*(2), 265-281. https://doi.org/10.1586/14760584.2015.973859.

Wolff, J. A., Malone, R. W., Williams, P., Chong, W., Acsadi, G., Jani, A., & Felgner, P. L. (1990). Direct gene transfer into mouse muscle in vivo. *Science (New York, N.Y.), 247*(4949 Pt 1), 1465–1468. https://doi.org/10.1126/science.1690918.

Yan, Y., Liu, L., Xiong, H., Miller, J. B., Zhou, K., Kos, P., Huffman, K. E., Elkassih, S., Norman, J. W., Carstens, R., Kim, J., Minna, J. D., & Siegwart, D. J. (2016). Functional polyesters enable selective siRNA delivery to lung cancer over matched normal cells. *Proceedings of the National Academy of Sciences of the United States of America, 113*(39), E5702-5710. https://doi.org/10.1073/pnas.1606886113.

Yan, Y., Zhou, K., Xiong, H., Miller, J. B., Motea, E. A., Boothman, D. A., Liu, L., & Siegwart, D. J. (2017). Aerosol delivery of stabilized polyester-siRNA nanoparticles to silence gene expression in orthotopic lung tumors. *Biomaterials, 118*, 84–93. https://doi.org/10.1016/j.biomaterials.2016.12.001.

Yanez Arteta, M., Kjellman, T., Bartesaghi, S., Wallin, S., Wu, X., Kvist, A. J., Dabkowska, A., Székely, N., Radulescu, A., Bergenholtz, J., & Lindfors, L. (2018). Successful reprogramming of cellular protein production through mRNA delivered by functionalized lipid nanoparticles. *Proceedings of the National Academy of Sciences of the United States of America*, *115*(15), E3351–E3360. https://doi.org/10.1073/pnas.1720542115

Yi, Y., Lagniton, P. N., Ye, S., Li, E., & Xu, R.-H. (2020). COVID-19: what has been learned and to be learned about the novel coronavirus disease. *International Journal of Biological Sciences, 16*(10), 1753.

Yokoo, H., Oba, M., & Uchida, S. (2021). Cell-penetrating peptides: emerging tools for mRNA delivery. *Pharmaceutics*, *14*(1), 78. https://doi.org/10.3390/pharmaceutics14010078.

Yu, A.-M., Jian, C., Allan, H. Y., & Tu, M.-J. (2019). RNA therapy: are we using the right molecules? *Pharmacology & therapeutics, 196*, 91-104.

Zeng, C., Zhang, C., Walker, P. G., & Dong, Y. (n.d.). *Formulation and Delivery Technologies for mRNA Vaccines* (pp. 1–40). Springer. https://doi.org/10.1007/82_2020_217.

Zhang, C., Maruggi, G., Shan, H. & Li, J. (2019). Advances in mRNA vaccines for infectious diseases. *Frontiers in Immunology*, *10*, 594. https://doi.org/10.3389/fimmu.2019.00594.

Zhang, N. N., Li, X. F., Deng, Y. Q., Zhao, H., Huang, Y. J., Yang, G., Huang, W. J., Gao, P., Zhou, C., Zhang, R. R., Guo, Y., Sun, S. H., Fan, H., Zu, S. L., Chen, Q., He, Q., Cao, T. S., Huang, X. Y., Qiu, H. Y., Nie, J. H., Jiang, Y., Yan, H. Y., Ye, Q., Zhong, X., Xue, X. L., Zha, Z. Y., Zhou, D., Yang, X., Wang, Y. C., Ying, B., & Qin, C. F. (2020, Sep 3). A Thermostable mRNA vaccine against COVID-19. *Cell, 182*(5), 1271-1283 e1216. https://doi.org/10.1016/j.cell.2020.07.024.

Zhao, Y., Moon, E., Carpenito, C., Paulos, C. M., Liu, X., Brennan, A. L., Chew, A., Carroll, R. G., Scholler, J., Levine, B. L., Albelda, S. M., & June, C. H. (2010, Nov

15). Multiple injections of electroporated autologous T cells expressing a chimeric antigen receptor mediate regression of human disseminated tumor. *Cancer Res, 70* (22), 9053-9061. https://doi.org/10.1158/0008-5472.CAN-10-2880.

Zhong, D., Jiao, Y., Zhang, Y., Zhang, W., Li, N., Zuo, Q., Wang, Q., Xue, W., & Liu, Z. (2013). Effects of the gene carrier polyethyleneimines on structure and function of blood components. *Biomaterials, 34*(1), 294–305. https://doi.org/10.1016/j.biomaterials.2012.09.060.

Ziemniak, M., Strenkowska, M., Kowalska, J., & Jemielity, J. (2013, Jun). Potential therapeutic applications of RNA cap analogs. *Future Med Chem, 5*(10), 1141-1172. https://doi.org/10.4155/fmc.13.96.

Chapter 16

Treatment of Autoimmune Diseases with Cancer Therapies and Treatment of Cancer with Autoimmune Disease Therapies

Serkan Yaşar*

Hacettepe University Institute of Cancer,
Department of Medical Oncology,
Ankara, Turkey

Abstract

Quite significant developments have recently occurred in both the treatment of autoimmune diseases and cancer, and new developments are also continuing to occur. There is evidence that anticancer drugs and drugs used in autoimmune diseases have been tried and used and even have been useful in cancer treatment. Researchers' interest and studies in this regard increase with each passing day. There are various bridging therapies between cancer treatment and autoimmune diseases, such as cytotoxic drugs, proteasome inhibitors, PIC3K/mTOR (mammalian target of rapamycin) inhibitors, and antimetabolic drugs. The biological agents developed for cancer treatment are another group of drugs that have also been demonstrated to be effective in the treatment of autoimmune diseases. Another issue of concern in this regard has been the immune system and cancer immunology, and as a result of the studies, very good responses have been achieved in resistant B-cell leukemia and lymphoma through chimeric antigen receptor cell therapies. At present, cell-based therapies such as CAR Treg or NK cells

* Corresponding Author's Email: dr.wetsiz@hotmail.com.

In: Autoimmunity and Cancer
Editors: Soner Şahin and Kenan Demir
ISBN: 978-1-68507-937-6

are attempted to be developed for tolerance induction and modified into both autoimmune diseases and cancer treatments (Kloss et al., 2020).

Keywords: cancer, autoimmune diseases, CAR T cell therapy, rheumatoid arthritis

Introduction

Cancer and autoimmune diseases are closely associated with each other and, nowadays, particular therapeutic agents are used to treat both diseases. When the complex structure and pathways of the immune system are taken into account, the fact that a disease with an immune system disorder is used in the therapeutic intervention in another type of immune system disorder, autoimmunity, or cancer is not very surprising (Kloss et al., 2020; Yasunaga, 2020). From very ancient times, understanding the effects of agents developed specifically for the treatment of cancer on the immune system has guided the research. Furthermore, cell-based therapies (adaptive T cell therapies) established with a better understanding of the immune system and a better use of technology have become another exciting advancement between cancer treatments and autoimmune therapies. A better understanding of cancer and the immune system, particularly autoimmune diseases, will enable us to set sail for new horizons in future bridging therapies (Kloss et al., 2020; Zmievskaya et al., 2021). In this chapter, the available agents in common treatments will be reviewed, and recent developments will also be addressed.

Alkylating agents, which are among the oldest agents in this field, were developed for solid and hematologic malignancies in the 1950s, and in the ongoing process, they started to be used in rheumatic diseases with the use of their immunosuppressive characteristics. *Cyclophosphamide*, a strong alkylating agent, has a wide usage area (Ponticelli et al., 2018). Cyclophosphamide is a prodrug and acts on the body through its conversion to inactive carboxycyclophosphamide, acrolein, and phosphoramide mustard. It adds alkyl groups to DNA nucleotides via a guanine base, forms crosslinks between DNA double strands, causes DNA breaks, and is used as an antineoplastic agent, especially by exhibiting these cytotoxic effects more in dividing cells. It is generally used in breast cancer, multiple myeloma, steroid-unresponsive nephrotic syndrome, and focal segmental glomerulosclerosis. In the ongoing process, it began to be commonly used in rheumatic diseases, and was used in cicatricial pemphigoid, rheumatoid arthritis, juvenile dermatomyositis, systemic sclerosis, interstitial lung disease, lupus vasculopathy, systemic vasculitis, and thrombocytopenic purpura associated with the resistant treatment of lupus (Teles et al., 2017). During those years, cyclophosphamide was quite commonly used, especially in hematologic malignancies, and also enabled clinicians to work more effectively with regard to therapeutic intervention both in this field and especially in systemic lupus and other rheumatic diseases. As is known, cytotoxicity was the most important side effect restricting its use (Ponticelli et al., 2018).

Methotrexate that was developed as an antimetabolite in the 1940s and achieved wide clinical use was used as an anticancer therapy in breast cancer, leukemia, lymphoma, lung cancer, osteosarcoma, and some other types of cancer. It was used in rheumatic diseases just like cyclophosphamide by taking into account subsequent studies and pharmacological drug properties. It was tried for the first time in psoriatic arthritis and psoriasis in 1951 and was demonstrated to be useful. Randomized controlled trials in patients with rheumatoid arthritis made it a standard treatment for rheumatoid arthritis (Gubner et al., 1951; Hagner & Joerger, 2010; Weinblatt, 2013). Methotrexate is a structural analog of folic acid that can competitively inhibit the binding of dihydrofolic acid (FH2) to the enzyme dihydrofolate reductase (DHFR). It also contributes to the anti-inflammatory effect by allowing the extracellular increase of adenosine, a potent autacoid (Morabito et al., 1998).

Rituximab, another bridging therapy in autoimmune diseases and cancer, was approved for the treatment of non-Hodgkin's lymphoma in 1997 (DiLillo et al., 2008). The combination of rituximab with chemotherapies has led to a considerable improvement in the prognosis of non-Hodgkin's lymphoma. In addition to an apoptosis-inducing effect, induction of effector pathways such as antibody-dependent cellular cytotoxicity, complement-dependent cytotoxicity, and antibody-dependent phagocytosis is involved in its mechanism. It is also known to increase susceptibility to chemotherapy and passive immunization (Oflazoglu & Audoly, 2010). After Edwards and Cambridge discovered in 1998 that autoreactive B clones are supported by macrophage activation and inflammation, clinical trials were started for rheumatoid arthritis (Edwards & Cambridge, 2006). It was based on the principle of suppression of pathological B cells that produce autoantibodies or activate T cells, and it began to be used to treat some autoimmune diseases (Du et al., 2017). It was licensed for use in rheumatoid arthritis in combination with methotrexate in 2006. Then it was licensed for severe refractory lupus and ANCA-associated vasculitis (Kloss et al., 2020). Rituximab is a chimeric immunoglobulin G1 antibody, which is expressed on the B cell surface and targets CD 20. It is observed to have long-term effects on immune cell function by causing the depletion of B cells (Cragg et al., 2005).

Bortezomib and *proteasome inhibitors* affect several pathways in cells and lead to apoptosis in cells and the bone marrow microenvironment and inhibition of cell cycle progression, angiogenesis, and proliferation. They carry out these events by targeting proteasome 26S. In oncology, they were included and approved for use in combination for initial, maintenance, and resistance conditions in both newly diagnosed and relapsed/refractory multiple myeloma. Furthermore, they are effective in other plasma cell disorders and non-Hodgkin's lymphoma (Tan et al., 2019). These changes in intracellular protein inhibit the immunoproteasome, which is a special form of proteasome expressed essentially in lymphocytes and monocytes, and consequently it changes the formation of antibodies, including autoantibodies. Eventually, plasma cells that have high protein turnover become susceptible to the inhibition of bortezomib.

It was observed to improve symptoms such as systemic lupus erythematosus, rheumatoid arthritis, myasthenia gravis, neuromyelitis optica spectrum disorder, and chronic inflammatory demyelinating polyneuropathy in various autoimmune diseases resistant to conventional therapies in different animal models. A phase 2 study including patients with systemic lupus erythematosus, rheumatoid arthritis, and myasthenia gravis was also conducted (Khalesi et al., 2021; Xi et al., 2019).

The *PI3K/AKT/mTOR* pathway is another treatment pathway that should be discussed. Irregularities in this pathway lead to the occurrence of many types of cancer. mTOR was described as a key kinase that functions in the downstream pathway of PI3K/AKT. On the basis of this pathway's function, inhibition of mTOR has enabled the development of treatment options for most cancers (Motzer et al., 2008). Everolimus, temsirolimus, and sirolimus (rapamycin) prevent cell proliferation by inhibiting the mTOR pathway. Advanced stage renal cell carcinoma is one of the most important cancers in which everolimus and temsirolimus are effective. Furthermore, everolimus received approval in gastroenteropancreatic neuroendocrine tumors, subependymal giant cell astrocytoma, and breast cancer (Kloss et al., 2020).

Recently, the mTOR pathway has also attracted attention in the treatment of rheumatic diseases, and relevant studies have been conducted, especially on lupus. Studies are available indicating that the mTOR pathway is activated in the liver of patients with systemic lupus and even starts before the clinical picture of lupus emerges (Oaks et al., 2016). A study demonstrated that the formation of sclerotic and crescentic glomeruli was inhibited in patients followed up due to lupus nephritis and receiving rapamycin therapy for 10 weeks. Based on the previous studies, it was considered that the success of rapamycin in nephritis was probably due to its anti-inflammatory properties. It achieves it by suppressing CD4+, CD8+ and doublet negative T lymphocytes and macrophages (Jacinto et al., 2006; Oaks et al., 2016). The positive results obtained from animal models in the literature paved the way for clinical studies, and phase 1 and phase 2 sirolimus studies were conducted with patients who were unresponsive to medical treatment or intolerant to treatments. The study demonstrated that progressive improvement was achieved in patients with active systemic lupus by improving the proinflammatory T cell clone specification (Lai et al., 2018).

In the studies, it was also attempted to answer the question of what effect it has on rheumatoid arthritis. mTOR activity did not increase in CD 4+ lymphocytes in rheumatoid arthritis, and the lack of an increase in this activity causes that these cells cannot obtain enough energy and cannot be protected from oxidative stress, and the process ends with autophagy (Messaoudi et al., 2006; Yang et al., 2013). Although mTOR activity does not increase in RA, there is some response to rapamin. Studies have demonstrated that it achieves this over fibroblast-like synoviocytes (FBS). Increased mTOR activity in fibroblast-like synoviocytes provides benefits by being inhibited by rapamycin (Bruyn et al., 2008; Foroncewicz et al., 2005). The mTOR pathway also leads to an increase in IL6, IL8 over another pathway. In brief, it acts in rheumatoid arthritis by causing a decrease in the invasive ability of IL 6, IL 8, fibroblast-like synoviocytes, and IL 9 activity. In conclusion, it was demonstrated that joint damage could be prevented and there was an improvement in arthritis (Bruyn et al., 2008; Foroncewicz et al., 2005; Lin et al., 2019).

In progressive systemic sclerosis (SSc), increased mTOR activation was shown in both patients with SSc and animal models, and in studies targeting mTOR, the effects of TGF-β (Transforming growth factor-beta) and PDGF (platelet-derived growth factor) were significantly suppressed, which was also promising for patients with SSc (Fried et al., 2008; Soypacaci et al., 2018).

Adoptive cell transfer therapies are another treatment modality developed through studies of the immune system and the more intensive use of technology. Adoptive cell transfer has become a promising approach, which started with the therapeutic application of tumor-infiltrating lymphocytes against melanoma and attracted clinicians' attention. Chimeric antigen receptor cell (CAR T cell therapy) therapies are the most obvious example of adoptive cell transfer technology. Chimeric antigen receptors are composed of two parts. The first part is an extracellular domain and the single-chain variable fragment (scFv) of a monoclonal antibody responsible for target recognition. The second part is intracellular and composed of a few signaling motifs that mediate T-cell activation (Zmievskaya et al., 2021).

Table 1. Characteristics of the drugs used for oncological and immunological indications (Kloss et al., 2020)

		Oncological Use		Immunological Use	
Drugs	Target	Indication	Potential mechanism	Indication	Potential mechanism
Methotrexate	Dihydrofolate reductase/thymidylate synthetase	Breast cancer, leukemia, lymphoma osteosarcoma	Antimetabolite, Precursor inhibition for DNA/RNA synthesis	Psoriasis, rheumatoid arthritis	Converting AMP to extracellular adenosine JAK1/2 kinase inhibitor
Rituximab Ocrelizumab	CD20	B-cell lymphoma Chronic lymphocytic leukemia	B cell suppression via apoptosis Antibody-associated cytotoxicity Complement-associated cytotoxicity	Multiple sclerosis (ocrelizumab) Severe refractory systemic lupus, ANCA-associated vasculitis, RA (Rituximab)	B cell suppression via apoptosis Antibody-associated cytotoxicity Complement-associated cytotoxicity
Bortezomib	Proteasome	Multiple myeloma	Inducing apoptosis, cell cycle, angiogenesis, and proliferation inhibition	Potential use for myasthenia gravis, Severe systemic lupus	Inducing apoptosis in plasma cells and suppressing cytokine production
PI3K/mTOR	Everolimus Temsirolimus Sirolimus	Advanced renal cell carcinoma, GEP NETs, subependymal giant cell astrocytoma, breast cancer	Inhibition of cell growth and proliferation by inhibiting the mTOR pathway	Prevention of rejection after kidney transplant	Inhibiting suppressor T cell proliferation via the mTOR pathway
IDH	Enasidenib	Acute myeloid leukemia	2HG synthesis inhibition	Not defined yet	

GEP NET: gastroenteropancreatic neuroendocrine tumor 2HG:2-hydroxyglutarate.

Significant responses have been achieved with revolutionary CAR-T therapy in specific hematologic malignancies such as acute lymphoblastic leukemia and large B-cell lymphomas, and currently, CAR-T cell-based therapies, Tisagenlecleucel and Axicabtagene ciloleucel, have been approved by the FDA (US Food and Drug Administration). Although they are used predominantly in hematologic malignancies at present, their use in solid tumors will be the next step. There are some obstacles to adapting these therapies to solid tumors (Ahmad, 2020). The promising improvements and the expanding targets in chimeric T cell therapies have caused scientists and clinicians to conduct studies suggesting that these therapies can also be used in other diseases (Zmievskaya et al., 2021).

It is considered that CAR T cells that act by targeting the surfaces of tumor-associated antigen-expressing cells can be used to treat autoimmune diseases by modifying them to target pathological cells that express pathological autoantigens and autoantibodies on their surfaces, similar to this treatment modality. It is possible to classify these therapies modified for autoimmune diseases as *chimeric autoantibody receptor T (CAAR-T) cell therapy and CAR Treg therapies* (Chen et al., 2019).

Many mechanisms in the occurrence of autoimmune diseases are not clear enough, but the pathogenesis in which loss of T cell tolerance plays a central role is indisputable. Loss of self-tolerance involves activation of autoreactive B cell clones that produce autoantibodies that promote tissue damage and suppression of regulatory or cytotoxic T cells (Zmievskaya et al., 2021).

The conversion of the cytotoxic T cell phenotype to regulatory T cells is included in Treg cell therapy because Treg cells are suppressed in autoimmune diseases. These CAR-Tregs recognize and regulate autoimmune T lymphocytes through anergy, immunological unresponsiveness, and clonal deletion (Tenspolde et al., 2019).

These developments were tried in preclinical studies. Ellebrecht et al. tried them in pemphigus vulgaris, an autoimmune disease with painful blisters and damage to the skin and mucosa. High efficiency was provided in mouse experiments both in vitro and in vivo. Likewise, these studies conducted by Parvathaneni et al. for patients with hemophilia A who have immunological intolerance to factor 8 and neutralizing anti-factor 8 antibody have been promising for future prophylaxis. There are also studies on CAR T cell therapy, focusing on type 1 diabetes mellitus. Likewise, multiple sclerosis, ulcerative colitis, generalized myasthenia gravis, systemic lupus erythematosus, neuromyelitis optica spectrum disease are the other disease groups studied (Zmievskaya et al., 2021).

Conclusion

Recent developments in both medicine and science and technology have led to a better understanding of disease-causing mechanisms and disorders at the molecular level in cancer patients and autoimmune diseases. Thus, researchers have made great efforts to better understand the disease and develop new treatment modalities in both fields based on previous treatments and on the new knowledge and experience they have acquired at the molecular level. At every stage, from the introduction of alkylating agents, one of the oldest treatments, and then their use in autoimmune diseases after their immunosuppressive properties were discovered, to CAR T cell therapies that were developed by making changes in the immune system with the latest technologies, the question of whether it could be a bridging therapy always came to mind and will continue to come to mind because the treatments developed are effective not only through one pathway but also through many pathways. In the future, perhaps more treatment modalities will be discovered that are intertwined and multidisciplinary study areas will be expanded.

References

Ahmad, A. (2020). CAR-T cell therapy. *Int. J. Mol. Sci.*, *21*(12). https://doi.org/10.3390/ijms21124303.

Bruyn, G. A., Tate, G., Caeiro, F., Maldonado-Cocco, J., Westhovens, R., Tannenbaum, H., Bell, M., Forre, O., Bjorneboe, O., Tak, P. P., Abeywickrama, K. H., Bernhardt, P., van Riel, P. L., & Group, R. S. (2008). Everolimus in patients with rheumatoid arthritis receiving concomitant methotrexate: a 3-month, double-blind, randomised, placebo-controlled, parallel-group, proof-of-concept study. *Ann. Rheum. Dis.*, *67*(8), 1090-1095. https://doi.org/10.1136/ard.2007.078808.

Chen, Y., Sun, J., Liu, H., Yin, G., & Xie, Q. (2019). Immunotherapy deriving from CAR-T cell treatment in autoimmune diseases. *J. Immunol. Res.*, *2019*, 5727516. https://doi.org/10.1155/2019/5727516.

Cragg, M. S., Walshe, C. A., Ivanov, A. O., & Glennie, M. J. (2005). The biology of CD20 and its potential as a target for mAb therapy. *Curr Dir Autoimmun*, *8*, 140-174. https://doi.org/10.1159/000082102.

DiLillo, D. J., Hamaguchi, Y., Ueda, Y., Yang, K., Uchida, J., Haas, K. M., Kelsoe, G., & Tedder, T. F. (2008). Maintenance of long-lived plasma cells and serological memory despite mature and memory B cell depletion during CD20 immunotherapy in mice. *J. Immunol.*, *180*(1), 361-371. https://doi.org/10.4049/jimmunol.180.1.361.

Du, F. H., Mills, E. A., & Mao-Draayer, Y. (2017). Next-generation anti-CD20 monoclonal antibodies in autoimmune disease treatment. *Auto Immun. Highlights*, *8*(1), 12. https://doi.org/10.1007/s13317-017-0100-y.

Edwards, J. C., & Cambridge, G. (2006). B-cell targeting in rheumatoid arthritis and other autoimmune diseases. *Nat. Rev. Immunol.*, *6*(5), 394-403. https://doi.org/10.1038/nri1838.

Foroncewicz, B., Mucha, K., Paczek, L., Chmura, A., & Rowinski, W. (2005). Efficacy of rapamycin in patient with juvenile rheumatoid arthritis. *Transpl. Int.*, *18*(3), 366-368. https://doi.org/10.1111/j.1432-2277.2004.00070.x.

Fried, L., Kirsner, R. S., Bhandarkar, S., & Arbiser, J. L. (2008). Efficacy of rapamycin in scleroderma: a case study. *Lymphat. Res. Biol.*, *6*(3-4), 217-219. https://doi.org/10.1089/lrb.2008.1006.

Gubner, R., August, S., & Ginsberg, V. (1951). Therapeutic suppression of tissue reactivity. II. Effect of aminopterin in rheumatoid arthritis and psoriasis. *Am. J. Med. Sci.*, *221*(2), 176-182. https://www.ncbi.nlm.nih.gov/pubmed/14799481.

Hagner, N., & Joerger, M. (2010). Cancer chemotherapy: targeting folic acid synthesis. *Cancer Manag. Res.*, *2*, 293-301. https://doi.org/10.2147/CMR.S10043.

Jacinto, E., Facchinetti, V., Liu, D., Soto, N., Wei, S., Jung, S. Y., Huang, Q., Qin, J., & Su, B. (2006). SIN1/MIP1 maintains rictor-mTOR complex integrity and regulates Akt phosphorylation and substrate specificity. *Cell*, *127*(1), 125-137. https://doi.org/10.1016/j.cell.2006.08.033.

Khalesi, N., Korani, S., Korani, M., Johnston, T. P., & Sahebkar, A. (2021). Bortezomib: a proteasome inhibitor for the treatment of autoimmune diseases. *Inflammopharmacology*, *29*(5), 1291-1306. https://doi.org/10.1007/s10787-021-008 63-2.

Kloss, S., Dehmel, S., Braun, A., Parnham, M. J., Kohl, U., & Schiffmann, S. (2020). From cancer to immune-mediated diseases and tolerance induction: lessons learned from immune oncology and classical anti-cancer treatment. *Front Immunol.*, *11*, 1423. https://doi.org/10.3389/fimmu.2020.01423.

Lai, Z. W., Kelly, R., Winans, T., Marchena, I., Shadakshari, A., Yu, J., Dawood, M., Garcia, R., Tily, H., Francis, L., Faraone, S. V., Phillips, P. E., & Perl, A. (2018). Sirolimus in patients with clinically active systemic lupus erythematosus resistant to, or intolerant of, conventional medications: a single arm, open-label, phase 1/2 trial. *Lancet*, *391*(10126), 1186-1196. https://doi.org/10.1016/S0140-6736(18)30485-9.

Lin, J., He, Y., Wang, B., Xun, Z., Chen, S., Zeng, Z., & Ou, Q. (2019). Blocking of YY1 reduce neutrophil infiltration by inhibiting IL-8 production via the PI3K-Akt-mTOR signaling pathway in rheumatoid arthritis. *Clin. Exp. Immunol.*, *195*(2), 226-236. https://doi.org/10.1111/cei.13218.

Messaoudi, I., Warner, J., & Nikolich-Zugich, J. (2006). Age-related CD8+ T cell clonal expansions express elevated levels of CD122 and CD127 and display defects in perceiving homeostatic signals. *J. Immunol.*, *177*(5), 2784-2792. https://doi.org/10.4049/jimmunol.177.5.2784.

Morabito, L., Montesinos, M. C., Schreibman, D. M., Balter, L., Thompson, L. F., Resta, R., Carlin, G., Huie, M. A., & Cronstein, B. N. (1998). Methotrexate and sulfasalazine promote adenosine release by a mechanism that requires ecto-5'-nucleotidase-mediated conversion of adenine nucleotides. *J. Clin. Invest.*, *101*(2), 295-300. https://doi.org/10.1172/JCI1554.

Motzer, R. J., Escudier, B., Oudard, S., Hutson, T. E., Porta, C., Bracarda, S., Grunwald, V., Thompson, J. A., Figlin, R. A., Hollaender, N., Urbanowitz, G., Berg, W. J., Kay,

A., Lebwohl, D., Ravaud, A., & Group, R.-S. (2008). Efficacy of everolimus in advanced renal cell carcinoma: a double-blind, randomised, placebo-controlled phase III trial. *Lancet*, *372*(9637), 449-456. https://doi.org/10.1016/S0140-6736(08)61039-9.

Oaks, Z., Winans, T., Caza, T., Fernandez, D., Liu, Y., Landas, S. K., Banki, K., & Perl, A. (2016). Mitochondrial dysfunction in the liver and antiphospholipid antibody production precede disease onset and respond to rapamycin in lupus-prone mice. *Arthritis Rheumatol.*, *68*(11), 2728-2739. https://doi.org/10.1002/art.39791.

Oaks, Z., Winans, T., Huang, N., Banki, K., & Perl, A. (2016). Activation of the mechanistic target of rapamycin in SLE: explosion of evidence in the last five years. *Curr. Rheumatol. Rep.*, *18*(12), 73. https://doi.org/10.1007/s11926-016-0622-8.

Oflazoglu, E., & Audoly, L. P. (2010). Evolution of anti-CD20 monoclonal antibody therapeutics in oncology. *MAbs*, *2*(1), 14-19. https://doi.org/10.4161/mabs.2.1.10789.

Ponticelli, C., Escoli, R., & Moroni, G. (2018). Does cyclophosphamide still play a role in glomerular diseases? *Autoimmun. Rev.*, *17*(10), 1022-1027. https://doi.org/10.1016/j.autrev.2018.04.007.

Soypacaci, Z., Gumus, Z. Z., Cakaloglu, F., Ozmen, M., Solmaz, D., Gucenmez, S., Gercik, O., & Akar, S. (2018). Role of the mTOR pathway in minor salivary gland changes in Sjogren's syndrome and systemic sclerosis. *Arthritis Res. Ther.*, *20*(1), 170. https://doi.org/10.1186/s13075-018-1662-4.

Tan, C. R. C., Abdul-Majeed, S., Cael, B., & Barta, S. K. (2019). Clinical pharmacokinetics and pharmacodynamics of bortezomib. *Clin. Pharmacokinet.*, *58*(2), 157-168. https://doi.org/10.1007/s40262-018-0679-9.

Teles, K. A., Medeiros-Souza, P., Lima, F. A. C., Araujo, B. G., & Lima, R. A. C. (2017). Cyclophosphamide administration routine in autoimmune rheumatic diseases: a review. *Rev Bras Reumatol Engl Ed*, *57*(6), 596-604. https://doi.org/10.1016/j.rbre.2016.09.008.

Tenspolde, M., Zimmermann, K., Weber, L. C., Hapke, M., Lieber, M., Dywicki, J., Frenzel, A., Hust, M., Galla, M., Buitrago-Molina, L. E., Manns, M. P., Jaeckel, E., & Hardtke-Wolenski, M. (2019). Regulatory T cells engineered with a novel insulin-specific chimeric antigen receptor as a candidate immunotherapy for type 1 diabetes. *J. Autoimmun.*, *103*, 102289. https://doi.org/10.1016/j.jaut.2019.05.017.

Weinblatt, M. E. (2013). Methotrexate in rheumatoid arthritis: a quarter century of development. *Trans Am. Clin. Climatol. Assoc.*, *124*, 16-25. https://www.ncbi.nlm.nih.gov/pubmed/23874006.

Xi, J., Zhuang, R., Kong, L., He, R., Zhu, H., & Zhang, J. (2019). Immunoproteasome-selective inhibitors: An overview of recent developments as potential drugs for hematologic malignancies and autoimmune diseases. *Eur J Med Chem*, *182*, 111646. https://doi.org/10.1016/j.ejmech.2019.111646.

Yang, Z., Fujii, H., Mohan, S. V., Goronzy, J. J., & Weyand, C. M. (2013). Phosphofructokinase deficiency impairs ATP generation, autophagy, and redox balance in rheumatoid arthritis T cells. *J. Exp. Med.*, *210*(10), 2119-2134. https://doi.org/10.1084/jem.20130252.

Yasunaga, M. (2020). Antibody therapeutics and immunoregulation in cancer and autoimmune disease. *Semin. Cancer Biol.*, *64*, 1-12. https://doi.org/10.1016/j.semcancer.2019.06.001.

Zmievskaya, E., Valiullina, A., Ganeeva, I., Petukhov, A., Rizvanov, A., & Bulatov, E. (2021). Application of CAR-T cell therapy beyond oncology: autoimmune diseases and viral infections. *Biomedicines*, *9*(1). https://doi.org/10.3390/biomedicines9010059.

Editors' Contact Information

Prof. Dr. Soner Şahin, MD

Faculty of Medicine,
Department of Neurosurgery,
Nisantasi University
İstanbul, Turkey
sahin.soner@nisantasi.edu.tr

Kenan Demir, MD

Health Sciences University,
Samsun Training and Research Hospital
İlkadım, Turkey
kenandemir@hotmail.com

Index

A

J

K

L

Q

R

U

V

W